POLITICS, POWER & POLICY MAKING

POLITICS, POWER & POLICY MAKING

The Case of Health Care Reform in the 1990s

Mark E. Rushefsky
Kant Patel

M.E. Sharpe
Armonk, New York
London, England

Library of Congress Cataloging-in-Publication Data

Rushefsky, Mark E., 1945–
Politics, power, and policy making : the case of health care
reform in the 1990s / by Mark E. Rushefsky and Kant Patel.
p.   cm.
Includes bibliographical references and index.
ISBN 1-56324-955-3 (c : alk. paper)
ISBN 1-56324-956-1 (p : alk. paper)
1. Health care reform—United States.   I. Patel, Kant, 1946–
II. Title.
RA395.A3R855   1997
362.1′0973—dc21   97-33625
CIP
Printed in the United States of America

The paper used in this publication meets the minimum requirements of
American National Standard for Information Sciences—
Permanence of Paper for Printed Library Materials,
ANSI Z 39.48-1984.

EB (c)   10   9   8   7   6   5   4   3   2   1
EB (p)   10   9   8   7   6   5   4   3   2   1

To my mother, Lillian Rushefsky
—M.E.R

To Brandy, Man's BEST FRIEND
—K.P.

CONTENTS

LIST OF TABLES AND FIGURES

Tables

Figures

PREFACE

The origin of this book can be traced to our previous one, *Health Care Politics and Policy in America* (1995). That book was completed before the conclusion of the 104th Congress with its concentration on budget reduction and health programs, such as Medicare, Medicaid, and insurance reform. Given the failures of that Congress with Medicare and Medicaid and the passage of health reform legislation, we thought it would be valuable to contrast the 1993–94 period, characterized by attempted expansion of health programs and presidential initiatives, with the 1995–96 period, characterized by attempted retrenchment and congressional initiative. Further, several books and a number of academic studies have focused on the earlier period, but not many on the latter period.

We presented this project to Patricia Kolb, the executive editor at M.E. Sharpe, but not as just another book on health policy. Instead, we saw the opportunity to use the mid-1990s attempts at health care reform to illustrate the workings of the policy process within the American political system. (Pat encouraged our efforts, demonstrating to us her insightfulness).

So this is not just another book on health policy; we already wrote that. The purpose of this book is much broader. It uses health care reform as a vehicle for understanding the potential and limits of American policy making as we approach the end of the twentieth century. The book examines a variety of factors and institutional venues that shape policy successes and failures. Individual chapters focus on the agenda-building process and the role of the president, Congress, interest groups, mass media, and public opinion in American democracy. Parties and elections factor into institutional deliberations and are interspersed throughout the book. Additionally, there is considerable discussion of health care policy proposals. Thus, *Politics, Power, and Policy Making: The Case of Health Care Reform in the 1990s* is appropriate not only for those interested in health care politics and policy but also for anyone interested in American politics and policy making in general. Each of our substantive chapters (2 through 7) considers the two periods (1993–94 and 1995–96) separately and then brings them together in the chapter conclusions. They should be thought of as extended comparative case studies.

This is our second project together. Despite our strong political and philosophical differences (Rushefsky is a Knicks fan and Patel roots for the Rockets), the first book survived the 1994 National Basketball Association finals. Since neither team made it to the 1997 finals, this project went more smoothly.

Apart from our mutual love of professional basketball, we also share a love of animals. One of us has a medium-to-large dog; the other has two small dogs and three cats. Like our differences in basketball attachments, lifestyle (one is married with two grown children, the other is single), and habits, our dogs also seem to reflect personality differences. The larger dog is friendly, welcoming all who enter the home. The smaller dogs act as if they graduated from police academy, barking at all sentient beings moving within a block or so of their house, welcoming only those who live there.

But somehow we have managed to be good friends for over a decade and worked well together. We have other projects in mind.

Acknowledgments

No person is an island, and no book is the product solely of its authors. We would like to thank Pauline Woods for her work on the bibliography and for proofreading parts of the manuscript. Tom Bliss, our graduate assistant, found articles for us and checked citations. He did a lot of the tedious work. We would also like to thank Patricia Kolb, executive editor at M.E. Sharpe, for her continued faith in us and Elizabeth Granda, program coordinator and Pat's assistant, for keeping us on track and on time. Thanks are also due to Steven Martin, production editor, and to his staff for the copyediting. Any remaining errors are the responsibility of the coauthor.

Mark E. Rushefsky
Kant Patel

POLITICS, POWER & POLICY MAKING

1 SETTING THE STAGE

Our story begins in April 1991 with the death of Pennsylvania Senator John Heinz in a small plane crash. It ends in November 1996, with presidential and congressional elections. In between were some of the most intensive attempts at reform of the health care system that the United States has seen.

While our focus is on health care, our purpose is much larger than that. Our goal is to use health care as the vehicle for exploring various aspects of American politics and government, such as the presidency, Congress, interest groups, and agenda building.

Recent books have also concentrated on the fascinating story of health care reform and the political changes of the mid-1990s. Balz and Brownstein (1996) look at the politics leading to the takeover of Congress by the Republicans in 1995. Elizabeth Drew (1996) chronicles the contentious relations between the Republican-controlled 104th Congress and Democratic president Bill Clinton, as does Maraniss and Weisskopf (1996). All three books touch upon the health reform battles.

Two other books look more explicitly at health care reform. Johnson and Broder (1996) thoroughly examine the health reform debates from 1993 to 1995. They use those debates as a prism to suggest that the American political system is breaking down. Skocpol (1996) examines how the conflict over Clinton's Health Security Act inadvertently fueled a growing antigovernment tide. We (Patel and Rushefsky 1995) have also made our contribution with a comprehensive examination of the health care system. So why another book on health care?

Our plan is to use health care reform to explore various theories and concepts in political science as a way of understanding how public policy is made or not made. We divide the health care reform battles into two parts. One part focuses on comprehensive reform proposals associated with presidential leadership. The second part focuses on more incremental, but still significant, proposals highlighted by congressional leadership. This comparison of the two periods (1993–94 and 1995–96) is the major organizing principle of the book. With this organizing principle, we can look at various aspects of the political system and see how they might differ. We do not suggest that the system has broken down, but we do highlight the difficulties of change.

Our purpose in this introductory chapter is to set the stage for the rest of the book. We first look at previous attempts at reform and look for explanations for what is a story of mostly failure and limited, but not unimportant, success. The chapter then finishes by outlining the rest of the book.

Prior Attempts at Reform

National health insurance (NHI) is not a new idea. The first such system was developed in Germany in the late nineteenth century. The German monarchy, having just created the German state, was facing unrest and challenge from the Socialist Party. The prime minister, Otto von Bismarck, saw social insurance, of which national health insurance was one part, as a means to decrease unrest and cement loyalty to the national government. As Starr (1982) points out, opposition from private interests forced Germany to adopt a fairly decentralized system based on sickness funds (somewhat related to what would be called health care alliances in 1993). Nevertheless, the precedent had been started. It was eventually adopted by almost all Western democracies, with Canada joining this group in 1971. Only the United States has not joined, though there were a number of attempts to do so prior to the 1990s. Starr makes the interesting point that social welfare policies were first adopted in the more authoritarian states, such as Germany, and adopted at a later point by liberal, democratic states, such as England. The United States, the most steeped in liberal democracy, is the most extreme example, coming to welfare policies at the federal level decades after the other countries and then only during a period of severe economic distress (the Great Depression).

Wilson and the Progressive Era

The Progressive movement in the United States began in the latter part of the nineteenth century and lasted until about 1920. Its focus was to make government efficient and to clean up political corruption. It also supported public regulation of corporations and social insurance measures. A key event was the election of 1912. The Progressives had largely identified with the Republican Party. William Howard Taft, however, running for reelection, was viewed as veering away from or not supporting the Progressive agenda. The Progressives left the Republican Party and supported the candidacy of a former two-term president, Theodore Roosevelt (Taft was Roosevelt's vice-president). Roosevelt strongly supported national health insurance as well as other Progressive reforms (workmen's compensation, child labor laws). But Roosevelt's candidacy split the Republicans and allowed the Democratic candidate, Woodrow Wilson, to win with less than 42 percent of the vote. Wilson was less committed to national health insurance. Starr (1982) notes that Roosevelt perhaps would have provided the presidential leadership to get national health insurance enacted.

The Progressives continued to push for national health insurance, and the momentum for it increased. At one point in 1917 the delegates of the American Medical Association (AMA) endorsed national health insurance. This did not reflect, however, the views of state medical societies. That vote was reversed. Further, the entry of the United States into World War I in 1917, against the Axis powers led by Germany, doomed NHI, which now became identified with the enemy (Huns). So attempt number one failed.

But the Progressive movement did have some successes that had an impact on further attempts to pass comprehensive national health insurance. These included such things as direct democracy mechanisms (referendum and initiative), nonpartisan local elections, an apolitical bureaucracy, and the direct primary election. The purpose of these kinds of reforms was to clean up politics and move away from the machine-oriented, city party machines that characterized the late nineteenth and early twentieth centuries. The impact of these and other changes in Congress was to fragment already diffused political power, thus making it more difficult, though not impossible, for policy changes to succeed (Steinmo and Watts 1995; see also Smith 1988).

The New Deal

The second attempt at national health insurance came during the New Deal and the Great Depression. The cost of health care was already an issue, and private insurance was beginning to emerge with the establishment of Blue Cross (covering doctor payments) and Blue Shield (covering hospital payments). The concern of the "Blues" was not so much controlling costs but enabling providers to be paid.

President Franklin Roosevelt created a task force, the Committee for Economic Security, to consider possibilities for a system of economic pensions for retired persons and insurance for health care. The committee developed the plan that eventually became Social Security, but reluctantly concluded that national health insurance could not be passed, largely because of the opposition of the American Medical Association. Further, though Congress was controlled by the Democrats, the power lay in the hands of southern conservatives, particularly those serving as heads of committees (Steinmo and Watts 1995). As was to be true later on, the Democratic Party in the 1930s was not unified behind a health care plan. Attempting to pass a package that included NHI with Social Security would doom Social Security. Roosevelt agreed with that assessment. The Social Security Act of 1935, the fundamental piece of social welfare legislation in the history of the United States, created the Social Security, welfare, and unemployment compensation programs that other Western industrialized nations had. But, unlike those others, health care was not a part of the program.

Truman and the Fair Deal

In 1945, Franklin Roosevelt died and his vice-president, Harry Truman, succeeded him. Truman ran for the presidency in 1948, a race he was widely expected to lose to the Republican nominee, New York Governor Thomas Dewey. As Starr (1982) points out, the Republicans, who had regained control of Congress in 1946, attacked national health insurance as socialist, a charge that was made from the beginning and continued into the 1990s. Truman, waging a populist campaign and attacking what he called a "do-nothing" Congress, supported NHI. The 1948 Democratic platform called for the enactment of such a plan. Truman's surprise victory created some momentum for the ambitious program. While the Democrats regained controll of Congress after the 1948 elections, southern conservative Democrats again held key positions of power. These Dixiecrats, combined with Republicans, thwarted efforts at passage of NHI (Maioni 1995). Because the president does not control Congress, opposition to his program, even from within his own party, contributed to the failure of national health insurance.

One other series of events is important here: the emergence of private health insurance. As we saw, the Blues were created in the 1930s with the goal of protecting the financial welfare of providers. During World War II, when wage and price controls were in effect, businesses found that they could increase compensation to their employees by offering nonwage fringe benefits, such as health insurance. The Internal Revenue Service allowed the costs of health insurance to business to be deducted as a business expense and then in 1954 issued a regulation that made the deduction permanent.

An Incremental Approach

Advocates of national health insurance were convinced by the 1950s that a comprehensive plan would not pass. They sought instead smaller, incremental changes, focusing on two groups that might win public sympathy, the elderly and the young (Marmor 1973).

Congress passed the Kerr-Mills bill in 1960. Under this law, states would get matching funds to pay providers and to help poor elderly people, though states were not required to establish such programs.

John Kennedy, the Democratic presidential nominee in 1960, advocated medical assistance for the elderly. His administration prepared a proposal to cover that group. When Lyndon Johnson became president in 1963, following Kennedy's assassination, he immediately embraced that program as well as others that came under the rubrics of the War on Poverty and the Great Society.

In 1964, Johnson won election with the largest popular vote in American presidential election history. Further, and equally important, Democrats won large majorities in both houses of Congress. Given the popular mandate, and despite AMA opposition, Congress combined the elderly program and the Kerr-Mills bill and created two new programs. One was *Medicare,* designed to cover the elderly. The other was *Medicaid,* to cover the medical needs of poor people. Both programs remain the mainstay of federal (and state in the case of Medicaid) efforts to provide health insurance. The cost of both programs soon exceeded the original projections, and attempts to control those costs played an important role in the 1993–94 and especially the 1995–96 debates over health care.

The Nixon Administration

The Nixon administration was faced with both a challenge and an opportunity to reform the health care system. The opportunity came with the development of a health maintenance strategy, which was to subsidize, promote, and regulate the growth of an alternative set of health provider institutions known as *health maintenance organizations,* or *HMOs.* The idea behind an HMO, which originated as prepaid group plans in the 1930s, was that an organization would receive a fixed set of payments for each member of the HMO in return for which the HMO would provide members with a comprehensive set of health care services. The HMO would receive no additional money for providing additional services, as is the case of a fee-for-service system. So the incentive for the HMO is to control costs and provide preventive services to its members. The strategy was incorporated into the 1973 Health Maintenance Organization Act and subsequent amendments. Growth of HMOs was relatively slow, and during the Reagan administration the program was eliminated for cost reasons. HMO growth has risen dramatically in the 1980s and 1990s, and HMOs are one of the legs of the managed care strategy that particularly marks the 1990s (Falkson 1980; Starr 1982; Patel and Rushefsky 1995).

The challenge came in 1970 when Senator Edward Kennedy (D-Mass.) proposed the Health Security Act, essentially a single-payer, universal national health insurance system. Kennedy became Congress's primary proponent of national health insurance, and his proposals recur during the Carter and Clinton administrations. Prior to that, the president of the United Auto Workers (UAW), Walter Reuther, called for the enactment of such a system. The problem for the Nixon administration was the challenge that such a program would cause to his reelection. The response in 1971 was the Comprehensive Health Insurance Plan (CHIP), mandating employer-provided health insurance, a less generous program than Kennedy's proposal to provide insurance for low-income people and cutbacks in Medicare. The plan would have left some 20 to 40 million people uninsured. A third proposal (by Senators Russell Long and Abraham Ribicoff) focused on covering only the more costly (catastrophic) medical expenses (Marmor 1994). None of the plans were enacted both because of continued opposition by the AMA and other interest groups, conservative opposition to NHI, the economic distresses of the period (largely inflation, which led to the wage-and-price control program from 1971 to 1974), and the at-best lukewarm attitude of the administration to the new social program.

The Late 1970s

Several developments occurred during the second half of the 1970s, though none proved to be lasting. The one with the greatest, though limited, impact occurred when Congress passed in the 1976 National Health Planning and Resource Development Act, an attempt to rationalize the expansion of health services and facilities through local and state reviews. The program was repealed during the Reagan administration.

The Carter administration proposed various measures to contain the increases in hospital costs. These included direct controls and a uniform hospital accounting system. Neither passed Congress.

In a replay of the early 1970s, Senator Kennedy introduced a modified version of the Health Security Act. By this time, the senator was challenging his party's incumbent president for the Democratic nomination and the bill was one part of that challenge (though Kennedy's sincerity in desiring national health insurance cannot be denied). The Carter response was to propose his own bill. Carter had promised a comprehensive bill during the 1976 campaign but was reluctant to make an actual proposal. Further, the economy during this period, especially during 1979–80, was in apparent distress (Rushefsky 1996; Schwartz 1988; Krugman 1994; Madrick 1995). The administration's response was to offer a version of the Nixon CHIP plan, but one that would go into effect only in 1983 and then only if the economy and budget were in good shape. Neither plan had a chance of passage, and Carter was defeated by Ronald Reagan.

The Reagan Era

The record of health care reform during the Reagan era was contradictory. It began with a series of large cutbacks in 1981 that reduced Medicaid eligibility and rolls. In 1982 Congress mandated, as part of a massive deficit reduction package (i.e., tax increases), a system for fixed hospital payments for Medicare. Under this system, known as *diagnostic related groups,* hospitals would know ahead of time how much they would receive to treat a particular medical problem; they would get no more money for longer treatments. The goal was to slow the increase in hospital costs for Medicare, and it was hoped that hospitals would then pressure doctors to reduce costs for their hospital patients. A similar program for doctors was enacted in 1989 during the Bush administration. As we have seen, the planning and health maintenance programs were eliminated.

But cutbacks and regulation were not the only things that happened during this time. Beginning in the mid-1980s, Congress slipped in small expansions in Medicaid coverage. And in 1988 Congress passed the Medicare Catastrophic Coverage Act, which provided for additional hospital stay coverage as well as coverage for prescription drugs. Because of opposition by more affluent senior citizens, however, the act was repealed the next year.

Explaining the Failure of Reform

Starr (1982) offers three explanations for the failure of health care reform. The first is ideology, which is, in an underlying manner, perhaps the most important of the explanations. *Ideology* may be defined as a "set of beliefs about what the world is like, values with which to appraise the state of the world (good/bad, satisfactory/unsatisfactory), and beliefs and attitudes about how to make the world conform to these values" (Rushefsky 1996, 28; see also Herson 1984). More simply, ideology is related to what might be called the *public philosophy*: questions about the appropriate role of government (see also Morone 1990). Should government be involved in a particular area and, if so, to what extent. Samuelson (1995b, 45; see also Starobin 1995, 3022) writes that a public philosophy is "a set of principles—and a restraining sense of tradition—that reserves the use of the federal government only for problems that are genuinely important and national in scope." Attempts at health reform, beginning in the early twentieth century, raise these questions.

The origins of the American Republic can be seen in this light. To a large extent, the American Revolution was a revolt against an intrusive government and should be seen as the first tax revolt (against things like the stamp tax and the tax on tea, the question of no taxation without representation) (see Makin and Ornstein 1994). Europe, which had a highly developed state apparatus, was familiar and comfortable with bureaucracy and public services. In the United States, big government developed in fits and starts, and then only in unusual circumstances (see Stillman 1991, especially chapters 1 and 2). The bias would always be against a government program.

The conflict between a limited government and a more activist one dates to the early years of the Republic. The debate can be simplified as one between the views of Alexander Hamilton, secretary of the Treasury during the Washington administration, and Thomas Jefferson, Washington's secretary of State and later third president of the United States (Spicer 1995; Stillman 1984). Hamilton argued for a strong, activist national or central government whose primary purpose would be to support the economic expansion and integration of the new country. Jefferson preferred a smaller national government with limits on its abilities, seeing the source of power of the country in the small farmer (though he was willing to take actions opposed to this philosophy when necessary, such as the purchase from France of the Louisiana territory). Government should do as little as necessary. As Stillman (1984) points out, in many ways we adopted the compromise position of James Madison, creating a government that could act but would also face checks on its powers (see below). Nevertheless, the Hamilton/Jefferson debate has continued throughout our history, with the Jeffersonian view prevailing until about the 1930s. Beginning in the 1980s, the view that government had overreached itself, trying to do too much, gained momentum, with the electoral victory of Ronald Reagan in 1980, continuing through the Contract with America in 1994 and President Clinton's statement in his 1996 State of the Union address that "the era of big government is over."

Consider what we have learned from the above very brief history. Social Security, welfare, and workmen's compensation at the federal level could come about only in the throes of the Great Depression. The Great Society programs of Medicare and Medicaid were enabled by a presidential assassination and an election victory (1964, both presidential and congressional) of historic proportions. Any time national health insurance appeared on the agenda, it was immediately cast as socialist (or communist during the Cold War) and intrusive. The public wanted health care reform but did not necessarily want an increase in government's role in the economy. This ambivalence characterizes much of the debate over national health insurance (see Jacobs 1993).

Another factor in the failure to pass national health insurance was the labor movement. In current times, the labor movement has been strongly supportive of comprehensive health care reform. A strong union movement in Europe also helped. As we have seen, the origin of national health insurance in the newly formed Germany was to prevent social unrest, the kind that unions might provide. In the United States, the unions originally opposed national health insurance (Starr 1982). Samuel Gompers, the founder of the American Federation of Labor (AFL, now the AFL-CIO), saw national health insurance (and other social welfare legislation, such as minimum wage, unemployment insurance, and pensions) as hurting the unions; he wanted the unions to provide those benefits. So a potentially strong supporter of national health insurance was missing from the early attempts. In later years, when big labor supported national health insurance, they were in decline. Union membership has decreased and, with that decrease, so has its political power.

The power of interest groups is another explanation. Business groups always opposed another burden on them, as well as expansions of government. Two groups stood out in opposition to NHI: insurance companies, which might lose business or be regulated under national health insurance; and doctors, embodied in the American Medical Association, who felt that their freedom to conduct their practices would be limited by national health insurance, which was correct given the experience with Medicare and hospital and doctor fee schedules instituted in the 1980s (see Marmor, Wittman, and Heagy 1983). The AMA was always the major roadblock to health care reform of various kinds (including health maintenance organizations, see Starr 1982). The interest groups opposing national health insurance were generally more numerous, better organized, and stronger than those supporting it. This has not changed. Indeed, as we later see, this disparity in the distribution of interest group support and opposition has intensified.

A fourth factor is the structure of government. The Founding Fathers were faced with a twofold task, well expressed by James Madison in *The Federalist Papers* #51:

> But what is government itself but the greatest of all reflections on human nature? If men were angels, no government would be necessary. If angels were to govern men, neither external nor internal controls on government would be necessary. In framing a government which is to be administered by men over men, the great difficulty likes in this: You must first enable the government to control the governed, and in the next place, oblige it to control itself.

The delegates to the Constitutional Convention had experience with a government that was too strong, English rule during the colonial period, especially after 1763, and government that was too weak to operate effectively under our first constitution, the Articles of Confederation. They wanted an effective government, but not one that was so strong as to infringe on our liberties. That is the dilemma framed by Madison in the quote above.

The solution was to create a structure of government that would make radical change difficult, but not impossible. This was done through the related principles of *separation of powers* and *checks and balances.* Separation of powers means that the three government powers, legislative, executive, and judicial, would be located in separate institutions: Congress, the president, and the courts. Checks and balances means that each of these three institutions would share some of those powers. Presidents could sign or reject legislation, legislatures had to approve executive and judicial appointments, courts could declare actions of the president and Congress as unconstitutional, legislatures could, to a certain extent, limit the actions of the judiciary, and so forth. The combination of these two principles creates a situation that is most accurately described as "separate institutions sharing powers" (Neustadt 1990, 29).

This argument is made most forcefully in health policy by Steinmo and Watts (1995) in a paper originally delivered in September 1993, the month that President Clinton introduced his Health Security Act to the public. They reviewed the history of health care legislation and pointed to the structural influences, such as fragmentation of power, the decline of political parties and the increase in campaign-centered elections, and checks and balances as reasons for the consistent failure of health care reform (with the partial exception of the Medicare/Medicaid programs). They predicted in the original version of their paper that health care reform would fail (for a critique, see White 1995; Smith 1995).

This constitutional, institutional structure that Steinmo and Watts describe makes changing public policy difficult enough, but it has more recently been combined with *divided government.* Divided government occurs when one party controls the presidency and the other party controls at least one house of Congress. This has been largely a post–World War II phenomenon. In forty-three elections between 1860 (with the birth of the modern political party system) and 1944, divided government occurred only 21 percent of the time. In the twenty-six post–World War II elections, 1946 to 1996, divided government has occurred 60 percent of the time. Many have argued that divided government makes compromise more difficult than if both parties controlled Congress and the presidency. Certainly, the record of the 104th Congress (1995–96) would support this statement. Budget resolutions were late, many appropriations bills were not passed until well into the fiscal year, little legislation was passed. On the other hand, attempts at national health insurance have failed under both divided and unified government, most recently in 1993–94, when Democrats controlled both branches. The essential point is that separate institutions sharing power makes significant change difficult, though not impossible (e.g., the Tax Reform Act of 1986); divided government may exacerbate that tendency (though Mayhew [1991] argues that significant legislation can be passed even during periods of divided government). In our two cases, 1993–94 and 1995–96, we have both situations, unified control in the first two years and divided control the second two years. Further, the attempted changes in 1993–94 were comprehensive, an overhaul that would have affected most components of the health care system. Under divided control in 1995–96, the contemplated changes were incremental, though still highly significant. The question is whether the outcomes were the same and whether structural/institutional factors made a difference in those outcomes.

Remainder of the Chapters

Our basic plan is to begin each chapter with a discussion of the concept or organization in question and then use to health care reform efforts as a comparative case study (1993–94, 1995–96) to show how that concept or organization works.

In chapter 2, our subject is agenda building. We begin by examining how public policy reaches the government agenda. After looking at the theoretical framework for agenda building, we explore our two periods to show how agenda building operates in the United States. The first period, 1991–93, is characterized by a recession, an increase in the number of those uninsured, continued increases in health care costs, and the elections of 1991–92. The second agenda-building period begins in 1994 with the failure of comprehensive reform, the Contract with America, and the Republican congressional electoral victories.

Chapter 3 focuses on the presidency and comprehensive reform. Here we look briefly at the evolution of the modern presidency and particularly the role of presidential leadership and rhetoric. We look at the formulation of the president's health reform proposal, briefly describe that proposal, and undertake a content analysis of President Clinton's statements on health reform from 1992 as candidate through 1994 as president. Our goal in this latter part is to show how presidential rhetoric is employed toward achieving policy ends and how that rhetoric changed over time. We also examine presidential actions in the 1995–96 period.

In chapter 4, we turn the spotlight on Congress. We trace the role of Congress and discuss its procedures and structure. We look at competing proposals, and examine congressional consideration of the Health Security Act and other reform proposals in 1994 and the changed policy agenda in 1995–96, focusing on proposed cuts in Medicare and Medicaid and proposals for insurance reform. We place this within the context of Congress's attempts to reshape federal policy through budget cuts and balancing the budget. We look at the impact of the 1994 and 1996 elections on congressional deliberations.

Chapter 5 turns its attention to interest groups. We look first at how interest groups were conceived by the Founding Fathers and then explore the growth of interest groups. There is a well-developed political science literature on interest groups dating back to the early years of the twentieth century. This includes examining some theories relating interest groups and types of public policies. This is followed by a discussion of the function of interest groups in the political system. We then look at some critiques of interest groups and how the group system has changed. The major portion of the chapter focuses on interest groups during the two sets of health debates. We discuss lobbying strategies, media ads, campaign contributions, and other ways that interest groups seek to achieve their goals. We also examine, particularly in the 1995–96 period, how congressional leaders sought to influence interest groups. This is a two-way street.

The media are the focus of chapter 6. Here we consider the role of the media, a role that was scarcely envisioned by the Founding Fathers. We look at the development of mass media and the role of the media in agenda setting. This is followed by an examination of political advertising in the media and then a focus on the media during the health care debates. We present some quantitative analysis of media attention to problems, policies, and politics in the 1991–96 period and look at the role of the media in shaping public opinion.

Democracy at its most basic means rule by the people. In a largely representative democracy such as ours, public opinion is an important consideration in making public policy. Chapter 7 is devoted to this concern. We begin by answering the question of what the role of public opinion should be and has been. We look at the issue of understanding what the public wants and how to interpret public opinion. The chapter also considers the critical issue of the relationship between public opinion and public policy. We then focus on public opinion and the health policy debates, noting especially its impact on policy.

Chapter 8 presents our conclusions and predictions based on the previous analysis. We review the successes and failures of the two attempts at health care reform, including what changes have been made. We look at the issue of fundamental versus incremental reform; never have two such attempts been so close together. We look at the role of the various political factors in accounting for these changes: agenda building, presidential leadership, congressional leadership and structure, elections and political parties, interest groups, the media, and public opinion. Finally, we outline what we see as needed changes in health care and the likelihood, given the above factors, that such changes will occur. We suggest that comprehensive health care reform, affecting such a large sector of the economy, can occur only under unusual and extraordinary circumstances. Given our political system, it will take a crisis for meaningful action to be taken.

Yet we also conclude that the political system is operating as designed. That is, it is reasonably responsive to the public, and change can and has occurred, even in the health care area. Change is difficult but not impossible.

2 HEALTH CARE REFORM RETURNS TO THE NATIONAL AGENDA: THE WINDS OF CHANGE

Health care reform returned to the national policy agenda in the early 1990s, opening a window of opportunity for a major overhaul of the U.S. health care system. No other issue dominated the national domestic policy scene and captured the public's attention and focus as much as this one. Public debate over the problems of the U.S. health care system and the kinds of reforms needed to address these problems took the front stage in both the public and the private sectors. The debate over health care reform gained prominence in the print (editorials, guest columns, letters to the editor, etc.) and electronic (national and local news, talk shows, special reports, etc.) media.

Before the 1990s, several major attempts to reform the U.S. health care system resulted in failure, as mentioned in chapter 1 (Marmor 1994b; Rothman 1993). What forces caused the issue of health care reform to reemerge on the national policy agenda in the United States in the early 1990s? The answer to this question requires some understanding of the policy cycle and its processes.

A policy cycle consists of a series of steps or stages. The first step in the policy cycle is *an agenda-setting* process. This includes the emergence and recognition of a public problem or issue and the placement of this problem/issue on the policy agenda of the government. The second step involves *policy formulation and adoption.* This step includes specification and consideration of available alternatives to address the problem(s) and the decision about whether to adopt a new policy or change existing policy. Successful policy adoption leads to the third step, *policy implementation.* This involves administration of a program or enforcement of a policy. The next step is *policy evaluation,* which provides feedback about the success or failure of the policy in addressing the public problem. This in turn requires decisions about continuation, termination, modification, or redefinition of the problem, leading to a new policy cycle. In this chapter, we address only the first two steps in the policy cycle with respect to health care reform: We explain why the issue of health care reform reemerged on the national policy agenda in the 1990s, leading to the opening of a window of opportunity for a major reform of the U.S. health care system.

Theories of Agenda Setting

For a long time, the agenda-setting process remained the least understood of the stages of the policy cycle, largely because this field of study was neglected by scholars. In the past twenty years or so, however, there has been a dramatic increase in the scholarly literature dealing with the process of agenda setting. Today, there is a plethora of scholarly articles and books dealing solely with the subject of agenda setting. Almost all the literature on agenda setting can be classified under the rubric of three subfields: media agenda setting, public agenda setting, and policy agenda setting (McCombs and Shaw 1993; Rogers, Dearing, and Bregman 1993; Kosicki 1993).

The *media agenda setting* literature examines the content of the media to determine how issues are defined, selected, and emphasized by the media. Such studies treat mass media news agenda as the main dependent variable. Most of the literature in this subfield of media agenda setting has grown primarily out of the disciplines of sociology and mass communication.

The *public agenda setting* literature deals with the link between issues as portrayed by the mass media and its relationship to the priorities the general public places on the issues. These studies treat the relative importance of issues to members of the general public as the main dependent variable. Most of the literature in this subfield came originally out of the disciplines of journalism and mass communication. In recent years, sociology, political science, and political psychology have also made some contributions.

Finally, the *policy agenda setting* literature examines how issues get on the agenda of governmental institutions. These studies treat issue agendas of governmental bodies or elected officials as the dependent variable. The main thrust of research providing such an institutional perspective has come from the discipline of political science. In this chapter, we focus on policy agenda setting. Public agenda setting and, to a lesser extent, media agenda setting are examined in chapter 6, which deals with the role of the mass media in the policy process.

Theories of Policy Agenda Setting

Where do public policy issues come from, and how do they get on the policy agenda of the government, that is, political system? Many early approaches used in political analysis did not deal directly with the topic of agenda setting but indirectly touched on some aspects of the agenda-setting process. For example, David Easton provides a *systems approach* for examining political life. He argues that the main task of a political system is to allocate authoritatively the valued resources in a society. This is referred to as the output of the political system, that is, laws, policies, and programs. According to Easton, the political system receives two kinds of input: supports and demands. Conversion of the demands into an issue can help elevate it to policy agenda status. Because of "gatekeepers", however, not all demands become issues and not all issues get elevated to the policy agenda of the political system. Gatekeepers are persons, groups, and institutions whose actions determine whether an issue achieves policy agenda status (Easton 1953, 1965a, 1965b). Because different individuals and groups have different amounts of resources, however, they have differential access to institutional gatekeepers (Bauer, Pool, and Dexter 1963).

Much of the *group approach* literature (Odegard 1958; Bentley 1908; Truman 1964) also provides valuable insight into the process of agenda setting. The interest-group literature falls under two subheadings: pluralist and elitist. The pluralist approach views policy agenda building as a fluid process. According to this approach, politics is a struggle between organized groups to have their issues placed on the policy agenda and have their preferences and interests reflected in policy outputs. But because no single group is powerful enough to dominate agenda setting and policy outcomes on every issue, the constellation of groups competing against each other changes depending on the issue. Policy outputs reflect the result of bargaining and compromises among these competing groups (Dahl 1956, 1961, 1967). This pluralist approach has been criticized for its failure to study "nondecisions"; prevailing community values often prevent certain issues from gaining policy agenda status, and not all groups have equal access to the political system (Bachrach and Baratz 1962, 1963; Schattschneider 1960). It has also been charged that American pluralism degenerates into a functional power system with each group exercising a "veto power" within its own functional (i.e., policy) area (Lowi 1979).

In contrast to the pluralist approach, the elitist approach argues that a well-defined, cohesive group of elites, through coordinated action, dominate the agenda-setting process. These groups include the most powerful individuals in society, who consistently manage to get their issues placed on the governmental policy agenda. The elitist approach presents a more hierarchical power structure in society with the top, that is, "the power elite," dominating the government's policy agenda (Mills 1956; Mosca 1939).

Finally, the *decision-making approach* views incrementalism as a form of agenda building. This approach argues that policy makers consider only those policy alternatives that are marginally different from existing policies or deviate only slightly from the status quo. Such disjointed incrementalism allows only a very limited number of new issues ever to get on the policy agenda of the government (Lindblom 1968).

One of the first major studies in political science that dealt directly with the policy agenda-building process was the work of Cobb and Elder (1982), originally published in 1972. They suggest that "an issue is a conflict between two or more identifiable groups over procedural or substantive matters relating to the distribution of positions or resources," (Cobb and Elder 1982, 82). How do issues get on the policy agenda? Cobb and Elder argue that various internal and external triggering devices help issues attain the policy agenda. *Internal triggering devices* include natural catastrophes, unanticipated human events, technological changes, imbalance or bias in the distribution of resources, and ecological changes. *External triggering devices* consist of acts of war or military confrontations, innovations in weapons technology, international conflicts, and changes in world alignment patterns (Cobb and Elder 1982, 84).

Cobb and Elder define two kinds of agendas: systemic and institutional. A *systemic agenda* "consists of all issues that are commonly perceived by members of the political community as meriting public attention and as involving matters within the legitimate jurisdiction of existing governmental authority," (Cobb and Elder 1982, 85). They define an *institutional agenda* as "that set of items explicitly up for the active and serious consideration of authoritative decision-makers" (Cobb and Elder 1982, 86).

One way to increase the chances of getting an issue on the policy agenda is through conflict expansion and through it, issue expansion. Another is through the use of symbols (Edelman 1964). Pritchard and Berkowitz (1993) specify two kinds of policy agendas: symbolic and resource. Symbolic agendas consist of issues that require visible but not necessarily substantive action on the part of policy makers. In contrast, resource agendas not only require substantive action but generally also allocation of resources by policy makers. An issue that is prominent on one agenda does not necessarily acquire prominence on the other agenda.

In recent years, John Kingdon has made one of the most important contributions to the policy agenda-setting literature (1995). He has provided a comprehensive framework for the study of the process of agenda setting and specification of policy alternatives. According to Kingdon, two categories of actors play a significant role in affecting agenda setting and specification of alternatives. One set of actors consists of *participants inside the government,* including the president, presidential staff and political appointees, bureaucrats or the civil servants, the Congress, and congressional staff persons. *Participants outside the government* consist of interest groups, academic researchers and consultants, the media, political parties, election campaigners, and public opinion.

Kingdon suggests that three major process streams help explain agenda setting: problem, policy, and political streams. To a large extent these streams develop and operate independently of one another. The *problem stream* focuses on how problems come to the attention of policy makers and get placed on the policy agenda of the government.

One of the crucial ways in which participants inside and outside the government recognize the existence of a problem is through examination of systematic *indicators,* such as government expenditure, crime, infant mortality, economic growth, and unemployment rates. Changes in those indicators signal the existence of a problem. For example, William Bennett's *Index of Leading Cultural Indicators* (1994) displays changes in such areas as teenage pregnancy, abortion rates, and crime. Changes in indicators can be in a positive or negative direction, and they can be interpreted differently by different individuals, leading to controversy (Stone 1996).

Furthermore, indicators often do not necessarily make problems self-evident (Kingdon 1995). A *focusing event,* such as a crisis or disaster, personal experiences, or the presence of powerful symbols, is often necessary to bring attention to the problem. A focusing event also needs an *accompaniment.* It needs to be accompanied by something else to carry it to the policy agenda. This helps reinforce some preexisting perception of a problem. Focusing events can often serve as an early-warning signal, and the accompanying events help convince policy actors that a problem exists. Finally, *feedback* about existing programs through public comments/complaints, evaluation studies, and the like can indicate the existence of a problem, which can help get the problem on the policy agenda. Just as problems emerge, problems may fade from prominence on the policy agenda because of the success or failure in solving the problem.

A *policy stream,* according to Kingdon, consists of proposals and policy communities. Policy communities are composed of specialists in a given policy area—health, environment, criminal justice, and so on. In any of these policy communities, policy specialists are scattered throughout the country, both inside and outside the government. They may be located in bureaucracy, congressional staff, academia, consulting firms, advocacy

groups, private companies, interest groups, and the like. These specialists constantly interact, both formally and informally, through professional conferences and social gatherings. They know one another's
research and policy ideas. The degree of fragmentation or cohesiveness
varies from one community to another. Some policy communities are
very diverse and fragmented, while others are cohesive and tightly knit.
This has important policy consequences. Fragmentation in a policy community leads to policy fragmentation and policy agenda instability. Cohesiveness in a policy community produces a common outlook, cohesive
policies, and agenda stability.

Members of policy communities are often advocates for various policy
proposals. Kingdon refers to these policy advocates as policy entrepreneurs.
They advocate policies to promote their own personal interests or values.
These policy ideas are floating around in the "policy primeval soup"
(Kingdon 1995) waiting for an opportunity to attach themselves to problems when they come along. Ideas in the policy community go through the
evolutionary process of mutation, recombination, and softening up. Some
ideas survive for a long time, while others fade away rapidly. The criteria
for survival include technical feasibility, value acceptability, and anticipa-
tion of future constraints. Consensus building in the political stream occurs
through the process of persuasion.

The *political stream,* according to Kingdon, is composed of things such
as the national or public mood, organized political forces or interest groups,
election results (change in administration, change in key personnel, turnover in Congress, and so forth), partisan and ideological distributions in
Congress, and questions of jurisdictions. Each of these has an impact on the
agenda-setting process. The national or public mood, whether measured by
public opinion polls, through mass media reports, comments from constituents and the like, can help put a problem on the policy agenda. Changes in
key personnel in the various branches of government, especially the executive and legislative branches, can also enhance or decrease the chances of
certain issues or problems getting on the policy agenda. Consensus building
in the political stream occurs through coalition building, bargaining, and
compromises.

The *policy window* provides an opportunity for the advocates of policy
proposals to push their ideas and solutions to the problems. Policy windows
open and close in the political system. Sometimes, windows open in a
predictable fashion, for example, during renewal of a policy or program or
during annual budget considerations; at other times, the opening of a policy
window is very unpredictable. When a policy window opens, it generally
stays open only for a short time. Thus, policy advocates, that is, policy

entrepreneurs, must seize this opportunity. The chances of a problem rising to the policy agenda increase dramatically if all three streams—problems, policy, and politics—are joined together at the same time. Successful coupling of the three streams provides an opportunity for fundamental changes in public policies. A policy window can also close very quickly, however, because of failure to act, lack of available alternatives, lack of a consensus about available alternatives, change in personnel, or because the participants feel that the problem is solved (Kingdon 1995).

Baumgartner and Jones (1993) have argued that even though the American political system is based on constitutional principles designed to limit radical changes, it continues to be swept by reforms. These changes alternate between incremental and more rapid, drastic shifts. According to the authors, an agenda-setting process implies that no single equilibrium exists in the American political system. Often, new ideas emerge that make prevailing policy monopolies unstable. Furthermore, they argue that issue definition and agenda setting are related and that agenda setting has important policy consequences. During periods of incremental changes, negative feedback dominates the process, while during periods of rapid changes, positive feedback dominates. Critical points that occur before the initiation of the positive feedback process are called *windows of opportunity*. The authors conclude that the American political system exists under structurally forced stability occasionally punctuated by dramatic change.

Health Care Reform, Agenda Setting, and the Window of Opportunity

This section examines why and how the issue of health care reform achieved policy agenda status, opening a window of opportunity for major changes in the U.S. health care system. We use the concepts of agenda-setting theories discussed above, and especially Kingdon's framework, to explain how the coupling of problem, policy, and political streams during the 1990s provided a window of opportunity for health care reform. We compare and contrast two different periods of reform. First, the years 1993–94 are examined. This reform period was characterized by presidential leadership and initiative advocating a major overhaul of the U.S. health care system, epitomized by President Clinton's proposed Health Security Act of 1993. The second reform period was characterized by congressional leadership and initiative advocating more modest or moderate reforms involving issues of health insurance, medical savings accounts, cuts in Medicaid and Medicare programs, and medical liability.

Health Care Reform: 1993–94

The Problem Stream

The U.S. health care system has been described as "scandalous" (Dentzer 1990), "sick" (Lewis 1991), a "disgrace" (Ehrenreich 1990), and "built for waste" (Taylor, H. 1990). There are many problems associated with the American health care system. Two of the most important are health care costs and access to health care. Most other problems of the U.S. health care system can ultimately be traced to these two things. An examination of systematic indicators in these two areas helps shed light on the nature of the problems.

The high cost of health care has been one of the most enduring problems facing the United States. As can be observed from Table 2.1, total national spending on health care jumped from $251.1 million in 1980 to $696.6 million in 1990. Health care costs continued to rise in the 1990s. By 1993, total health care spending amounted to $884.3 million a year. Similarly, as Table 2.2 indicates, per capita national health care expenditure jumped from $1,068 in 1980 to $2,686 in 1990. By 1993, national per capita spending had increased to $3,294. The United States spends 40 percent more money per capita on health care than any other Western industrialized nation. Most of these countries provide basic universal health coverage to their people with lower levels of spending (Canaham-Clyne 1995). The United States, despite its high level of spending on health care, remains the only industrialized nation in the world that does not provide a basic health benefit package to all its citizens.

As Table 2.2 demonstrates, by 1993 U.S. national health care expenditures as a percentage of gross domestic product amounted to 13.9 percent compared to only 9.3 percent in 1980. Ironically, even though the United States spends proportionately more money on health care than all other Western industrialized nations, it ranks low on many health care indicators. For example, the United States has a higher infant mortality rate (9.7 per 1,000 live births) and a lower life expectancy rate at birth (71.5 years for males) compared to France, Canada, Germany, Japan, and Britain ("A Survey of Health Care" 1991).

Both the public and the private sectors in the United States have experienced these spiraling health care costs. During the 1970s, the business community was not very concerned about rising health care costs. By the early 1990s, this had changed: private-sector health care spending increased from $145.8 billion in 1980 to $410.0 billion in 1990; by 1993, it had risen

Table 2.1

National Health Expenditure Amounts, Percentage Distribution, and Average Annual Growth Rates, by Sources of Funds: Selected Calendar Years 1980–1995

Sources of funds	1980	1990	1991	1992	1993	1994	1995 (projected)
			(In billion $)				
All sources	251.1	696.6	755.6	820.3	884.2	938.3	1,007.6
Private	145.8	410.0	432.9	462.9	496.4	518.1	552.7
Public	105.3	286.5	322.6	357.5	387.8	420.2	454.9
By program							
Medicare	37.5	112.1	123.3	138.3	154.2	171.4	190.0
Medicaid	26.1	75.4	93.9	108.0	117.9	128.5	138.4
Other	41.6	99.0	105.5	111.2	115.7	120.3	126.5
By government level							
Federal	72.0	195.8	224.7	254.3	280.6	306.7	334.1
State and local	33.3	90.7	98.0	103.2	107.3	113.5	120.8
			(Percentage distribution)				
All sources	100.0	100.0	100.0	100.0	100.0	100.0	100.0
Private	58.1	58.9	57.3	56.4	56.1	55.2	54.9
Public	41.9	41.1	42.7	43.6	43.9	44.8	45.1
By program							
Medicare	14.9	16.1	16.3	16.9	17.4	18.3	18.9
Medicaid	10.4	10.8	12.4	13.2	13.3	13.7	13.7
Other	16.6	14.2	14.0	13.6	13.1	12.8	12.6
By government level							
Federal	72.0	195.8	224.7	254.3	280.6	306.7	334.1
State and Local	33.3	90.7	98.0	103.2	107.3	113.5	120.8

(continued)

Table 2.1 *(continued)*

			(Average annual percentage change from previous year)					
All sources	—	10.7	8.5	8.6	7.8	6.1	7.4
Private	—	10.9	5.6	6.9	7.2	4.4	6.7
Public	—	10.5	12.6	10.8	8.5	8.3	8.3
By program							
Medicare	—	11.6	10.0	12.2	11.5	11.1	10.9
Medicaid	—	11.2	24.5	15.0	9.2	9.0	7.7
Other	—	9.1	6.5	5.5	4.1	4.0	5.2
By government level							
Federal	—	10.5	14.8	13.2	10.3	9.3	8.9
State and local	—	10.5	8.0	5.3	3.9	5.8	6.4

Source: Burner and Waldo (1995, 234–35).

Table 2.2

Selected National Indicators, 1980–1994

Selected indicators	1980	1990	1991	1992	1993	1994
National health expenditure (per capita)	$1,068	$2,686	$2,875	$3,086	$3,294	$3,463
Gross domestic product (GDP) (in billions)	$2,708	$5,546	$5,725	$6,020	$6,343	$6,735
National health expenditure as a percentage of gross domestic product	9.3	12.6	13.2	13.6	13.9	13.9
Consumer Price Index (all items)	—	130.7	136.2	140.3	144.5	148.2
Medical Care Price Index	—	162.8	177.0	190.0	201.4	211.0
Unemployment rate (all workers)	—	5.5	6.7	7.4	6.8	6.1
Federal budget deficit (in millions)	$73,835	$221,384	$269,169	$290,403	$255,140	$203,169

Sources: Burner and Waldo (1995, 234–235); Donham, Sensenig, and Heffler (1995, 252–253); U.S. Office of Mangement and Budget (1995, 174–175).

to $496.4 billion. A national survey of 1,955 employers indicated that the average company spent 21.6 percent more in 1990 to provide doctor and hospital care for its employees than it did in 1989. From 1989 to 1990, the cost to employers of providing employee health benefits rose 46.3 percent. Thus, by the early 1990s, the private sector had become very interested in controlling rising health care costs and finding solutions to this problem (Swoboda 1991).

The public sector was also feeling the pinch of rising health care costs. Health care spending by the public sector increased from $105.3 billion in 1980 to $286.5 billion in 1990, and by 1993 the spending was up to $387.8 billion. The federal government's spending increased from $72 billion in 1980 to $280.6 billion in 1993. During the same period, state and local governments' spending on health care increased from $33.3 billion to 107.3 billion.

The most visible impact of rising health care costs can be seen in Medicare and Medicaid programs. Medicare is a federal program designed by the federal government to meet the health care needs of the elderly (65 and over) population. The cost of Medicare increased from $37.5 billion in 1980 to $154.2 billion in 1993. Medicaid, a joint federal-state program established to meet the health care needs of the poor, also experienced dramatic increases. Total Medicaid program costs increased from $26.1 billion in 1980 to $117.9 billion in 1993. State governments were increasingly feeling the impact of Medicaid program cost, as it was taking up an ever larger share of state budgets. Thus, by the early 1990s, there was a recognition by both the federal and state governments that some new approaches were needed to contain rising health care costs. Past efforts at cost containment in the form of health care planning through a health systems agency (HSA), professional standards review organization (PSRO), certificate of need (CON), and others had failed to stem the rising tide of health care costs (Patel and Rushefsky 1995).

Many factors have been cited as responsible for rising health care costs. These include increased expectation by the public, increased demand and utilization, advances in health care technology, the perception of health care as a right, the third-party payment system, a medical arms race among hospitals, general price inflation, and labor-productivity changes (McGregor 1981; Latham 1983; Virts and Wilson 1984; Ginzberg 1990). While there may be disagreement about which factors are most responsible for rising health care costs, there is little disagreement among policy makers, health care practitioners, researchers, and health care consumers and purchasers that health care costs too much. By the early 1990s, the focus in the health care policy debate shifted from "should we contain costs?" to "how should we contain costs?" (Grumbach and Bodenheimer 1990)

Another major problem facing the U.S. health care system is the issue of access to health care services. Despite the fact that the United States spends more money on health care than any other Western industrialized nation, millions of Americans either do not have access to health care or have a very limited access. Several factors have contributed to this situation. One major reason is that in the United States a large majority of persons receive health coverage and benefits through an employer as part of their fringe benefit package. Elderly retirees are provided health care coverage through the Medicare program, while the very poor are provided health protection under the Medicaid program. Nevertheless, it is important to keep in mind that in the Medicaid program, eligibility requirements, coverage provided, and benefit levels vary significantly from state to state because it is a joint federal-state program, and states enjoy a great deal of discretion in establishing eligibility rules and benefits. Despite all these programs, many people fall through the social programs' "safety net." Many persons who are unemployed and cannot afford to buy private health insurance are left without any health insurance. Persons who are between jobs often go without health insurance, and many more are denied health insurance coverage due to preexisting medical conditions or are dropped from coverage once they are afflicted with a catastrophic illness. Small employers do not provide health insurance to their workers, leaving them uninsured. Young persons working in a small company at a minimum wage often cannot afford or prefer not to buy insurance. Uninsured persons are less likely to have access to health care, and when they do it is more likely to be in an emergency situation, further escalating health care costs (Patel and Rushefsky 1995). The number of uninsured persons is another major indicator of the problems in the U.S. health care system.

As Table 2.3 shows, the number of uninsured persons in the United States grew from 33.4 million in 1989 to 39.7 million in 1993. The percentage of the uninsured in the total population rose from 13.6 percent in 1989 to 15.3 percent in 1993. While these numbers are significant, they do not tell the whole story; they provide only a snapshot of one point in time. Some have argued that many more people go without insurance than the numbers indicate. They argue that many people lose insurance for short periods of time (e.g., for a few months during the year while in transition from one job to the other) and that such individuals are not reflected in the aggregate annual number of uninsured persons. According to one estimate, about 25 percent of the population was without health insurance at some point during 1990–92 (Pear 1994). According to another estimate, some 51.4 million Americans were without health insurance for some time during 1993 (Rowland, Lyons, Salganicoff, and Long 1994). Six percent of people

Table 2.3

Total Population, Number, and Percentage of Uninsured Persons in United States, 1989-93

	Total population (in millions)	Total uninsured (in millions)	Total uninsured (percentage)[a]
1989	246.2	33.4	13.6
1990	248.9	34.7	14.0
1991	251.4	35.7	14.2
1992	256.8	38.6	15.0
1993	259.8	39.7	15.3

Source: Health Insurance Association of America (1995, 13)
[a]Figure is calculated from columns 1 and 2.

who worked in companies that offer health insurance were without it because they were not eligible for insurance. Fifty-four percent of these workers worked only part-time, and another 14 percent had not been on the job long enough to qualify for health insurance (Long and Marquis 1993).

Who are the uninsured? Table 2.4 sheds some light on this question. Above all, poverty emerges as one of the main factors that contribute to the lack of health insurance. The incidence of lack of insurance also seems to be higher among young persons, part-time workers, workers who worked full-time only part of the year, and nonwhites. The likelihood of being uninsured decreases as the level of education rises. The number of uninsured persons also varies from state to state (Bennefield 1995).

Related to access issues are problems of equality and equity. Equality refers to the notion that we should treat everyone as equal and not discriminate on the basis of such factors as race, age, religion, sex, ethnic group, or national origin. The concept of equity in the context of health care implies that everyone should have equal access to health care resources and services. From this standpoint, some have argued that minorities and women are treated differently by the U.S. health care system and that they do not have the same level of access. It is important to keep in mind, however, that since these are the two groups that are most likely to suffer from poverty, it is difficult to figure out whether it is race and gender or poverty that directly contributes to the problems of equality and equity in the U.S. health care system. Minorities, and African Americans in particular, consistently rank lower than whites on many health care indicators, such as premature birth, low birth weight, and infant mortality. Hispanics display the same characteristics (U.S. Department of Health and Human Services 1991; Valdez, Morgenstern, Brown, Wyn, Chao, and Cumberland 1993; Trevino, Moyer,

Table 2.4

Characteristics of Persons without Insurance, 1994

	All persons (percentage)	Poor persons (percentage)
Total	15.2	29.2
By gender		
Male	16.6	33.5
Female	13.7	25.8
By age		
Under 18	14.2	21.8
18 to 24	26.7	39.6
25 to 34	22.0	41.4
35 to 44	16.0	41.0
45 to 64	13.3	36.6
65 and over	00.9	3.7
By race		
White	14.0	30.7
Black	19.7	23.2
Hispanic origin[a]	33.7	39.8
By education		
No high school diploma	21.7	31.0
High school graduate	14.9	33.1
Some college, no degree	12.8	32.6
Associate degree	10.8	34.3
Bachelor's degree or higher	7.6	37.9
By work experience		
Worked during the year	16.5	44.9
Full-time	15.6	47.1
Part-time	19.5	41.7
Did not work	13.4	26.4

Source: Bennefield (1995, 2)
[a]Persons of Hispanic origins may be any race.

Valdez, and Stroup-Benham 1991a, 1991b). Some have suggested that the American health care system shares the same characteristics as that of South Africa's health care system under apartheid. While the South African system was based more on explicit racial segregation, the American system is based more on socioeconomic differences (Brooks, Smith, and Anderson 1991).

It has also been argued that the U.S. health care system treats women differently from men. Medicare tends to cover diseases that are more common among men (e.g., heart attacks), rather than chronic diseases that are more prevalent among women. Men also receive more preventive services than women. Women are also likely to have more unnecessary surgeries than men, such as cesarean births and radical mastectomies. It has also been alleged that there is a bias in the medical research agenda with more resources devoted to research on male medical problems than female medical problems (Muller 1990; Clancy and Massion 1992; Hafner-Eaton 1993).

Both the major problems of the U.S. health care system—costs and access—were well recognized by many policy makers as significant problems that needed to be addressed. As Kingdon suggests, however, mere recognition of a problem does not place it on the policy agenda of the government. Democratic presidential candidate Michael Dukakis tried to make health care reform an issue in the presidential election of 1988, but it failed to catch on as a major campaign issue (Kosterlitz 1991). Similarly, Senator Kennedy (D-Mass.) in 1989 held hearings around the country to call attention to the health care crisis hoping to set the congressional policy agenda for 1990. But nothing materialized, despite the fact that health care costs and the number of uninsured had been climbing for much of the 1980s.

But, as mentioned earlier, indicators do not necessarily make problems self-evident. They often require a focusing event. The focusing event that helped push health care reform on to the national policy agenda was the election of Democrat Harris Wofford to the U.S. Senate on November 5, 1991. He defeated a very popular Republican, Richard Thornburgh, a former Pennsylvania governor and a former U.S. attorney general, in the Pennsylvania Senate race, after trailing by as many as 45 points in the polls. Wofford's main campaign issue was health care reform; his slogan suggesting that if criminals have a right to a lawyer, all Americans ought to have a right to health care resonated with the Pennsylvania electorate. He promised that, if elected, he would work hard to reform the U.S. health care system through the establishment of national health insurance. His victory made the Washington establishment take notice. Wofford became a symbol to the Democrats of what they could achieve in the 1992 congressional and presidential elections (Peterson 1992, 570). His dramatic come-from-behind victory helped propel the issue of health care reform on to the national stage (Brown 1992).

A number of other events came together to push health care reform on the policy agenda during 1992 and 1993.

1. The context of pursuing health care reform in the 1990s had been set in the 101st Congress (1989–90). A consensus was developing that the U.S. health care system was in need of reform. This was reflected in the establishment of the Pepper Commission in 1988 (Peterson 1992).
2. The recession of 1990–91 led to increased unemployment, raising the number of uninsured. This also created a great deal of insecurity

and fear among the middle class about the prospects of losing one's job and thus one's health insurance.

3. By mid-1991 decreasing international tension as a result of the end of the Cold War made domestic issues far more salient in the election of 1992 (Marmor 1994).

4. The percentage of Americans who thought that the health care system needed fundamental changes grew from 75 percent in 1982 to 92 percent in 1991. Indeed, health care reform had become the second most important issue for the electorate, after jobs (Navarro 1995a). This was an important public feedback about the U.S. health care system.

5. All Democratic presidential candidates during the party's primaries endorsed some version of health care reform.

6. By 1992 the nature of interest-group politics surrounding health care had changed dramatically, with various groups clamoring for change in the health care system (Baumgartner and Talbert 1995).

7. After winning the Democratic Party's nomination for president, Bill Clinton made health care reform a cornerstone of his presidential campaign.

8. There was increasing and expansive media coverage of the health care reform issue during 1992 and 1993 (Peterson 1992, 569–70).

9. A March 1993 opinion poll gave reforming the health care system the second highest priority. Eighty-eight percent of the public believed that it would be a serious failure if President Clinton did not keep his promise to control health care costs, while 69 percent said they would consider it a serious failure if he broke his promise to ensure that everyone had health insurance coverage (Blendon, Hyams, and Benson 1993).

The issue of health care reform had, without a doubt, taken a prominent place on the national policy agenda by the end of 1992 and the beginning of 1993.

The Policy Stream

The health policy community consists of specialists and experts in the health care field. They may be located inside the government or in the private sector. They act as policy entrepreneurs advocating their ideas and solutions to the perceived problems. Thus, at any given point, ideas and solutions are floating around in the policy community waiting to attach themselves to the problems when they come along. Such was the case in the 1990s.

During much of the 1960s and part of the 1970s, ideas based on regulatory strategies to contain health care costs dominated the health policy community. The regulatory strategy was based on certain key assumptions. One of the most important assumptions was that the health care market suffered from too many imperfections and that government regulation could help improve the performance of the market. The second assumption was that the health care market was different from all other economic markets. The third assumption was that government regulation promoted important public values of political accountability, public access to information, and public participation (Ball 1975; Altman and Weiner 1978; Vladeck 1981; Weiner 1982). The failure of many of the government regulatory strategies to contain health care costs, such as the certificate of need (CON), planning and health systems agency (HSA), and Professional Standard Review Organizations (PSRO), led to increased criticisms of the regulatory strategy (Noll 1975; Breyer 1979; Goodman 1980; McClure 1981; Durenberger 1982). To the critics of the regulatory strategy the answer is a competitive market strategy.

Several policy entrepreneurs began to develop and test their market-based solutions in the health policy community. Dr. Paul Ellwood had been pushing the idea of "health maintenance strategy" since the late 1960s and early 1970s (1971, 1975). The idea was to rely on already existing prepaid group plans (PGPs) to establish a capitation system for health care providers. He advocated establishment of *health maintenance organizations* (HMOs), which would enroll subscribers who would pay monthly premiums. Those premiums would constitute an HMO's budget. Providing more services would not produce more revenue because subscribers paid the same monthly premiums regardless of the services they received. The incentive would be not to overtreat patients. Furthermore, such an alternate health care delivery system would provide competition to the traditional fee-for-service plans, forcing all health care providers to look at their costs. Ellwood's ideas were picked up by the Nixon administration and became embodied in the 1973 Health Maintenance Organization Act. The HMO became the prototype of managed care organizations during the 1990s (Falkson 1980).

Alain Enthoven took the concept of competitive strategy further by suggesting a complete reorganization of the U.S. health care system. During the 1970s and 1980s he advocated a Consumer Choice Health Plan (CCHP), a form of a national health insurance system. According to this plan, providers and insurers would be organized into competitive health care plans. Each plan would determine the premium it would charge. The plan entailed an open enrollment period, community rating, and limits on out-of-pocket expenses. Consumers would be free to choose among the competing plans that best met their needs. The federal government would estimate the average cost of care in various geographic regions of the country and pay a percentage of that cost through a tax credit or pay 100 percent of the average cost for the poor via vouchers (Enthoven 1978a, 1978b, 1980; see also Rushefsky 1981).

Competition plans created some interest but little action in the late 1970s and early 1980s. For example, Congressmen Richard Schweiker (R-Pa.) and David Stockman (R-Mich.) offered health bills based on the CCHP, without much success. But several developments helped further movement in the direction of a competitive strategy. One was the fact that the American Medical Association (AMA), which in the past had strongly opposed the concept of group medical practice, lessened its opposition. Second, the state of California established a plan, California Public Employees' Retirement System (CalPERS), which was based on the Federal Employees Health Benefits Program (FEHBP). CalPERS is a purchasing cooperative that negotiates a variety of different plans that include HMOs, preferred provider organizations (PPOs), and traditional fee-for-service plans. Public employees are free to choose from among these competing plans.

By the late 1980s and early 1990s, Enthoven refined his ideas and advocated the concept of *managed competition* (Enthoven 1988, 1991, 1993a, 1994; Enthoven and Kronick 1989a, 1989b). Around this time, Ellwood moved from Minnesota to Jackson Hole, Wyoming, and formed a working group to develop a strategy for change based on the concept of managed competition. This working group and its guests included "academics, public officials and leaders of the insurance and health industry" (Reinhold 1993).

The managed competition proposal was designed to meet two major goals: to provide financial protection from health care expenses for everyone; and to promote development of economically efficient financing and delivery arrangements (Enthoven and Kronick 1989a). Managed competition is a complex concept involving several key features.

1. Consumers of health care would be organized into large purchasing groups. They could be large employers or a combination of small employers and individuals who join together to form a purchasing cooperative or an alliance.
2. Health insurers and health care providers would merge into a variety of organizational forms such as HMOs and PPOs that offer a variety of health plans.
3. Employers or sponsors would negotiate with qualified health plans for the best price.

4. The employer's contribution would be 80 percent of the average of the price of plans offered.
5. Those not covered by employer plans, such as self-employed persons, would pay into public-sponsored plans.
6. Individuals would be required to pay more out-of-pocket money (i.e., increased deductibles and co-payments), creating incentives for them to join low-cost plans and make them conscious of the cost of health care.

Thus, the idea of managed competition advocated by the Jackson Hole group (Enthoven 1993b) came to be perceived as a viable solution to the problems of the U.S. health care system. The idea of managed competition had emerged in the late 1970s and had gone through the evolutionary process of mutation, recombination, and softening up. By the early 1990s, the idea of managed competition was floating around in the policy primeval soup, Kingdon's (1995) mctaphor, waiting for an opportunity to attach itself to reform proposals when they come along.

In reaction to the Jackson Hole group, a number of political scientists in 1993 joined forces to comment on the claims and counterclaims about health care reform. The group was known informally as the "No Hole Group" and included such well known political scientists as Larry Brown of Columbia University, Mark Peterson of the University of Pittsburgh, Deborah Stone of Brandeis University, James Morone of Brown University, Tom Oliver of the University of Maryland, Larry Jacobs of the University of Minnesota, and Theodore Marmor of Yale University. What role this group will come to play, if any, remains to be seen (Marmor 1994).

The Political Stream

The political stream, as we have seen, is composed of such things as the national or public mood, organized political forces or interest groups, election results (change in administration, change in key personnel, turnover in Congress, etc.), and partisan and ideological distribution in Congress. Questions of congressional committees' jurisdictions also have important influence on the agenda-setting process (Kingdon 1995). All these factors came together in the political stream during 1993–94 to elevate the issue of health care reform to the national agenda.

There is strong evidence that the national mood, as measured by public opinion polls, had changed significantly by the early 1990s. The public's perception of the American health care system had changed in a more negative direction. A study examining the public's feeling about the health care system found that of the ten countries included in the study, the lowest degree of satisfaction with a health care system was in the United States and the highest was in Canada (Blendon, Leitman, Morrison, and Donelan 1990). Public opinion polls by the *Los Angeles Times* in March 1990, NBC in 1989, and Louis Harris & Associates in 1988 showed that majorities of at least 61 percent of those polled supported establishing a Canadian-style health care system (Freudenheim 1990). In fact, seven polls between 1989 and 1993 showed that a majority of the American public (68 to 77 percent, depending on the poll) favored the establishment of a government-funded national health program (Navarro 1995a).

Ironically, polls also showed that Americans want more health care and not less. About half of all Americans believe that the United States spends too little on health care. Polls also indicate that the public does not believe that increased health care costs have been matched by similar increases in the quality of treatment. In fact, many Americans think that they are not getting their money's worth when it comes to health care (Morin 1990).

Those who are dissatisfied with the health care system cited the high cost of care and lack of access as primary reason for their dissatisfaction (Jajich-Toth and Roper 1990). Polls also showed that Americans saw health care costs as a problem that threatens them and their families personally and were most concerned by the rising out-of-pocket costs and frightened by the prospect of losing their health insurance benefits (Blendon, Hyams, Stelzer, and Nemson 1993). One-third of those questioned in 1992 indicated that they worried a lot that a family member would lose health insurance coverage (Princeton Survey Research Associates 1993; see also the discussion in chapter 7). The recession of 1991 and the resulting high unemployment rate, which jumped from 5.5 percent in 1990 to 7.4 percent in 1992, contributed to such concerns on the part of the public. As mentioned earlier, health care reform was the second most important issue for the electorate in 1992, after jobs (Navarro 1995a). Clearly, this suggests a major shift in the national mood, with an overwhelming majority of Americans expressing their support for health care reform.

Another major development in the political stream was the position of organized interests on the issue of health care reform. In the past, one of the pet answers to the question why the United States does not have national health insurance was that organized groups such as the American Medical Association, the insurance industry, and big business used their political and economic muscles and strong rhetoric (socialized medicine, threats to American freedom, etc.) to capitalize on deep-rooted American suspicions of government action to defeat any major reform of the U.S. health care system (Morone 1994). By the early 1990s, this had changed. As Baumgartner and Talbert (1995) argued, in the decade leading to the 1990s there was an explosion in the number of interest groups, especially in the field of health care. Many of these groups supported change in the health care system. An impressive variety of interest groups—Blue Cross and Blue Shield, the American Medical Association, the American Hospital Association, the national Chamber of Commerce and many others—produced white papers and task force reports to demonstrate their support for health care reform (Brown 1992). It is important to keep in mind, however, that while all kinds of interest groups, which in the past had vetoed any reform measures, were now supporting change does not mean that all major players were in agreement on the nature of the change or that they were willing to seek solutions that would distribute benefits and burdens in an equitable manner (Judis 1995).

Finally, perhaps the most important development within the political stream was the election in November 1992 of President Bill Clinton, who was strongly committed to the establishment of a national health insurance program. As a candidate for the Democratic Party's nomination for the presidency, Clinton endorsed a major overhaul of the U.S. health care system. At the Democratic Party's convention, candidate Clinton called for the establishment of a national health program that would provide for universal coverage. During the general election, Clinton ran as an agent of change advocating a comprehensive domestic agenda. He successfully made health care reform a major campaign issue in the 1992 elections. Upon his election as president, he promised to deliver on his campaign promise by sending to Congress legislation that would overhaul the U.S. health care system and establish a national health insurance program that would guarantee universal coverage. This was a major change in the policy stance of the executive branch of government. Previous Republican presidents, Ronald Reagan and George Bush, never demonstrated a genuine commitment to major health care reforms. President Bush supported modest reform during the 1992 campaign, in response to candidate Clinton's call for a major reform, including medical malpractice reform and more private-sector initiatives.

A Window of Opportunity

As the above discussion has demonstrated, by 1993 all of the three streams—problem, policy, and politics—had flowed together to open a window of opportunity for major reform in the U.S. health care system. President Clinton, in January 1993, established the National Health Care Reform Task Force, chaired by the first lady, Hillary Clinton, with Ira Magaziner as executive director. This task force held public hearings in different parts of the country, and discussed, debated, and revised their plan until they came up with the final draft of the proposed legislation. In a September 1993 nationally televised address to a joint session of Congress, President Clinton outlined the major features of his plan. In the weeks following his speech he sent to Congress his proposed 1,300–page legislation—the Health Security Act of 1993—designed to overhaul the U.S. health care system and establish a national health insurance program. The Health Security Act of 1993 was conceptually based on managed competition, incorporating many of the features advocated by the Jackson Hole group. Competing plans were introduced in Congress, ranging from the most dramatic (i.e., single-payer system) to those that were moderate and incremental in nature.

None of these plans passed Congress. Indeed, no votes were taken on any of the plans, including the president's proposal, on the floor of either house of Congress. The window of opportunity for major reform of the U.S. health care system under presidential initiative and leadership had closed for 1993–94. The main provisions of the competing plans and the reasons for their failure are discussed in the various chapters that follow.

Health Care Reform: 1995–96

The congressional elections of 1994 brought about a dramatic shift in the distribution of partisan and ideological alignment in Congress, and it ushered in a new era of divided government with the White House occupied by a Democrat and both houses of Congress controlled by Republican majorities. What did this mean for health care reform?

Problem Stream

By the end of 1994, some of the problems in the health care system showed signs of abatement while others had intensified. On the positive side were the following. First, as Table 2.2 shows, even though medical price inflation continued to be much higher than the overall inflation rates, both appeared to be easing. Overall inflation dropped from 5.4 percent in 1990 to 2.6 percent in 1994. During the same period medical inflation declined from 9.1 percent to 4.8 percent. Second, the unemployment rate decreased for two successive years, from a high of 7.4 percent in 1992 to 6.8 percent in 1993 and 6.1 percent in 1994 (see Table 2.2). Third, as Table 2.1 indicates, despite the fact that overall national health care expenditures continued to climb, the average annual growth rate in spending was declining. This was true of both the public and the private sector. The decline was much more significant in the private sector, however, where it had dropped from 10.9

percent in 1990 to 4.4 percent in 1994. In the public sector the decline in the growth rate was much smaller, from 10.5 percent in 1990 to 8.3 percent in 1994. These developments eased some pressure, especially in the private sector, for comprehensive reform of the U.S. health care system.

Despite these positive developments, several problems were getting worse. The fact remained that overall health care spending (total dollar amounts) was still rising in both the public and private sectors (see Table 2.1). As Table 2.2 demonstrates, overall national health care expenditures in 1994 still amounted to 13.9 percent of the gross domestic product (GDP), higher than other industrialized nations with a national insurance system.

One of the areas where the problem grew worse was the number of persons lacking health insurance. The total number of uninsured persons climbed from 34.7 million in 1990 to 39.7 million by 1993. This represented 15.3 percent of the total U.S. population in 1993. In 1990, 14 percent of the population was uninsured. One of the major reasons for this is "downsizing" in the private sector ("Downsizing of America" 1996). U.S. Labor Department statistics indicate that more than 36 million jobs were eliminated in the country between 1979 and 1993. An analysis by the *New York Times* puts the number at 43 million through 1995. According to a report prepared by Challenger, Gray and Christmas, a firm that tracks layoffs, between 1992 and 1996, AT&T eliminated 128,000 jobs, representing 30 percent of its workforce. IBM eliminated 122,000 jobs, 35 percent of its workforce. Other major companies that engaged in downsizing included General Motors, Boeing, Sears, Roebuck & Co., Digital Equipment, Lockheed, BellSouth, and McDonnell Douglas ("People Trends," 1996).

While it is true that far more jobs are being added to the economy than are lost, many of the new jobs are in small companies that offer less pay and few benefits. Others are part-time positions or temporary jobs that provide few or no benefits. Small companies generally do not provide health insurance coverage to their workers as a part of benefit packages. Similarly, part-time and temporary workers do not receive health insurance coverage from their employers, and most cannot afford to buy private health insurance (Uchitelle and Kleinfield 1996).

Another significant dimension to the problem of the uninsured is that the number of children without health insurance coverage continued to increase, reaching 10 million in 1994, the highest since 1987 (U.S. General Accounting Office 1996). What makes this problem even more serious is the fact that although Medicaid provided health coverage for 16 million children in 1994, more than 60 percent of those children had a working parent. This trend placed a significant strain on public resources because taxpayers ended up either paying for Medicaid coverage or for hospital subsidies to provide acute care for the uninsured (U.S. General Accounting Office 1996).

This brings us to the problems associated with two of the largest public health care programs—Medicaid and Medicare—that came to the forefront during 1995–96. The bipartisan Commission on Entitlement and Tax Reform, in its interim report to the president in August 1994, concluded that the nation cannot continue to allow entitlements to consume an ever increasing share of the federal budget and that any attempt to control long-term entitlement growth must take into account the projected increases in health care costs. According to the report, if health care costs are not controlled, federal spending on Medicaid and Medicare is projected to triple as a percentage of the economy by 2030 (Bipartisan Commission on Entitlement and Tax Reform 1994).

Medicaid is a state-administered program that operates under federal guidelines. The federal government establishes basic requirements for eligibility and benefits, but states enjoy considerable discretion and flexibility in setting eligibility requirements and benefit packages beyond the minimum requirements. The federal government pays at least one-half of the cost of Medicaid, while the states pay the balance. The share of federal cost varies from a low of 50 percent to a high of 80 percent, depending on the per capita income of the state. The program was created to meet the health care needs of the poor. Today, millions of Americans rely on the Medicaid program for health and long-term-care services that they could not afford. Medicaid helps with nursing home costs, which are not covered by Medicare. Medicaid is the only source of health insurance for children of low-wage working parents. Medicaid also provides highly specialized health care services for about 4.9 million children and adults with serious disabilities ("Hurting Real People" 1995).

In recent years, Medicaid has gone through some turbulent times. Table 2.5 shows that even though the annual average growth rate of Medicaid expenditures slowed, it still grew at about a 9 percent rate during 1993 and 1994. The recent decline in the growth rate partly reflects measures taken by state governments, such as moving away from the traditional fee-for-service system of reimbursement to a managed care, capitated system of reimbursement. The most dramatic increase occurred in 1991, a 24.5 percent increase in expenditures from the previous year. This was largely due to congressional mandates expanding the Medicaid program to cover more women and children during the late 1980s. Of the 33.4 million Medicaid recipients in 1993, pregnant women and children living on incomes up to 133 percent of the federal poverty level accounted for 71 percent (23.7 million) of the total recipients (Liu 1996).

The data in Table 2.5 reveal some disturbing trends in the Medicaid program. The number of Medicaid recipients increased from 25.3 million in 1990 to 33.4 million in 1993. Total Medicaid expenditures increased from $75.4 billion in 1990 to $117.9 billion in 1994. This represents a significant increase for both the federal and state governments. Total federal Medicaid payments to state and local governments increased from $41.1 billion to $75.8 billion between 1990 and 1993, while the per capita federal Medicaid aid increased from $166.96 to $295.07. Federal Medicaid aid amounted to 30 percent of total federal aid to state and local governments in 1990. By 1993, this had increased to 39 percent.

The situation, in many ways, is worse for state governments. Even with the decline in the growth rate, Medicaid remains the fastest-growing budget item for state governments. In the last few years Medicaid spending has displaced higher education as the second most expensive budget item. On average, the Medicaid program accounts for 18.4 percent of the state budget. This is second only to the 21.2 percent devoted to primary and secondary education (Lemov 1995). For many state governments, Medicaid has become a financial time bomb waiting to explode. Many have argued that unless significant reforms are adopted, states will face a heavy increase in spending and increasingly larger proportions of their revenue will be taken up by Medicaid expenditures. Under these circumstances, states will be either forced to increase taxes, divert money from other programs, or cut Medicaid spending (Beach 1995). Despite innovative and often aggressive cost-containment policies pursued by state governments, the fact remains that states are stuck with the demographic realities of an aging population and the high cost of long-term care (Beach 1995).

Over the past three decades, Medicare has successfully provided economic security and access to health care for millions of the nation's elderly and disabled population. Persons eligible to receive Medicare benefits include those sixty-five and over who are eligible for Social Security benefits, persons under the age of sixty-five who have been receiving disability insurance for at least two years, persons of any age with end-stage renal disease (ESRD), and persons age sixty-five and over who are otherwise not eligible but elect to enroll by paying a monthly premium.

Medicare is based on the concept of "social insurance." The Hospital Insurance (HI) Trust Fund is used to finance Part A of the Medicare program. Current employees and their employers each pay 1.45 percent of a worker's salary to the trust fund. Self-employed workers pay 2.90 percent. The HI Trust Fund, contrary to expectations, is not accumulating a large surplus for future years. Instead, it operates on a "pay-as-you-go" basis. Benefits provided under Part A include inpatient hospital care, inpatient

Table 2.5

Medicaid Expenditures by Source of Funds, Number of Recipients, and Federal Payments for Medicaid to State and Local Governments

	Total Medicaid expenditures (in billion $)	Average annual percentage change from previous year	Medicaid recipients (in millions)	Total federal aid to state and local governments (in billion $)	Total federal payment for Medicaid to state and local governments (in billion $)	Medicaid payment as percentage of total federal aid to state and local governments	Federal Medicaid aid to state and local governments (per capita)
1994	128.5	9.0	—	193.7	75.8	39%	$295.07
1993	117.9	9.2	33.4	178.1	67.8	38%	$269.76
1992	108.0	15.0	31.2	154.6	52.5	34%	$211.06
1991	93.9	24.5	28.0	135.4	41.1	30%	$166.96
1990	75.4	11.2	25.3	91.5	14.6	16%	$62.54
1980	26.1	—	21.6				

Sources: Burner and Waldo (1995, 234–35); Health Care Financing Review, Medicare and Medicaid Statistical Supplement (1993, 161).

psychiatric care, skilled nursing care, home health care, and hospice care.

Part B of the program is financed through the Supplementary Medical Insurance (SMI) Trust Fund. SMI is financed by premiums paid by enrollees (about 25 percent of the costs) and from general revenues (about 75 percent of the costs). Some of the major benefits provided under Part B include 80 percent of physician and outpatient services after a certain deductible amount, laboratory and other diagnostic tests, X rays, and other radiation therapy. Even though Part B of the program is voluntary, an overwhelming majority of Medicare beneficiaries opt to enroll in Part B (see Table 2.6). Not included in Part B are services such as outpatient prescription drugs, routine physical examinations, hearing aids, eyeglasses, and most long-term care in nursing facilities. Many elderly purchase a "Medigap" policy to fill the gaps left by Part A and Part B. The cost of a Medigap insurance policy has been rising rapidly, however, creating hardships on the elderly who are dependent on a fixed income (Morrow 1996).

Many indicators in recent years have suggested problems for the program. The number of enrollees in HI and/or MSI programs increased from 28.5 million in 1990 to 36.3 million in 1993. Medicare expenditures jumped from $112.1 billion in 1990 to $154.2 billion in 1994. As Table 2.6 shows, the growth rate in expenditures has averaged in double-digit numbers since 1990. Medicare spending has grown in real terms (i.e., inflation adjusted) by an average of 6.5 percent annually.

Medicare poses immediate and long-term financial problems (Iglehart 1995). The program is projected to grow at an average rate of around 10 percent per year in the near future, and it is estimated that spending may reach $450 billion by the year 2005 (National Academy on Aging 1995). As the size of the elderly population increases and Americans live longer, Medicare will have to finance the care of an even older and frailer group of enrollees. In 1995, one in ten Medicare recipients was over the age of eighty-five and another one in ten was a disabled person under the age of sixty-five. It is not surprising, then, that Medicare patients have high rates of chronic and acute diseases requiring extensive and costly medical care (Davis 1995). The sickest 10 percent of Medicare recipients account for 70 percent of program expenditures (Moon and Davis 1995). By the time the baby-boom generation reaches retirement age, around 2010, the number of elderly (sixty-five and over) will increase dramatically. By 2030, Medicare will become responsible for covering nearly 20 percent of the population, compared to the 12.8 percent currently covered. Medicare costs are likely to continue to grow at a rapid pace.

The focusing event that helped place the issue of Medicare reform on the policy agenda was the 1995 Annual Report of the Social Security and

Table 2.6

Medicare Program: Total Expenditures, Annual Average Percentage Change, and Number of Enrollees by Type of Coverage

Year	Total expenditures (in billion $)	Annual average percentage increase from previous year	Number of enrollees: HI and/or SMI (in millions)	Hospital insurance (HI) Enrollment (in millions)	Supplementary medical insurance (SMI) enrollment (in millions)
1994	154.2	11.1	—	—	—
1993	154.2	11.5	36.3	35.9	34.6
1992	138.3	12.2	35.6	35.1	33.9
1991	123.3	10.0	34.9	34.4	33.2
1990	112.1	11.6	34.2	33.7	32.6
1980	37.5	—	28.5	28.0	27.4

Source: Burner and Waldo (1995, 234–35); Health Care Financing Review, Medicare and Medicaid Statistical Supplement (1995, 161).

Medicare Trust Funds by the Board of Trustees. According to the report, the SMI Trust Fund, which is financed on a year-by-year basis, was adequately financed. But the report concluded that the HI Trust Fund will be able to pay benefits for only about seven more years and will run out of money by 2002. Further, it concluded that, under adverse conditions, the HI Trust Fund could run out of money as soon as 2001. The HI Trust Fund, according to the Board of Trustees, faced serious problems both in the short- and long-run. The report concluded by stating that

> we strongly recommend that the crisis presented by the financial condition of the Medicare Trust Funds be urgently addressed on a comprehensive basis, including a review of the program's financing methods, benefit provisions, and delivery mechanisms. (Social Security Administration 1995)

Despite the failure of health care reform during 1993–94, many changes were taking place in the U.S. health care system. State governments and the private sector were working aggressively to contain health care costs. HMOs and managed care plans began to take root, and the number of individuals enrolled in HMOs or some type of managed care increased dramatically. In 1995, about 590 HMOs were enrolling about 53.3 million individuals, and the number is projected to grow to 103.2 million by the year 2000. The HMO revolution is transforming Marcus Welby–style medicine into a Wal-Mart model of health care (Spragins 1996). More and more Medicare and Medicaid patients are enrolled in managed care plans. Because of this, the growth rate of health care expenditures, especially in the private sector and the Medicaid program, has experienced some decline. Many companies that five years ago faced double-digit inflation in health care costs saw their costs go flat (Starr 1995). Some of these positive developments (accompanying events) helped reduce the pressure for a major overhaul of the U.S. health care system during 1995–96. Overall health care expenditures, however, continued to climb. The number of uninsured continued to increase, as did the number of Medicaid recipients. Both Medicaid and Medicare experienced serious problems, demanding policy makers' attention.

The Policy Stream

During the reform period of 1995–96, the concept of managed care still dominated discussion and debate within the policy community. President Clinton's Health Security Act of 1993, designed to overhaul the U.S. health care system, was based on the concept of managed competition, but it also included a heavy regulatory role for the government. It was a soft or less pure version of managed competition (Navarro 1995b). Its failure signaled the need for an incremental approach to address specific problems and solutions that were more market driven with less or no government involvement. This brought the conservative agenda for incremental reform to the forefront. Some of the ideas and proposed solutions originated from conservative think tanks such as the Heritage Foundation and the Cato Institute.

The main idea advocated by purely market-oriented policy entrepreneurs is consumer choice. Proposals to develop a consumer-choice health care system start on the premise that today's employment-based health care system is failing because the normal producer-consumer relationship is undermined by the employer's role as a quasi consumer due to the current tax code. Employees enjoy a large tax break for health care, but the employer determines each worker's coverage, which is paid out of funds that otherwise would be part of the worker's cash compensation (Butler 1995). Critics charge that the current tax treatment of employment-based health insurance fuels higher health care costs; it hides the true cost of health care due to a third-party payment system, and it leads to "job lock" and uninsurance. Lower-income individuals and families are helped least by the current system (Liu and Moffit 1996).

A consumer-based health care system would establish a new economic relation. Under such a system, the consumer (i.e., the household) would own his or her own plan and would determine how much of his or her compensation would be devoted to health care coverage and the type of coverage (i.e., benefits). Such a plan would require tax reform, giving households the freedom to choose their own plan and coverage. According to proponents, such a plan would bring economic rationality back in to the health care marketplace by encouraging consumers to make rational economic choices (Liu and Moffit 1996). Such a plan would restore power and accountability to individuals. It would put power in the hands of the patients (Lindsey 1993; Goodman and Musgrave 1994).

One way to establish a consumer-based health care system is through the creation of a *medical savings account* (MSA), which represents a relatively new solution to the health care cost problems of the current system. A medical savings account would elevate the role of the individual above that of the system. MSAs would be personal funds established by individuals to pay current out-of-pocket medical costs and accumulate funds for future expenses. MSAs would give individuals, rather than managed care professionals or third-party payers, complete control over how resources are allocated for health care services. Many of the proposals also call for such accounts to be combined with high deductible or catastrophic health insurance policies that would cover certain medical expenses once the insured person spends beyond a substantial deductible. The establishment of MSAs would require changes in tax laws, allowing individuals to deduct their contribution to MSAs from their taxes. The concept of MSAs has been criticized by some and defended by others (Tanner 1995; Ferrara 1996; Moon, Nichols, and Wall 1996).

Some have advocated similar ideas for reforming Medicare. They argue that the Medicare program cannot continue in its present form for three reasons: First, America is growing older. The older people become, the more services they consume, and the services they consume are more expensive. Second, new medical treatments and technologies are costly, contributing to rising costs. Third, the Medicare program suffers from the inherent problem associated with a third-party payment system. Individuals consume more and consume more expensive services because someone else is paying the cost. Under such a system, a consumer has very little incentive to avoid unnecessary expenses. Increasing payroll taxes or premiums, or reducing reimbursement rates, are not the solutions to the problem. The only real solution is to change the incentive structure by raising deductibles and eligibility ages and allowing the elderly to opt out of the system by providing them with vouchers that they can use to buy private insurance or HMO coverage or to make contributions to a medical savings account (Bandow and Tanner 1995).

The Heritage Foundation has advocated using the Federal Employees Health Benefit Program (FEHBP) as a model for reforming the Medicare program. This system allows almost 400 private insurance carriers nationwide to compete for the personal business of members of Congress, their staffs, and millions of federal employees. Once a year, these consumers make their own personal choices. The application of such a model to Medicare would mean that Medicare beneficiaries would be given a choice. They could stay under the present system, if they wanted, or they could choose from a wide range of private health care plans. This would allow senior citizens to get better value for their money because of the competitive nature of the health insurance market. It would require reforming the tax code by adopting a flat tax or by providing a tax credit or a voucher for the purchase of health insurance and services (Liu 1995; Butler 1996; Liu and Moffit 1996).

Other solutions advocated to address the problems of the U.S. health care system include turning Medicaid into block grants to states and giving them greater latitude in setting eligibility and benefit requirements, adopting medical malpractice reforms, improving the insurance coverage to address the problem of the uninsured by making insurance portable, and prohibiting insurance companies from denying coverage for preexisting conditions.

Political Stream

The political stream for 1995–96 was significantly different from the political stream of the 1993–94 reform period. As part of their election year strategy, Republicans produced a document consisting of various campaign promises, the Contract with America, which was signed by 367 Republican candidates. Among other things, Republicans promised to deliver a balanced budget amendment, a line-item veto for the president, welfare and criminal justice reforms, middle-class tax relief, term limits for members of Congress, limits on product liability, and reduced spending. The themes stressed were individual liberty, economic opportunity, personal responsibility, and limited government (Gillespie and Schellhas 1994). While the Contract with America did not directly mention health care reform, it did discuss cutting government spending, particularly spending for entitlement programs. The Republicans also used the Health Security Act to portray President Clinton as a proponent of big government.

The 1994 congressional elections on November 8 brought about dramatic changes in the partisan alignment in Congress. The Democratic Party suffered major losses in congressional and gubernatorial races. In a stunning electoral victory the Republican Party gained a majority in both houses of Congress, ushering in a period of divided government. This also brought about significant changes in the chairmanships of important committees in the Congress. Conservative Republicans took over as chairpersons of crucial committees dealing with health care issues.

There was also a detectable change in the national mood. According to a national survey of 1,200 voters conducted on election day by the Henry J. Kaiser Foundation and the Harvard School of Public Health, President Clinton's failed plan to reform the health care system was a major reason Democrats suffered at the polls (Iglehart 1995). A second survey of voters conducted by President Clinton's own pollster confirmed the same results. Perhaps even more important, the Kaiser-Harvard survey also reported that survey respondents strongly opposed comprehensive health care reform. They favored instead an incremental approach to solving problems of the national health care system. This was a dramatic turnaround from the early 1990s when a strong majority supported comprehensive reforms (Iglehart 1995).

Finally, the consensus that had emerged before the 1993–94 reform period among various organized groups on the need for reform quickly dissipated after the elections (Judis 1995). By 1995–96, no consensus could be found about even the need for comprehensive reform of the system.

A Window of Opportunity

The joining of the problem, policy, and political streams again forced open a small window of opportunity for modest, incremental reform during 1995–96. There was a recognition on the part of the policy makers that specific problems of the uninsured and the Medicare and Medicaid programs needed to be addressed without trying to overhaul the whole system. A number of piecemeal reform proposals were introduced in Congress. Some of the major reform proposals were the Kassebaum-Kennedy health insurance legislation designed to address the problems of the uninsured, legislation to create medical savings accounts, product liability reforms, and proposals to cut Medicare and Medicaid programs. Chapter 4 provides a detailed analysis of the outcome of these proposals.

Conclusion

This chapter has examined the process of policy agenda setting. We looked at why the issue of health care reform returned to the national policy agenda during the early and mid-1990s. During this time frame, the issue of health care reform moved from a systemic agenda to an institutional agenda. One might say that before the 1993–94 reform period, if polls are any indication, the American public was not merely supporting a major overhaul of the health care system but demanding it. By 1995–96, though the support for a comprehensive reform had declined, support from the general public for an incremental approach to reform remained strong. During both reform periods, a number of internal and external triggering devices helped the issue of health care reform reach policy agenda status.

One of the reasons all previous efforts at comprehensive health care reforms, especially for the establishment of a national health insurance system, had failed in the twentieth century (discussed in chapter 1) was the fact that powerful organized interests with access to institutional gatekeepers prevented this issue from achieving a policy agenda status or exercised their "veto power" once the issue had reached the policy agenda. The result often was a "nondecision" on the part of policy makers. At least in the beginning of the 1993–94 reform period, however, this situation changed. Most organized interest groups came to recognize the need for reform, even though they ultimately could not agree on the precise nature of the reforms. Even during 1995–96, most organized interests came to recognize that something needed to be done about the problems of the uninsured, Medicare, and Medicaid.

During both reform periods, many indicators pointed to a significant number of problems in the U.S. health care system, and policy makers came to recognize them as problems. Within the policy streams, policy entrepreneurs were advocating a variety of solutions to the problems. Finally, the political stream was characterized by a supportive national mood, initial support by organized groups for the reform effort, and changes in administration, key personnel, and/or partisan alignment in the Congress. A large number of individuals, both inside and outside government, played a major part in the process of agenda setting and alternative specifications. Finally, during both reform periods, the joining of all three streams—problem, policy, and political streams—opened a window of opportunity for reforms. A significant number of reform initiatives were introduced in Congress. As Kingdon points out, however, windows of opportunity remain open for only a short period within which major policy changes can take place. In the chapters that follow we analyze what happened to these reform initiatives and attempt to illuminate factors that influence the process of agenda setting, alternative specifications, and policy making.

3 PRESIDENTIAL LEADERSHIP AND POLICY MAKING

The American constitutional system of government, with its separation of powers and checks and balances, reflects a strong antimonarchical conviction and distrust of a strong leader. Thus, it was designed to keep its leader, the president, in his place ("The Search for the Perfect President" 1995). It is no surprise then that the American Constitution does not assign a significant role to the president and that his powers are stated very briefly. The Constitution makes him the commander-in-chief, yet he is not given the power to declare or finance war. He is given the power to negotiate international treaties and appoint ambassadors, federal judges, and other high-level executive officials with the advice and consent of the Senate, and he may grant pardons for crimes committed against the United States. Finally, the Constitution states that "he may from time to time give to the Congress Information on the State of the Union, and recommend to their consideration such Measures as he shall judge necessary and expedient" (Constitution of the United States, Art. II, sec. 3). This suggests a very limited role was intended for the president in the policy-making process.

Yet presidents have intermittently been cast in the role of legislative leader. Especially in the twentieth century the president has been expected to act as chief legislator. He is expected to propose legislative initiatives, and Congress is expected to react and act on these initiatives. The conventional wisdom states that "the president proposes and Congress disposes." Presidential success in securing congressional approval for major legislative initiatives, such as Roosevelt's New Deal and Johnson's Great Society, has come to be regarded by some as the norm for presidential leadership in policy making. Others, however, have argued that such leadership expectations are too excessive and that examples of great presidential successes are rare, representing an unusual convergence of opportunities and presidential abilities.

In this chapter we first examine various theories of presidential leadership, rhetoric, and performance. Next, we utilize the ideas and concepts outlined in these theories to analyze the role played by President Clinton regarding the health care reform initiatives during 1993–94 and 1995–96. The primary focus of this chapter is President Clinton's leadership role in 1993–94, during which time he undertook a major legislative initiative to overhaul the U.S. health care system, the Health Security Act of 1993. A secondary focus is placed on the examination of President Clinton's role during the 1995–96 reform period, when initiatives for health care reforms mainly came from Congress. Finally, the chapter concludes with an assessment of President Clinton's leadership during the two reform periods and a general discussion of the role of the president in policy making in the American political system.

Theories of Presidential Leadership, Rhetoric, and Performance

The Constitutional and Cultural Setting

Richard Ellis and Aaron Wildavsky (1989), in *Dilemmas of Presidential Leadership*, suggest that each presidency's basic character is shaped by the particular culturally induced dilemmas it faces. They argue that the American political culture is characterized by three competing political cultures: individualism, egalitarianism, and hierarchical. Individualism emphasizes personal autonomy and minimizes the need for authority; an egalitarian culture is antiauthority and stresses the diminishing differences between individuals (i.e., equality); and the hierarchical culture welcomes a leadership hierarchy and views authority flowing from structurally ordered positions. Conflicts between the first two cultures, that is, individualism and egalitarianism, and the third, hierarchical, and between individualism and egalitarianism produce many dilemmas for presidents.

Ellis and Wildavsky further argue that the structural factors related to the Constitution make America much more difficult to govern compared to parliamentary democracies. Constitutional checks and balances are reinforced by the antihierarchical ethos of the American society and the polity (Ellis and Wildavsky 1989, 13). Both of the predominant cultures (individualism and egalitarianism) are antihierarchical in nature. This, combined with a uniquely independent Congress, makes strong presidential leadership very difficult. This constitutional hamstringing of presidential leadership often stops the president from getting what he wants.

The two authors further argue that too much is made of personality, politics, personal weaknesses, flaws, and political errors in explaining presidential failures. Failure comes more from each president's inability to overcome the cultural dilemmas facing him, and the key to presidential success or failure lies more in what followers expect or demand than in what the president does. Ellis and Wildavsky conclude that presidential leadership should be evaluated on how well presidents provide solutions to their particular cultural dilemmas, and that success depends on how well a president builds and sustains cultural coalitions to confront particular dilemmas.

The presidency has changed significantly since the mid-twentieth century (Pika and Thomas 1992). In addition to the constitutional constraints imposed on the presidency, the frequency of divided government (different political parties controlling the White House and Congress) since mid-century has created new challenges for a president's ability to lead the nation. James Sundquist (1988) argues that since 1969, "party government and presidential leadership" have been replaced by a system of "forced coalition governments" to contend with the outcome of electoral processes that have produced divided governments (1988). According to Charles O. Jones (Jones 1991, 1990, 1989), the original constitutional formation of "separation of power," better understood as "separated institutions sharing powers," needs to be reformulated as "separated institutions competing for shared powers" for the contemporary period.

The Hidden-Hand Presidency

Ellis and Wildavsky suggest that overcoming the difficulty of presidential leadership in an antileadership system that subordinates hierarchy to individualism may require the president to mask a strong leadership role or to cast the leadership role in antihierarchical terms. This is often called the *hidden-hand presidency*. The authors point to a number of presidents in U.S. history as hidden-hand presidents. They view Thomas Jefferson as an adroit hidden-hand president. They also point out how Andrew Jackson justified taking power in order to empower the majority, not himself. Similarly, Ronald Reagan, like Jackson, sought greater power in order to reduce the size and scope of the federal government. In recent years, further credence is lent to the notion of the hidden-hand presidency by Fred Greenstein's study of President Eisenhower's leadership (1994a). Greenstein argues that on the surface Eisenhower appeared to be a president who was lacking in political skills and motivation, an epitome of a nonleader. Nevertheless, the author argues that a detailed and in-depth analysis reveals a president who was politically very astute.

In most democracies, two separate roles—the head of state and the head of government—are held by separate individuals. For example, in Great

Britain the monarch, as head of the state, represents the entire nation and reflects national values that transcend partisan politics. The head of government is the prime minister. In the United States, both of these contradictory roles are combined into the single office of the president. Thus, in the United States a president must be both ecumenical and divisive. As head of the nation, the president must represent the nation as a whole yet at the same time advance policies favored by his party and thus part of the nation. This partly explains why presidents often enter the office in a glow of national approval that soon turns to disapproval. Greenstein (1994a) asserts that Eisenhower succeeded in resolving the contradiction inherent in the office by being an effective head of state in public and by being a prime minister (head of government) in private. He rarely showed his hand or engaged in political maneuvering in public. The hidden hand was central to his leadership. In fact, a recent study compares Eisenhower's leadership to that of Abraham Lincoln and suggests that both presidencies reflected or symbolized the hidden-hand presidency (Turner 1994).

Presidential Power

More then three decades ago, Richard Neustadt examined the issue of presidential power, authority, and influence (1960). At that time, presidential power was thought of primarily in terms of constitutional rights, constraints, and institutional arrangements and functions. Neustadt added a human dimension that was left out of the analysis of the dynamics of presidential power and leadership. He argued that in a constitutionally constrained presidency, true presidential power is not the power to command but the power to persuade. True presidential power lies in the president's ability to persuade others that what he wants from them is in their own self-interest, that is, persuade others to follow where he wants to lead them. A president's ability to bargain depends on his ability to persuade. He can enhance his ability to persuade by minimizing the uncertainties of noncompliance (i.e., making sure that everyone understands the consequences of noncompliance). Over the years Neustadt has added new chapters to the original book, which provide a more rigorous and systematic analysis of the issues of presidential leadership and power (1990).

Others have suggested that the amount of importance a president attaches to particular policy outcomes influences his ability to persuade. When a president attaches great importance to a particular policy outcome, one would expect him to be heavily involved in persuading others of his viewpoint, and vice versa. Presidential involvement and activity may also vary depending on the amount of consensus that is present among other important participants in the policy- or decision-making process. Presidential involvement in the policy-making process should be very high when there is a strong lack of consensus on how to proceed (Silvia 1995).

Personality, Character, Values, and Motives

Another approach to the study of presidential leadership is to combine the issue of presidential power with that of presidential character, values, and motives. For example, James McGregor Burns calls for examining power and leadership in the context of complex human relationships. He argues that moral leadership involves "relating leadership behavior—its role, style, commitments—to a set of reasoned, relatively explicit, conscious values" (1978, 13). The moral leader is able to motivate his followers to rise above the mundane. Unfortunately, Burns suggests that most leadership tends to be transactional. A transactional leader has very little independent influence. His main role is to sift through and broker competing demands. Such a leader is mainly interested in staying afloat, drifting with the tides of history (Oliver 1991). In contrast, a transformational leader operates in a world of bounded rationality. In such a world of bounded rationality,

> policies are often the result of circumstantial coupling of problems, proposals and political priorities of elites than a direct response to discernible demand from the public. Decisions in this world of bounded rationality are arrived at despite ambiguous public preferences, a limited set of policy options and unpredictable consequences of actions. (Oliver 1991, 161).

A transformational leader creatively shapes the public's perception of social conditions and designs responses to these perceived problems and opportunities (Oliver 1991).

James David Barber develops a model of presidential character based on two dimensions: level of activity and the positive or negative elements of a president's character. He classifies presidents into one of four categories. Active-positive presidents exhibit a high level of activity and positive orientation. They are interested in results and accomplishments. They actively involve themselves in the policy process. Active-negative presidents exhibit a high level of activity but have a negative view of themselves and the world. They do not take criticism well, and they tend to be rigid and self-destructive. The passive-positive president exhibits a low level of activity but has a positive outlook, while the passive-negative type exhibits a low level of activity as well as a negative outlook (Barber 1972).

Numerous other studies have attempted to measure presidential leadership and performance based on concepts of character, values, and styles.

For example, Robert Shogan (1991) argues that how successfully a president meets the challenges he confronts depends on his ideology, values, and character. Another study argues that presidential effectiveness depends on the president's personality and charisma and not solely on his control of bureaucratic structure. The authors of that study conclude that 66 percent of the variability in a measure of direct presidential action may be explained by motives, behavioral charisma, institutional age, and crises (House, Spangler, and Woycke 1991). Still another study concludes that as much as 59 percent of the variance in measures of presidential performance may be explained by individual differences in power, affiliation, and number of *nots* appearing in presidential speeches and letters (Spangler and House 1991).

Presidency at the Margins

George C. Edwards III (1989) points to the paradox between the mythic expectations for presidential leadership and the less than impressive performance of many past presidents. He argues that this paradox is an important feature of U.S. political culture. It forces presidents into an active leadership role. Yet, at the same time, his efforts are complicated by the failure to provide reliable support and insistence that the president be all things to all people. Edwards develops a contingency analysis of presidential leadership in Congress. He argues that the president's strategic position derives from three prime sources of presidential influence on Congress: nominal party leadership and attendant partisan support, public opinion, and legislative skills. But his examination of these resources leads him to conclude that the resources and tools available to presidents for use in persuading Congress to follow their leadership are only of marginal utility, effectiveness, and reliability. Presidential leadership efforts operate at the margins of congressional decision making. Edwards also dismisses the notion of "two presidencies," the notion that we in fact have one president for foreign affairs and one for domestic affairs and that presidents are much more successful in getting what they want from Congress in foreign affairs than in domestic policy matters. He argues that presidents do not enjoy any special bipartisan support or congressional deference regarding foreign affairs. He further states that winning a mandate election can provide a president with an edge on leadership and governance. Mandate elections are characterized by a "combination of change, a substantial defeat of the leading opponent, and a sense of new directions in policy" (Edwards 1989, 161). Edwards concludes by suggesting that skillful presidents can recognize and exploit opportunities in a changing environment and that their exercise of leadership, even only at the margins, can turn opportunities into significant accomplishments. Presidents are better thought of as facilitators than as directors. This sounds very close to Neustadt's description of presidential leadership as the ability to persuade and bargain.

The Public Presidency and Presidential Rhetoric

Lowi (1985) has described the modern presidency as a "plebiscitary," which means that the president is viewed as the property of the citizens. Voters invest the president with authority and power to govern. Presidents work hard to keep the initiative and/or control over the policy agenda within the White House. Presidents want their proposals to dominate congressional debate. In order to accomplish this, presidents have relied on communication with Congress, press conferences, speeches, and public appearances. Presidents can have more legislative success by shaping the overall policy agenda through the use of such means (Lowi 1985).

Kernell (1986) argues that bargaining provides an insufficient answer to the contemporary problem of presidential leadership. Using the example of the Reagan presidency, he argues that presidents need to go to the public more often to galvanize support for their policy agenda and to build winning coalitions. "Going public" represents a new style of presidential leadership in which the president sells his programs and leadership skills directly to the American public. Richard Rose (1991) argues that modern presidents continue to perfect the art of going public because of the declining influence of political parties as an effective means of political communication with the electorate. One of the consequences of "going public" is that public opinion can play an important role in a president's effectiveness as a leader or his success as a policy maker (Brace and Hinckley 1992).

Confronted by crisis and controversy, presidents such as Johnson, Nixon, and Carter used rhetorical tools to mobilize public support for their presidencies (Zernicke 1990). History shows that U.S. presidents who engage in fiery rhetorical language have been able to win the sympathy of people and display a sense of moral leadership (Geldeman 1995). Political circumstances invite presidents to make rhetorical choices, each of which has political consequences (Smith and Smith 1994). Presidential rhetoric can have a positive impact on public agenda building. The more attention presidents give to policy areas in their speeches, such as the State of the Union address, the more concerned the public becomes with those policy areas. Thus, presidents can use public rhetoric to build support for their policy agenda (Cohen 1995).

Jeffrey Tulis (1987) draws our attention to presidents' expanded use of public rhetoric to legitimize the use of the inspirational leadership pioneered by Theodore Roosevelt (Dorsey 1995). Woodrow Wilson advocated an active and continuous presidential leadership of public opinion as a way of providing the political system with requisite energy (Tulis 1987). Woodrow Wilson saw a president's role as interacting directly with the public and responding to, as well as influencing and shaping, its desires. Jimmy Carter, since leaving office, has used "humility" and "virtue" as central concepts in his public rhetoric to shape the public memory of his presidency (Lee 1995).

In recent years, President Reagan was very successful in "going public" and converting his standing with the public into political influence in Washington. President Reagan restored the public image of the office as "a place of popularity, influence and initiatives, a source of programmatic and symbolic leadership," (Neustadt 1990, 269). Reagan used his professional skills as an actor and television spokesman to exploit fresh opportunities for influence (Neustadt 1990; Conti 1995). Reagan employed public rhetoric to change what he believed was a flawed metaphor that had become dominant in American politics and culture. The flawed metaphor was the life-as-a-footrace metaphor that depicted a society in which there were countless losers. President Reagan and his speechwriters developed an alternate metaphor of "partnership" to depict the American society. Reagan's public language was laced with terms such as spirit, freedom, and progress to drive home the metaphor of American society as a partnership (Muir 1992).

Presidential Leadership in a Pluralist Society

Peter Drucker (1981, 1990) argues that ours is a highly pluralist society (i.e., a fragmented society made up of single-purpose factions). A faction is a group of true believers who are strongly committed to a narrow issue, interest, or ideology. They prefer confrontation over consensus and combat over compromise. They do not hesitate to use dirty politics or dirty means to pursue their ends ruthlessly. The roots of dirty politics lie in the anxiety created by the threatened survival and loss of identity. Drucker claims that the role of the leader is to face up to the challenges of managing in today's pluralist society. The main question that a leader has to deal with is how a pluralist society can create a unity of purpose out of the conflicting diversity of institutions, interests, and values. In other words, how can a society get its act together, that is, be able to act together out of diversity. This is what Tocqueville (1988) called "habits of acting together."

President Clinton and Health Care Reform: 1993–94

The 1993–94 health care reform period was dominated by presidential initiative and leadership. It was during this time that President Clinton initiated and proposed to Congress his Health Security Act of 1993, designed to overhaul the U.S. health care system. By August/September 1994, however, no congressional action was forthcoming. The Health Security Act of 1993 was declared dead and laid to rest. In this section we examine President Clinton's initiative and his leadership role in his attempt to reform the U.S. health care system.

The Presidential Election of 1992

On June 5, 1991, a major salvo was fired in the debate on health care reform that set the stage for the 1993–94 reform period. It was on this day that Democratic Senators Mitchell, Kennedy, Riegle, and Rockefeller announced to the press and the public the introduction of S. 1227, their plan for comprehensive reform of the U.S. health care system called "Health America." The major features of the plan included universal coverage, cost containment, national expenditure targets, and negotiated provider reimbursement rates. The plan was to be financed by a pay-or-play incentive structure. It would require employers (employer mandate) either to offer their employees health benefits or to pay into a new public program called AmeriCare, which would supplement Medicaid while retaining the Medicare program (Peterson 1992).

Senator Robert Dole (R-Kans.), the Senate minority leader, asked Senator John Chafee (R-R.I.) to chair the Senate Republican Health Care Task Force and instructed the task force to produce an initiative designed to counter the Democrats. In November, Senator Chafee and others formally introduced S. 1936, Senate Republicans' response to the Democrats. This plan was modest and incremental in nature. The main features of the plan included tax incentives to encourage the purchase of private insurance, insurance market reforms, medical liability reforms, and giving states greater flexibility to address the problem of the uninsured (Peterson 1992). President Bush, in February 1992, introduced his health care reform plan, a very modest plan that relied on tax incentives and medical malpractice reforms. All these developments helped set the stage for the 1992 elections.

On November 5, 1991, in a special election for the U.S. Senate, Democrat Harris Wofford soundly defeated a popular Republican, Richard Thornburgh, in Pennsylvania after starting far behind in the polls. The centerpiece of his campaign was a call for a national health care plan. The Wofford election gave credence to the prevailing wisdom that Democrats could capitalize on middle-class resentment in the coming general elections by focusing on health care costs and coverage. It was believed that focusing on these issues would make them concrete to the voters, many of whom were afraid of losing their jobs and thus their health insurance coverage. The number of uninsured people had already increased from 34.7 million in 1990 to 38.6 million in 1992, roughly about 15 percent of the U.S. population (see Table 2.3). Furthermore, many national polls taken from 1990 to 1992 indicated that a large number of Americans viewed cost to them personally as the main health care issue (Blendon, Hyams, and Benson 1993). Thus, it is not surprising that all major Democratic contenders for the party's nomination for the president pledged support for health care reform (Brown 1992). Upon winning the Democratic Party's nomination for the presidency, Bill Clinton made health care reform a centerpiece of his campaign for the presidency. The presence of a Democratic challenger in the 1992 presidential race who was committed to reforming the American health care system helped move health care problems onto the front pages (Marmor 1994c). In a speech to the American Nurses Association in Pittsburg, California, on August 15, 1992, candidate Clinton stated that,

> the crisis we face in health care has a deeply human face and a stark economic reality. The truth is we can not make America the place it ought to be for all our people until we finally join the ranks of other advanced nations and provide a basic package of comprehensive but affordable health care for all.

He went on to say that

> in the first hundred days of our administration, Al Gore and I will send to the United States Congress an attempt to pass a program that finally will bring America in line with the rest of the world; with a plan for a comprehensive, affordable health care for every citizen in this country as a right, not a privilege.

The basic philosophy and structure of the Clinton health care plan began to emerge in early 1992. During the New Hampshire Democratic primary, Clinton was attacked by his two Democratic rivals for the nomination, Bob Kerrey of Nebraska and Paul Tsongas of Massachusetts, for his failure to produce any specific health care reform proposal. Senator Kerrey (D-Neb.) had introduced his own version of a comprehensive health care reform plan in July 1991, which bore close resemblance to the "single-payer" system of Canada. Senator Paul Tsongas's (D-Mass.) reform plan relied on the concept of "managed competition" developed by Stanford University economist Alain C. Enthoven, who was working with other academics and business people in Jackson Hole, Wyoming, the vacation home of managed care proponent Paul Ellwood.

During the Nixon administration (as we saw in chapter 2), Ellwood was instrumental in getting the administration to encourage the development of health maintenance organizations as alternative health delivery organizations that would compete with traditional organizations in the health care market. The theory of managed competition came to be known as the Jackson Hole Plan and the people who helped develop it as the Jackson Hole Group. This plan mainly relied on the market forces of supply and demand and envisioned a very small role for government in the health care market.

If Clinton were to pitch himself successfully as a new Democrat to the American voter, he had no choice but to search for a policy that was distinct and that would occupy a middle ground between Kerrey's heavy reliance on big government and Tsongas's heavy reliance on a restructured marketplace. Thus, he initially came to favor Senate Democrats' "play-or-pay" plan and issued a health care reform position paper on January 19, 1992, that was based on this plan. Over the next eight months Clinton continued to refine his views as rival groups of presidential campaign advisers and policy entrepreneurs tried to get their ideas and themselves accepted by the man who might become president (Johnson and Broder 1996).

By June 1992, with the Democratic nomination in his hand, Clinton was under pressure to spell out his general election campaign proposals. The battle was on to influence and shape Clinton's proposal for reforming the health care system. It was a contest between the "Blueberry Donut Group" representing the views of the Democratic Washington establishment (i.e., play-or-pay approach) and the Cambridge-California alliance led by Ira Magaziner, which was attracted to the new theory of managed competition.

Bruce Reed, an analyst on Clinton's campaign staff, and Ira Magaziner teamed up to draft a plan that relied on cost savings through reduction in paperwork and the application of managed competition. It envisioned cost savings by organizing the health care market into provider and purchaser cooperatives designed to produce economic efficiency in the health care market (Thomas 1995). Another campaign staffer, Atul Gawande, brought with him to Little Rock, Arkansas, the managed competition concepts he had developed while working with Congressman Jim Cooper (D-Tenn.). Magaziner and Gawande hoped to form a merger of Democratic positions from the left and right and to shed the play-or-pay label, which had come under increasing Republican attack. The Bush administration attacked the play-or-pay plan associated with Democratic leaders in Congress as a government takeover scheme for "socialized medicine," and as a threat to business because of the payroll taxes this approach would necessitate (Skocpol 1996). Gawande prepared a memorandum that summarized the internal campaign agreements on policy. This became the basic text for briefing and preparing Clinton for his first presidential debate with George Bush on September 22, 1992.

The key elements of the new approach included the following: All workers and their families would receive health insurance through their jobs, with employers paying most of the premiums; small businesses would receive direct subsidies to subsidize their costs; universal coverage for those outside the workforce would be paid for by the government; networks of hospitals, physicians, and other medical professionals would be organized in every community that would compete in the marketplace and charge a flat fee for a standard benefit package; states would organize health insurance purchasing alliances through which small groups, the self-insured, and others could buy a policy; and, finally, the national government would set an overall national health budget. "The Clinton campaign had given birth to its version of managed competition" (Johnson and Broder 1996, 87). This new plan was very much influenced by *The Logic of Health Care Reform* (1992), a book written by Paul Starr, a sociologist at Princeton University.

Bill Clinton's campaign strategy was designed to position the Democratic Party at the center of American politics (Canaham-Clyne 1995). The strategy worked, and Bill Clinton was swept into the office of the presidency with an electoral vote landslide (370 electoral votes out of a possible 538), though he received only 43 percent of the popular vote. George Bush received 37.4 percent of the popular vote and Ross Perot 19.6 percent.

A Kaiser Family Foundation/Harris poll, taken after both political conventions in the summer of 1992, showed Clinton holding a 55 to 27 percent edge over President Bush when voters were asked which candidate would do more to provide affordable health coverage for all Americans. By early October, Clinton had widened his health issue margin over Bush from 28 points in late August to 42 points. On election day Clinton enjoyed a 34 point lead on the health care issue. But voters ranked health care only third in importance to them, after the economy and the budget deficit. Public support for the Clinton plan was very shaky. Public opinion was split, with one-third of those polled favoring Bush's subsidy plan and another third favoring a single-payer plan; only 28 percent favored Clinton's managed competition plan. Robert Blendon's analysis of the poll result was prophetic. He said that Clinton had a mandate for health care reform that would expand coverage and contain costs; however, he did not have a mandate for any specific plan and would find it very difficult to create a consensus on any specific reform plan (Johnson and Broder 1996).

President's Task Force on National Health Care Reform

Upon his election and inauguration, President Clinton moved quickly to fulfill his campaign promise of delivering a comprehensive health care reform plan. The health care transition team, headed by Judith Feder, had been working on health care reform. Immediately following the inauguration, Ira Magaziner presented to President Clinton a twenty-three-page document entitled "Preliminary Work Plan for Interagency Health Care Task Force," which became an organizational blueprint for a multipronged task force approach followed by President Clinton to devise his plan for national health care reform (Skocpol 1996).

On January 25, 1996, Clinton announced the formation of the President's Task Force on National Health Care Reform. He named his wife, Hillary Rodham Clinton, as the head of the task force and Ira Magaziner, his long time close friend, as the chief coordinator. This advisory task force also included six cabinet ministers and several other White House officials. Additionally, President Clinton announced the creation of an interdepartmental working group responsible for gathering information and developing various options and alternatives for health care reform. The members of this group were divided into many subgroups. Ultimately, the size of the group grew to more than 500 persons drawn from various government agencies, the private sector, and academia (Thomas 1995–96).

The naming of Hillary Clinton to head the task force signaled to Congress and everyone else the importance the president attached to the issue of health care reform. Nevertheless, it also immediately limited how far cabinet secretaries would go in pressing their own views and their disagreements with the first lady. As one official opined, "the person who is in charge shouldn't sleep with the president, because if you sleep with the president, nobody is going to tell the truth" (Johnson and Broder 1996, 101).

The first formal and only public meeting of the task force was held on March 29, 1996. The public's one and only opportunity to comment and provide input into the formulation of the administration's reform plan came on this day. The task force very carefully controlled public access during this thirteen-hour meeting. Each witness was given only three minutes to deliver a prepared statement. Groups invited to testify at the public hearings included representatives of physicians, insurers, hospitals, pharmaceuticals, and consumers. The only other opportunity to address the task force by the public was through submission of written comments. In addition, the public never had an opportunity to address the Working Group, which was developing various options. The Clinton administration initially even refused to provide a list of the members of the Working Group. Ultimately, the administration released the list on March 26, 1993 (Thomas 1995–96).

The administration came under significant criticisms for its attempt at maintaining secrecy surrounding the task force and the Working Group. In the spring of 1993, organizations representing physicians and consumers filed a lawsuit in federal court challenging the secrecy of the process. The suit claimed that since the first lady was not a federal employee, and since the task force was an advisory committee, all its meetings should be open to the public under the requirements of the Federal Advisory Committee Act (Thomas 1995–96). The U.S. District Court ruled in favor of the plaintiffs on the ground that the first lady was not an employee of the federal government. On appeal, the Court of Appeals for the District of Columbia ruled that the task force was not an advisory group subject to requirements of the Federal Advisory Committee Act, but criticized the Clinton administration for its penchant for secrecy. Faced with determined plaintiffs, the administration capitulated and revealed the information that plaintiffs sought (Thomas 1995–96).

Despite the secrecy surrounding the work of the task force, it is important to note that the task force went out of its way to hear a variety of viewpoints. While it is true that there were no representatives of organized outside interests on the task force, the task force met frequently with outside groups to solicit their views. According to the *Congressional Quarterly*, the task force met with 572 separate organizations, and the headline on the May 22, 1993, issue of *Congressional Quarterly* read, "Clinton Task Force All Ears on the Subject of Overhaul" (Fallows 1995).

The theoretical framework of the task force began as the purest form of managed competition, based on the work of Alain Enthoven, Paul Ellwood, and other members of the Jackson Hole Group. According to this school of thought, Americans are not conscious about health insurance because their coverage is paid for by their employers and not out of their own pockets. As a result, Americans are overinsured and overuse health services and health care resources. This tendency is encouraged even further by fee-for-service providers who benefit economically by overconsumption.

To make consumers cost conscious, their cost sharing should be increased. Employers would pay 8 percent of the cheapest available plan, and the government would tax all benefits over and above this basic plan. The insurance industry would discipline providers by making them work in insurance-controlled provider networks or managed care plans. Health care providers would become employees of insurers, or contract their services to them. Consumers would have to enroll in one of these insurance-controlled plans. According to this version, managed competition would lead to vertical integration of the health industry under the control of insurance companies. This came to be called the hard version of managed competition and was favored by the staff of Democratic Congressman Cooper and members of the Jackson Hole Group (Navarro 1995b).

There also emerged a soft version of managed competition (a degenerate version according to the Jackson Hole Group) that was concerned with cost controls. This version was primarily theorized by Paul Starr and Walter Zelman, deputy insurance commissioner of the state of California. The soft version of the managed competition plan shared many of the main features of the hard version, but it advocated insurance premium caps and a regulatory role for the government, such as establishing a global budget designed to control costs. Large employers would be allowed to stay out of the alliances (Navarro 1995b). The final version of the plan put forth by the Clinton administration resembled the soft version.

The task force disbanded on May 30, 1993. The members of the Working Group met in private to fill in the details of the policy decided by the task force. Participants experienced delays and/or cancellations of meetings and a lack of communication due to the emphasis on secrecy. A Justice Department lawyer described the whole process as "an anonymous horde or a leviathan" operating in a state of "creative chaos" (Thomas 1995–96, 89). Another participant described the process as a "four-alarm fire," while still another participant indicated that "the policy making process was unusual, exhilarating, disorienting and rather bizarre" (Thomas 1995–96, 89).

Despite the best intentions and the campaign promise to present to Congress a comprehensive health care reform plan in the first 100 days, it was not until September 1993 that the administration produced a draft bill. It was November 1993 before the Clinton administration sent the proposal, a comprehensive, 1,300-page bill called the Health Security Act of 1993, to Congress. This points out very clearly how quickly events often spin out of control and the president can lose control of his agenda. The Clinton administration had started off very badly on the issue of gays in the military. This was quickly followed by a prolonged battle with Congress over the budget and the economic stimulus package; ratification of the North American Free Trade Agreement (NAFTA) was also given priority by the administration. By the fall of 1993, the budget battle was over. All these other agendas helped push back the president's timetable for health care reform.

The Health Security Act of 1993

In his nationally televised address to the joint session of Congress President Clinton stated that

> this health care system of ours is broken and it is time to fix it. Despite the dedication of literally millions of talented health care professionals, our health care system is too uncertain and too expensive, too bureaucratic and too wasteful. It has too much fraud and too much greed. (*Public Papers* 1994)

In the remainder of the speech President Clinton outlined the major principles and features of his proposal to reform the U.S. health care system known as the Health Security Act. He specifically outlined six major underlying principles: security, simplicity, savings, choice, quality, and responsibility. Security meant that those who did not have health insurance coverage would have it (i.e., universal coverage), and for those who had it, it could never be taken away. Simplicity meant that our health care system must be less complex for both patients and health care professionals with less complicated rules and less bureaucratic paperwork. A reformed health care system must produce savings in the health care system to combat spiraling health care costs. At the same time, reform must preserve and maintain the high quality of medical care. Patients must continue to have freedom of choice in selecting their own health plan and their own doctors. The sixth and final principle was one of responsibility. Everyone—patients, health care providers, insurers, and others—must act and behave responsibly in the health care market (*Public Papers* 1994).

As discussed above, the president's proposed health care reform plan was based on the concept of managed competition. Everyone would belong to a health alliance, a purchasing cooperative set up by states. Large companies (5,000 or more workers) could set up their own health alliance. Insurers and providers would establish health care plans. The alliances and health care plans would negotiate and offer subscribers a minimum of three health care plans to select from. One plan would be a health maintenance organization that would provide all services to subscribers. A second plan would offer consumers traditional fee-for-service system with higher premiums and co-payments. The third plan was a hybrid of the first two versions. This would include a preferred provider organization. In such a plan, subscribers could get a discount if they used providers from the approved list.

Employers would be required to pay 80 percent of the premiums for their employees (employer mandate), while the workers would pay the remaining 20 percent. Small employers with less than fifty employees would receive a government subsidy to offset their costs. Self-employed workers would pay their own health premiums up to a point—$1,800 for individuals and $4,200 for families—and all premiums would be fully tax deductible.

The unemployed would also receive a government subsidy to cover their insurance premiums. The Medicaid program would be eliminated. Federal and state governments would pay premiums for the poor; however, poor individuals would be restricted to the low-cost health plan. The Medicare program would remain intact, though it would face some spending cuts, and the federal government would pay the premiums for retired persons over the age of sixty-five.

The minimum benefit guaranteed by the health care plans must include the following services with certain restrictions: hospital, emergency, physician, clinical preventive, family planning, pregnancy related, mental health and substance abuse, home health care, hospice, extended care, ambulance, outpatient laboratory and diagnostic, outpatient prescription and biologicals, outpatient rehabilitation, durable medical equipment, preventive dental services for children, vision and hearing, and health education classes.

The Health Security Act also focused on cost controls. It was anticipated that managed competition and managed care would result in cost control. It was also argued that reduced administrative (i.e., paperwork) requirements would help contain costs. In addition, a series of regulatory mechanisms would be used if managed competition and managed care failed to produce sizable cost savings. These included a cap or a ceiling on the growth of insurance premiums and a national global budget for health care.

The plan President Clinton sent to Congress was a softer version of managed competition that included several regulatory tools. Despite the months of deliberation in the preparation of the plan, what is most surprising is that the plan submitted to Congress, presumably after several months of discussion, debate, and deliberation by the President's task force on National Health Care Reform, was almost identical in its main features to the reform plan ideas advocated by President Clinton during the presidential campaign of 1992.

The reform plan as envisioned under the Health Security Act was a complex one, and it was based on a combination of several different ideas. The proposed bill itself was 1,300 pages long! It advocated universal coverage, a generous basic package of services, managed competition, managed care, health care alliances, employer mandates, elimination of the Medicaid program, reduced and simplified paperwork, government subsidies to small employers and the unemployed, and a host of regulatory mechanisms such as a cap or ceiling on insurance premiums and a global budget. The plan explicitly rejected a single-payer approach yet permitted states to establish a single-payer system if they wished.

During the deliberations over health care in 1993–94, a number of competing reform plans, Democratic and Republican, were offered in Congress. One was a single-payer plan, some were modifications of the Clinton approach, while others relied more on voluntary mechanisms. A few were bipartisan, including a Senate coalition plan offered in the waning days of the health care reform debate. These proposals are described in detail in chapter 4.

Death of the Health Security Act

After his nationally televised address to the Joint Session of Congress on September 22, 1993, President Clinton had planned to spend most of the month of October traveling and speaking about his health care plan to generate public support. Instead, he ended up spending most of the month dealing with the death of American soldiers in Somalia and the debate over ratification of NAFTA. This again underscores how events beyond the president's control, or unanticipated events, can undermine his ability to control the policy agenda.

The presence of numerous health care reform plans did not translate into congressional support and action on any of the competing plans. As these various plans moved through different committees in the House and the Senate during 1994, it became obvious there was no clear consensus on any of the plans or approaches for reforming the U.S. health care system. If anything, the earlier consensus on the need for reform began to break down. Furthermore, with the passage of time and increased lobbying by proponents and opponents, public support for reform also declined considerably.

Despite the fact that the Democratic Party enjoyed a majority in both houses of Congress, Democrats were unable to create a majority coalition behind any of the plans, including President Clinton's Health Security Act. Republicans, on their part, were convinced that given the disunity within the ranks of the Democrats, by working together they could defeat President Clinton's ambitious plan to reform the U.S. health care system and use the failure to their advantage in the 1994 congressional elections.

By the late summer of 1994, with congressional elections approaching in November, it was clear that no health care reform bill was likely to pass Congress. By fall 1994, the issue of health care reform was dead and buried and with it were President Clinton's Health Security Act and all other reform bills. Not a single health care bill was voted on by either house of the 103d Congress.

Presidential Leadership and Failure of Health Care Reform: 1993–94

What factors account for the failure of health care reform in general and the Health Security Act of 1993 in particular? A variety of explanations have been offered in the literature. Some have attributed the failure of health care reform solely or partially to the institutional and structural features of the American political system (Steinmo and Watts 1995; White 1995; Smith 1995; Morone 1995). Some have blamed the public for contributing to congressional gridlock on health care reform (Brodie and Blendon 1995), while others have argued that the general public does not deserve the blame for the failure of health care reform (Jacobs and Shapiro 1995; Peterson 1995). Still others have argued that attempts at health care reform failed because of business and various interest groups (Martin 1995; Baumgartner and Talbert 1995; Judis 1995), failure to appeal to the preferences of critical voters in both the House and the Senate (Brady and Buckley 1995), and the nature of class relations in American society (Navarro 1995b). Finally, some have placed the blame on President Clinton and his administration (Rockman 1995). In this section our discussion is confined to the leadership role of President Clinton in dealing with health care reform. The chapters that follow examine the failure of health care reforms to examine in detail the role played by institutions, interest groups, public opinion, and the mass media.

One of the factors that contributed to the failure of health care reform was that the Clinton presidency got off to a very rocky start, and much of the blame must rest with the president and the White House. During the 1992 campaign, Clinton portrayed himself to the American electorate as a New Democrat and an agent for change. But some of the earliest initiatives undertaken by the Clinton administration (minor as they might have been perceived by the White House), such as the issue of gays in the military, quickly destroyed any credibility he might have enjoyed as a new kind of Democrat. This, combined with the prolonged battle with Congress over his proposed budget with large tax increases, allowed Republicans to portray him as just another tax-and-spend liberal who favored big government acting as big brother. To put it very simply, the health care issue gave way to other priorities, such as the economy and the budget.

A second reason for the failure of health care reform can be attributed to the significant delay in presenting the administration's plan to Congress. Clinton, during the campaign, had promised to deliver a comprehensive plan to reform the U.S. health care system within the first 100 days of his administration. But it was not until September 1993 that the Clinton administration finally produced its plan, the outline of which the president presented to a joint session of Congress on September 23. Instead of capitalizing on the goodwill and a honeymoon period between the president and Congress that usually characterizes the first three months of a new presidency, crucial time was lost by the administration in developing its plan (Fallows 1995). Six weeks after the inauguration, Magaziner wrote a memo to Bill and Hillary Clinton warning them that if health care reform legislation was not presented and passed immediately, it might not be possible to pass it during Clinton's first term in office (Fallows 1995). The fact that the plan was associated with President Clinton also generated a great deal of partisanship (Starr 1995). The actual plan, the Health Security Act of 1993, as it was presented to Congress, was 1,300 pages long. It was a very detailed and complex plan that combined elements of market reform in the form of managed competition with government regulatory schemes such as a global budget and caps on insurance premiums. This again allowed the Republicans to attack the plan as representing big government and big bureaucracy. Having increased taxes in its hard-fought first budget, the administration could not propose major tax increases to finance the reform. It had to rely on selling the plan for its cost savings, a very hard sell.

Both of these factors can be related directly to President Clinton's personality and leadership style. As Fred Greenstein argues, the leadership style of Clinton is neither unitary nor layered. Instead, over time it alternates between two basic modalities. One is a no-holds-barred style striving for many policy outcomes at the same time without paying much attention to establishing priorities or accommodating to political realities. The other style is more measured and pragmatic, focusing on a limited number of policy goals and attending closely to the politics of selling the program (Greenstein 1994b). Many of Clinton's personality traits, under some circumstances, combine to form an undisciplined, have-it-all approach, and under other circumstances converge in a more focused and accommodating style (Greenstein 1993).

There is little doubt that during the first two years of his presidency Clinton displayed the first leadership style, characterized by a lack of discipline and a too ambitious policy agenda without any clear priorities. Clinton often seemed to suffer from an absence of self-discipline, experiencing difficulty narrowing his goals, prioritizing his efforts, and devising strategies for advancing and communicating his goals. He also had a tendency to take on too many personal responsibilities and failed to establish a structure of delegation. The result was a paradox. On the one hand, he overloaded the national policy agenda; on the other hand, his administration had difficulty operating on more than one track at a time (Greenstein 1994b).

Clinton's ambition and self-confidence often led him to policy initiatives that were sweeping in their scope and complexity. His health care reform program and his early economic program (first budget) were examples of this. Furthermore, his policy initiatives came so rapidly that it left little time for public institutions to appreciate the implications of these policies. Not surprisingly, he often fell short of his grand policy aspirations (Renshon 1994).

The lengthy health care reform proposal can also be explained by the fact that Clinton brings to his leadership a passionate interest in public policy, particularly domestic policy; he can be called a "policy wonk." He was preoccupied and fascinated by not just the general policy goals but also by the specific details (Greenstein 1994b). His speeches often had a ring of a public policy graduate school rather than the political arena (Greenstein 1993). He could spend hours and days debating the finer points of every policy angle, but he had great difficulty making up his mind and making decisions. He is a political animal in the sense that he is willing to change his positions based on the responses of the public, who also enjoys the art of persuasion and cajolery (Greenstein 1994b). Thus it is not surprising that his enemies accused him of being wishy-washy on issues and critics charged that on the issue of health care reform he caved in too much too frequently.

A third factor that helped explain the failure of the health care reform was that Clinton failed to win an electoral mandate in the 1992 presidential election. He won 43.6 percent of the popular vote, making him a minority president. Thus, when he assumed the office of the presidency, he was unable to claim that his election represented the mandate of the public for his policy agenda.

Even on the issue of health care reform there were troubling signs. Although a poll conducted on election day showed that there was strong support for reforming the U.S. health care system, the voters ranked health care only third in importance to them, after the economy and budget deficit. Public support for the Clinton plan was even weaker. While Clinton had a mandate for health care reform that would expand coverage and contain costs, he did not have a mandate for any specific plan and found it very difficult to create a consensus on any specific reform plan (Johnson and Broder 1995). As George C. Edwards III (1989) has argued, winning a mandate election can provide a president with a leadership and governance asset. Clearly, President Clinton did not have this asset at his disposal.

A fourth reason for the failure of health care reform was that President Clinton's ability to persuade and bargain with members of Congress was severely constrained. As Richard Neustadt has argued, the president has two basic resources beyond his executive power to help him accomplish his purposes and to use as bargaining chips. These resources are the president's reputation with other policy makers as a skilled and determined player and their perception that he has the support of the public. These resources give the president his true power—the power to persuade (Neustadt 1990). President Clinton managed to diminish both resources during his first few months in office. He was perceived by other policy makers in the political community as inconstant and disingenuous (Greenstein 1993).

He could have overcome this problem if he was seen as having strong public support behind him. But such was not the case. Even though he enjoyed a 55 percent approval rating during a very early point in his presidency, it was in sharp contrast to the very high approval ratings enjoyed by other presidents at similar points in their presidencies. President Truman enjoyed an 87 percent approval rating, Eisenhower 74 percent, Kennedy 83 percent, Johnson 75 percent, Nixon 61 percent, Carter 61 percent, Reagan

67 percent, and Bush 58 percent. Clinton's approval level at the traditional 100-day marker was lower than that of eight of his nine immediate predecessors. A June 5–6, 1993, survey showed his approval rating reached a low of 37 percent (Greenstein 1993). Throughout the first two years of his presidency, Clinton's approval rating fluctuated dramatically. This significantly reduced his ability to persuade and bargain with members of Congress about his health care reform plan because he had very few, if any, bargaining chips left to bargain with.

By the spring of 1994, Republicans in Congress had no reason to accept a deal. They were already anticipating major midterm electoral gains, and killing health care reform in the 103d Congress made perfect sense to them. Indeed, Republican strategist Bill Kristol's advice to the Republicans about any attempt at arriving at a compromise proposal was "sight unseen, oppose it" (Starr 1995).

The fifth and the final factor that contributed to the failure of President Clinton's attempt to overhaul the U.S. health care system was his inability to communicate his objectives and his rationale for the proposed reform to the American public and generate strong public support for it. Samuel Kernell (1986) argues that bargaining provides an insufficient answer to the contemporary problems of presidential leadership and that presidents need to go to the public more often to cultivate public support for their policy agenda and to build winning coalitions. History shows that presidents who engaged in fiery rhetoric were able to get the sympathy of people and display a sense of presidential moral leadership. Such a rhetorical president was Theodore Roosevelt, who called the office a "bully pulpit" (Gelderman 1995). President Clinton tried to do this but was not very successful. As Table 3.1 indicates, President Clinton gave over 110 speeches dealing with health care reform during 1993. From August through October 1993 alone, he gave fifty-four speeches on the topic of health care. From February to August 1994, in an attempt to build a momentum for his health reform plan, he gave about seventeen speeches a month. Yet he failed to galvanize support for his health security plan or any other reform proposals.

President Clinton has a fluency with words and a craftsmanship with sentences that his predecessor, President Bush, lacked (McMannus 1993). Clinton has exceptional verbal intelligence and an effortless ability to elaborate at length about his policies. Yet, as articulate as he is, his record of communicating his goals to the public has been very poor. Ironically, his fluency with language serves him poorly because he often deluges the public with details. He has difficulty communicating broad policy principles and values without communicating policy mechanics (Greenstein 1994b). His difficulties are the result of his failure to come to grips with "the

Table 3.1

Number of Speeches on Health Care Delivered by President Clinton, 1993–94[a]

1993		1994	
January	3	January	5
February	6	February	16
March	6	March	16
April	6	April	15
May	6	May	18
June	9	June	21
July	7	July	18
August	11	August	16
September	24	September	2
October	20	October	6
November	7	November	5
December	6	December	1
Total	114	Total	139

Sources: Public Papers of the Presidents of the United States—William J. Clinton—1993, vols. 1 and 2 (Washington, D.C.: Government Printing Office, 1995).
[a]Includes speeches, town hall meetings, media interviews, and statements to Congress in which health care reform, the Health Security Plan, or health insurance were discussed.

rhetorical presidency" (Gelderman 1995). President Clinton gave 600 speeches in 1993. In his first year as president he spoke publicly three times as often as President Reagan did in his first twelve months in office. This very strategy undermined his message. Too much presidential talk cheapens the value of presidential rhetoric (Gelderman 1995).

There also seemed to be a great deal of emphasis in the Clinton administration on selling its policy instead of educating the public about the merits and limitations of other policy alternatives and explaining the rationale for the policy chosen (Renshon 1994). Clinton relied on political consultants and pollsters to a great extent, and they are often more concerned with image making than speechwriting. Modern presidents have also become too dependent on polling data, and President Clinton was no exception. He made matters worse by trying to get on track with speeches that play to public opinion, which creates a disconnect between his past words and the present ones. This lessens the impact of his speeches.

The classic example of this is provided by his discussion of "universal coverage" in the debate over health care reform. First, he started out insisting that any health care reform bill that Congress passed must provide for universal coverage and that if Congress passed a health care reform bill that did not provide for universal coverage he would veto such a bill. He soon retreated, however, stating that he could accept 95 percent coverage as an acceptable goal, only to go back to insisting on universal coverage. He explained his retreat from universal coverage by stating that he had not thought about how this would be interpreted by those who were waiting to see the first sign of a cave-in (Thomas 1995–96). Needless to say, many of his opponents saw this as a sign of cave-in and became more resolute in their opposition to his plan.

In summary, a variety of reasons contributed to the failure of health care reform during 1993–94. We have discussed only a few of the major reasons related to presidential leadership. Some of the reasons were within the president's control, while others were beyond his control.

President Clinton and Health Care Reform: 1995–96

During 1995–96, initiatives for reform of the health care system came from the Congress. In this section we examine the congressional election of 1994, health-related initiatives undertaken by Republican majorities in Congress, President Clinton's response to these initiatives, and his leadership role during this period.

The Congressional Elections of 1994

> The Republicans enjoyed a double triumph, killing reform and then watching jurors find the president guilty. It was the political equivalent of the perfect crime. (Starr 1995, 20–21)

Starting a few weeks after Clinton's election in 1992, Republicans won some important Senate seats in Georgia and Texas, governorships in Virginia and New Jersey, and mayoral races in New York and Los Angeles. With the defeat of President Clinton's Health Security Act, Republicans were very optimistic about their prospects in the 1994 congressional elections. The first sign of the tide turning in favor of Republicans came on the evening of May 24, 1994, when, in a special election for a vacant House seat in a mostly rural congressional district in Kentucky, a little-known Republican candidate, a minister named Ron Lewis who operated a Christian bookstore and had not run for office in more than twenty years, beat his well-known Democratic rival, Joe Prather. Two weeks earlier, the Republicans won another special election for a congressional seat in Oklahoma, where the Republican candidate, Frank Lucas, defeated his Democratic opponent, Dan Webber Jr., labeling him as a creature of the liberal Washington establishment.

With Clinton's legislative agenda, especially health care, pronounced dead and buried and his popularity sinking in the polls, Republican leaders like Newt Gingrich (House), Bob Dole (Senate minority whip), and Haley Barbour (Republican National Committee chairman) were feeling increasingly optimistic about their chances of wresting control of Congress from the Democrats. By the spring of 1994 they saw a chance to capitalize on the public's anger toward big government, its frustration over the problems of rising crime, declining schools, the breakdown of traditional values, and the lack of trust and confidence in governmental institutions. Newt Gingrich and his closest political adviser, Joseph Gaylord, prepared a battle plan for the fall campaign. The plan called for a three-pronged strategy: (1) develop a positive governing agenda and communicate this agenda to the public in a language that the voters could understand, (2) derail Clinton's agenda for the rest of the year and frame the election around Clinton's failures, and (3) amass a large campaign war chest to make sure that no viable Republican candidate lost because of lack of resources (Balz and Brownstein 1996). Gingrich proposed writing a vision statement that could be converted into a campaign document to nationalize the fall elections.

The result was the Contract with America, a ten-point platform issued by the Republicans in the fall of 1994, which helped unify Republican candidates around a sweeping set of policy proposals and energize the party's key constituencies. It promised to bring these ten policy matters to a vote within the first 100 days of the new Congress. The policy items included a balanced budget amendment and line-item veto for the president, a crime bill, welfare reform, a family tax cut, parental rights in education, strong national defense, a rise in the Social Security earnings limit, regulatory reforms, legal reforms to prevent frivolous lawsuits, and term limits for members of Congress (Gillespie and Schellhas 1995). The selling and marketing of the Contract with America began with an ad in TV Guide at a cost of about $265,000 underwritten by the Republican National Committee and continued with polls, focus groups, other commercials, and conservative talk shows on radio and television.

In Washington, the 103d Congress adjourned after ugly partisan fights over health care reform, campaign finance reform, and the crime bill. In the face of united Republican opposition and deep divisions within the ranks of the Democrats, Democratic leaders in Congress pulled the plug on the health care reform plan in late September 1994. On September 27, 1994, more than 300 Republicans—157 incumbents seeking reelection and 185 challengers—gathered in the West Front of the Capitol and one by one marched to the front of the table to sign the Contract with America.

Even though reforming health care was not part of the Contract, it was a key part of the Republican campaign strategy. In their speeches and campaign ads, Republican candidates for Congress denounced the Clinton plan as the symbol of big government, a bureaucracy run amok, and a threat to the American way of life. They played on the fears and mistrust of government and used health care reform as a symbol of the failings of the liberal welfare state (Johnson and Broder 1996). By Tuesday, November 8, 1994, election day, the Democrats knew from their private polls that they were in trouble. By that evening, as the polls closed, it was clear that their worst fears had come true.

The voters had delivered the worst midterm repudiation of a president since Harry Truman in 1946. It signaled the largest shift in the role and direction of government since Franklin Roosevelt and the New Deal. It broke the forty-year hold of Congress by the Democrats and installed Republicans in power at all levels of government. The Republican victory was strong, complete, and historic (Johnson and Broder 1996). Republicans gained 52 seats in the House, the biggest midterm gains by either party since 1946, giving them a 230–205 majority. In the Senate, the Republicans captured eight more seats, giving them a majority in the Senate. Interestingly, one of the two incumbent Democratic senators swept out of office was Harris Wofford of Pennsylvania, who was elected to office in the special election on November 5, 1991, in one of the most stunning victories against a well-known Republican, by promising to work for the establishment of a national health insurance. Republicans won eleven new governorships, giving them a total of thirty, including governorships in eight of the nine largest states. Republicans also gained an additional 484 state legislative seats, which gave them control of 50 legislative chambers. Finally, and perhaps most impressive, was the fact that not a single Republican senator, member of the House, or governor was defeated in the general election (Balz and Brownstein 1996).

Congressional Health Care Initiatives and President Clinton's Response

Some voters viewed the failure of health care reform as another example of Clinton's misguided belief in a liberal, activist government; others saw it as the breakdown of the entire political system. A postelection survey by Clinton pollster Stanley Greenberg identified the health care plan as the single item that most directly linked Clinton with big government (Balz and Brownstein 1996). According to a survey of voters conducted on election day, President Clinton's failure to reform the health care system was a major reason Democrats suffered at the polls (Iglehart 1995). According to a national survey of 1,200 voters conducted by the Henry J. Kaiser Family Foundation and the Harvard School of Public Health, respondents strongly opposed comprehensive health care reform and instead favored incremental solutions to the nation's health care problems (Iglehart 1995). Polls indicated that most voters in 1994 congressional elections wanted Congress to initiate moderate health care reform. Voters in two surveys deemed health care the top priority for the new Congress and 41 percent supported congressional approval of modest health care reforms (Blendon et al. 1995).

During the campaign, President Clinton came to the defense of Medicare, Social Security, and veterans' benefits. The Republican Party committed itself to shrinking the size of government, balancing the budget, and relying on market forces to allocate medical resources. It was clear that the victorious Republicans in the 104th Congress would battle President Clinton and his defeated Democratic Party over these issues during 1995–96. The fact that Congress would be setting the agenda and Clinton would be responding to that agenda is reflected in the smaller number of speeches on health given by the President during this period (see table 3.2).

President Clinton's 1995 State of the Union address acknowledged the message of the 1994 congressional elections. Twice during his address he declared that the era of big government was over. Nevertheless, he also warned that we cannot go back to the times when citizens were left to fend for themselves and stressed that there was still a role for the government (Koszczuk 1996). He indicated his support of Medicare by stating that he would oppose any attempt to cut Medicare to pay for the tax cut Republicans had advocated. On the issue of health care reform he seemed to acknowledge the message of the 1994 elections when he said:

> I still believe our country has got to move toward providing health security for every American family. But I know that last year, as the evidence indicates, we bit off more than we could chew. So I am asking you that we work together. Let's do it step by step. Let's do whatever we have to do to get something done. Let's at least pass meaningful insurance reform so that no American risks losing coverage for facing skyrocketing prices. That nobody loses their coverage because they face high prices or unavailable insurance, when they change jobs, or a family member gets sick.

Attempt to Reform Medicare and Medicaid

President Clinton further staked out his position on Medicare, Medicaid, and Social Security in February 1995 when he unveiled the administration's fiscal year 1996 budget. The proposed budget allocated $716 billion to the

Table 3.2

Number of Speeches on Health Care Delivered by President Clinton 1995–96[a]

1995		1996	
January	2	January	7
February	2	February	9
March	2	March	5
April	9	April	6
May	7	May	7
June	16	June	8
July	6	July	8
August	8	August	13
September	14	September	7
October	8	October	6
November	4	November	4
December	10	December	1
Total	88	Total	81

Sources: Public Papers of the Presidents of the United States—William J. Clinton—1995, vols. 1 and 2 (Washington, D.C.: Government Printing Office, 1996); Public Papers of the Presidents of the United States—William J. Clinton—1996, vols. 1 and 2 (Washington, D.C.: Government Printing Office, 1997).

[a]Includes speeches, town hall meetings, media interviews, and statements to Congress in which health care reform, the Health Security Plan, or health insruance were discussed.

Department of Health and Human Services, an increase of 7.5 percent over fiscal year 1995. The major share of this increase was allocated for Medicare, Medicaid, and Social Security. His budget projected no savings in Medicare, no new health care proposals, and no balanced budget.

Health care reform was not a part of the Contract with America. Republican majorities in Congress, especially in the House under the leadership of Speaker Newt Gingrich, were busy trying to adopt the ten-point plan during the first 100 days as they had promised. House Republicans succeeded in passing all but one—a term-limits constitutional amendment—of the items in the Contract. Many of these proposals got stalled in the Senate, however, which had more moderate Republicans and was led by the Senate majority leader, Bob Dole, who planned to make a run for the Republican Party's nomination for the presidency in 1996.

As soon as the Republicans turned to writing their own budget in April 1995, health care reform emerged as an important issue. Their campaign agenda promised a balanced budget, a tax cut for the middle class, and shrinking the size of the federal government. They knew that they could not provide a large tax cut and at the same time balance the budget without addressing the problem of entitlement programs, especially Medicare and Medicaid. Medicare posed both an immediate and long-term financial problem for policy makers. The program's Board of Trustees projected that its hospital insurance trust fund (Part A) would be bankrupt by 2001. Medicare spending had grown in real (inflation-adjusted) terms by an average of 6.5 percent annually, as compared with a 4.7 percent increase in health care spending in the private sector (Iglehart 1995).

After a series of compromises among various House and Senate committees, the Republican budget plan, that is, the budget resolution adopted by Congress for FY 1996, included the following major provisions: It promised to balance the budget within seven years (i.e., by the year 2002). It called for $245 billion in tax cuts. The plan also included reducing projected spending (growth rate) on Medicare by $270 billion over the next seven years (Starr 1995; Iglehart 1995). Finally, the plan called for reducing Medicaid spending by $182 billion over the next seven years. This represented about a 30 percent average cut in Medicaid payments to the states. The budget resolution made no explicit assumption about how the $182 billion in Medicaid savings would be realized (Mann and Kogan 1995). After seven years, Medicaid would be converted to block grants and turned over to the states. The proposed reductions in projected spending in the Medicare and Medicaid programs were criticized by many as unworkable (Rasell 1995; Mann 1995; "New Republican Medicaid Bill" 1996).

Republicans argued that managed care and health maintenance organizations would make the system more efficient and less costly. Thus, a considerable amount of savings could be achieved in Medicare and Medicaid. This in itself was very ironic because President Clinton tried to make the same argument two years previously about cost savings in his health care reform plan and Republicans had rejected it as unrealistic. Furthermore, President Clinton fought hard in 1993 to get a deficit-reduction budget through Congress. He succeeded by one vote in both the House and the Senate without any Republican support (Johnson and Broder 1996).

Republicans had now stepped into a political hornets' nest. A year after they killed the president's health care reform plan, which had given them their greatest victory in the 1994 elections, they now faced the same problem—trying to convince the public that their plan would save and strengthen, not weaken and destroy, the public-sector health care system.

Democrats went on the offensive. They charged that the Republicans were calling for the largest Medicare cut in history to pay for a tax cut for the wealthy. Republicans tried to launch a counteroffensive by arguing that they were trying to save and preserve Medicare from the bankruptcy it faced. Democrats were united and continued to hammer Republicans for trying to destroy Medicare. The attacks were working because polls showed a sharp decline in public approval for the new Republican congressional majority.

On June 13, 1995, President Clinton announced that he would favor a ten-year period to balance the budget, which would cause less hardship. He said that the Republican plan to balance the budget in seven years would require draconian measures. Medicare would be cut by $124 billion, Medicaid by $54 billion. President Clinton's support for a balanced budget was partly orchestrated with an eye toward the 1996 elections to prevent any challenge to his nomination from the conservative wing of the Democratic Party. This in turn allowed the president to portray himself as fiscally responsible, a defender of the poor and elderly, fighting excessive cuts in health care and other programs. The debate over the budget continued in Congress into the fall of 1995 and became more heated with the passage of time. The Republican Medicare and Medicaid plans passed the House on October 18, followed by passage in the Senate a few days later, largely along partisan lines. President Clinton vetoed the bill as he had promised.

As 1995 neared an end, a crisis was in the making. There was no budget. House Speaker Newt Gingrich raised the stakes even higher by adding a new threat. He stated that if Clinton did not satisfy Republicans' demand for a balanced budget and a tax cut, they would refuse to raise the federal debt ceiling (which was rapidly approaching the $5 trillion statutory limit), leading to a shutdown of the federal government and forcing the U.S. government to default on its debt for the first time in history.

This was a major calculated gamble. It was based on the assumption that President Clinton would either accept the Republican's budget, or, if he refused, the public would blame the president for the resulting shutdown of government. But a *Wall Street Journal*/NBC poll published the morning after Gingrich's threat showed a sharp drop in public support for the Republican revolution. Congressional approval rating dropped from a positive rating in the spring to a very negative rating; 58 percent disapproved of the job Congress was doing (Johnson and Broder 1996). Clinton was determined not to cave in to the Republican demands. Such poll numbers further strengthened his resolve. After the temporary extension of funding expired and no new budget was in sight, the first shutdown of major parts of the federal government came in mid-November. A new, temporary spending bill was passed, due to expire on December 15, 1995. Clinton accepted the Republican goal of balancing the budget by 2002, though with smaller Medicare, Medicaid, and taxes than Republicans desired. This December 15 deadline also passed without a budget, leading to the second shutdown of the federal government. After a series of continuing resolutions, President

Clinton and the Republicans in Congress agreed to continue funding the government through an omnibus reconciliation resolution. No action was taken on the proposed reductions in spending for Medicare and Medicaid. The controversy over the Medicare and Medicaid programs was left up to voters to resolve in the 1996 elections. The political system had again failed to reform the public-sector health care programs.

Welfare Reform and Its Impact on Medicaid

The Republicans had vowed to end the entitlement to Medicaid and welfare (Aid to Families with Dependent Children [AFDC]). The 1995 legislation passed by Congress dealing with the FY 1996 budget included provisions converting both programs into block grants to be administered with few conditions by the states. As mentioned earlier, President Clinton vetoed the legislation. Republican leaders promised to continue their fight. In 1996 legislation on the FY 1997 budget, the Republican leadership again proposed block grants to replace the Medicaid and AFDC programs. Clinton was firm in his insistence that he would not sign any legislation that turned Medicaid into a block-grant program. But the president did support welfare reform, promising in his 1992 campaign to end welfare in its current form. For a time, congressional leadership tried to keep both block-grant proposals in the same bill, but Clinton twice vetoed welfare-reform legislation. Some House Republicans wanted to pass a welfare-reform bill before the 1996 elections and began to pressure the leadership to drop a proposal to block-grant Medicaid in the welfare-reform bill. Rather than risk yet another presidential veto and be left with no welfare reform, Republican leadership in Congress finally relented and dropped the provision of turning Medicaid into a block-grant program. The welfare-reform bill easily passed the House and the Senate and President Clinton signed the bill. The new law, the Personal Responsibility and Work Opportunity Act of 1996, includes changes in welfare, supplemental security income, child-support enforcement, immigration, child care, food stamps, social services, earned income tax credit, and Medicaid. The main feature of the law is a new welfare program called Temporary Assistance to Needy Families (TANF) under which states are given a block grant to design their own welfare program. The Medicaid program was left virtually intact. The structure of the program, the benefit package, federal and state financial obligations, and so forth, all remain the same. Eligibility also remains the same with some exceptions (Waxman and Alker 1996; "An Analysis of the AFDC-Related Medicaid Provisions in the New Welfare Law" 1996).

Health Insurance Reform

Despite the partisan acrimony that dominated the 104th Congress during 1995 and 1996 over the issues of a balanced budget, Medicare, Medicaid, welfare reform, and other conservative agenda items ushered in by the 1994 Republican revolution, Congress did succeed in accomplishing one important piece of health care reform dealing with health insurance.

A recurring and legitimate concern among millions of working Americans who currently have employment-based health insurance is the fear of losing their insurance when they lose or change their jobs or try to get insurance coverage when they have a preexisting health condition. In a large majority of cases, employers and their dependents are covered by an employer-based insurance policy only as long as they remain with the same employer and for a very short time afterward. Workers and their dependents can be left without insurance if they are laid off or quit their job unless they find another job or buy private insurance. Private insurance may be difficult to get if workers or their dependents have a preexisting medical condition. If a worker joins a firm that does not provide group insurance and if the worker buys his own coverage, he receives no tax breaks for purchasing that policy. Thus it is no surprise that today's employment-based health insurance system has been a major source of worker anxiety.

Senator Nancy Kassebaum (R-Kans.), chair of the Senate's Labor and Human Resources Committee and the ranking minority member, Senator Edward Kennedy (D-Mass.), cosponsored an insurance reform bill designed to address this specific concern (Liu 1996). In March 1996 the House of Representatives passed a GOP health insurance reform bill, followed by Senate approval the next month. The Senate version did not include any provisions for the establishment of medical savings accounts (MSAs) that conservative Republicans insisted on, while the House version did include such a provision. Critics of MSAs argued that they would provide a tax break for the wealthy and result in less health care coverage for many workers ("Bipartisan Consumer Health Bill" 1996). President Clinton threatened to veto the legislation if MSAs were included. There were also differences over the issue of mental health and substance-abuse coverage (Bowermaster 1996). The Senate version required that benefits for mental health and substance abuse be comparable to medical benefits. The House version did not have such a provision. The legislation got tied up in the conference committee until the differences could be worked out. Late in July, the House and the Senate finally reached a compromise on the issue of MSAs that would allow a limited number of MSAs in a demonstration program beginning in 1997 on a trial run of four years. After four years, there would be no expansion of MSAs unless Congress voted to extend and expand the program. Furthermore, MSAs are to be limited to the self-employed, the uninsured, and workers in businesses with fewer than fifty employees. Under intense lobbying from the business community, mental health provisions were taken out of the conference negotiations.

The final version of the bill, S. 1028, the Health Insurance Reform Act, was adopted by the House on August 1, 1996, with only two dissenting votes. On August 2, the U.S. Senate unanimously approved the bill. The major provisions of the act include the following:

- Prohibits insurers from denying coverage or imposing preexisting condition exclusions for more than twelve months for any condition diagnosed or treated in the preceding six months. This twelve-month exclusion is a lifetime limit. No additional preexisting conditions may be imposed on anyone who maintains continuous coverage (i.e., no more than a sixty-three-day gap in coverage).
- Insurers must offer individual coverage to people who leave jobs, voluntarily or involuntarily, and for their dependents. This provision applies only to those who had maintained coverage for the preceding eighteen months.
- Prohibits insurance companies from denying coverage or charging higher premiums to individuals in group plans who are in poor health. Insurers may charge more for groups that include many people with preexisting conditions or groups with higher health costs.
- Makes long-term care deductible for federal income tax purposes.
- Prohibits excluding pregnancy as a preexisting condition.
- Encourages development of a system for electronic transfer of health insurance information. It also allows for the transfer of confidential medical information about Medicare and Medicaid beneficiaries and the privately insured ("Kassebaum-Kennedy Health" 1996)

Critics argued that the bill falls far short on several counts. First, the guarantee of continued insurance coverage is meaningless if workers who lose their jobs cannot afford to purchase coverage. Second, limits on preexisting conditions apply only to those who have been previously enrolled in group plans. Third, mental health coverage was not protected, though it would be included in later legislation. Fourth, the legislation does nothing to help the millions of uninsured Americans who are not covered by their employers or any public program and are unable to afford private insurance ("Kassebaum-Kennedy Health" 1996).

President Clinton signed the Health Insurance Portability and Accountability Act into law in August 1996. The signing ceremony was a bipartisan event. President Clinton celebrated the legislation as an example of what Democrats and Republicans could do when they put the nation's interest first. Both Senators Kennedy and Kassebaum paid tribute to President Clinton for his prodding of Congress in his 1995 State of the Union address to pass a health insurance reform bill. Congress adjourned in early October 1996 to prepare for the 1996 elections.

Throughout the 1996 campaign, Clinton and other Democrats and their allies (such as labor unions) talked about preserving Medicare and Medicaid (as well as education and environmental programs) from the clutches of congressional Republicans. The result of the elections was a second term for Clinton, a narrowing of the Republican majority in the House, and an increase in the Republican majority in the Senate. Though Clinton's 1996 popular vote was larger than his 1992 popular vote, he was denied a majority vote. The state of the economy (in its fifth year of expansion) undoubtedly helped. The 1996 elections were a personal victory for Clinton and the theme of protecting the two federal government programs. But the message from voters was mixed. Protecting those programs was fine, but there was no mandate for an activist agenda.

President Clinton's Leadership and Health Care Reform: 1995–96

> Americans see him as a slippery character, charming and not quite trustworthy, but born to listen and effective enough to respond. He is just like us, a pleaser in a crowded nation of pleasers—a work in progress (Fineman and Turque 1996).

There is no denying the fact that the last two years of President Clinton's first term in office were very different from the first two years. Clinton's leadership style alternated between two basic modalities. One style was a no-holds-barred style of striving for many policy outcomes at the same time without paying much attention to establishing priorities or accommodating to political realities. The other style was a measured, pragmatic style that focused on a limited number of policy goals and attended closely to the politics of selling the program (Greenstein 1994b). Many of Clinton's personality traits combined to form an undisciplined, have-it-all approach, while others converged in a more focused and accommodating style (Greenstein 1993).

As we discussed earlier, the first two years of the first term can only be characterized as discontinuous and episodic (Renshon 1994). There is little doubt that during the first two years of his presidency, Clinton displayed a basic lack of self-discipline and offered too ambitious a policy agenda without any clear priorities. He had difficulty narrowing his goals, prioritizing his efforts, and devising strategies for advancing and communicating his goals. The result was a major policy failure with respect to comprehensive health care reform, though there were successes in other areas.

Clinton's second, more disciplined, more pragmatic, and more focused mode of leadership came into play only when outside forces humbled him. He resists self-discipline until some outside agent forces it on him. His record as governor of Arkansas demonstrated this vividly. During his first term as governor he launched a very large and ambitious policy agenda, and he was defeated in his bid for a second term. This humiliation taught him a lesson; he became more focused and self-disciplined and went on to serve as the governor of Arkansas for ten more years. The humiliating defeat of the Democratic Party in the 1994 congressional election again served as an outside force to restrain him. It was as if a cold slap of repudiation had brought him to his senses.

Clinton is a very ambitious person (Maraniss 1995a, 1995b, 1995c). Nevertheless, the irony of his successful career is that the style and substance of his character have been shaped more by rebuke than acclaim. Repudiation is a theme that characterizes his political career and his rise to power (Maraniss 1994). Clinton is also self-confident, determined, and resilient, with a strong need for validation and affirmation (Renshon 1994). The redeeming traits that have served him well in the long run are his pragmatism and his capacity to admit to his failings (Greenstein 1994b).

The last two years of President Clinton's first term represented the second modality of leadership. The repudiation he suffered at the hands of the voters in the 1994 elections taught him a lesson. It taught him self-discipline. He became more focused, and his policy agenda less ambitious. As we discussed earlier, in his 1995 State of the Union address he admitted to his failures, especially with respect to his ambitious plan to reform the U.S. health care system. He declared that the era of big government was over, adopted the 2002 balanced budget goal, politically moved to the right, and took a more centrist approach on issues of crime and welfare, among others. He also demonstrated his determination and pragmatism by calling on Congress to adopt health insurance reform. He was also more accommodating and open to negotiations and bargaining with the Republican leadership in Congress. After the disaster of the 1994 elections, Clinton was advised that he had to quit playing legislator-in-chief. He had to be above the fray, president of all America and not just the Democratic Party (Fineman and Turque 1996). Clinton acted on this advice for the remainder of his first term. In fact, his reelection campaign—his speeches, the party convention, his acceptance speech, his debates with Republican nominee Bob Dole— were so well orchestrated that many media commentators referred to him as the most disciplined politician in the campaign!

Clinton's leadership during 1995–96 came to be defined more by what he stood against than by what he stood for. During 1993–94, a major initiative for reforming the U.S. health care system came from President Clinton in the form of the Health Security Act of 1993—a battle that he lost badly. During 1995–96, initiatives in the area of health care reform came from Congress. Instead of being an advocate of his policy initiatives, his role became one of responding to the policy initiatives of a Congress dominated by conservative Republicans. He took on the role of a fighter, standing up to Newt Gingrich and defending against the draconian policy measures initiated by Republicans with respect to Medicaid and Medicare. He became the protector of the elderly and the poor. He also took on the tobacco and gun lobbies, winning most of those battles. He even successfully prodded Congress into passing a health insurance reform law.

Whether President Clinton ultimately turns out to be a transformation leader or a transactional leader remains to be seen. Thus far, he gives every indication of being a transactional leader who has very little independent influence. Such a leader is mainly interested in staying afloat, drifting with the tides of history. A transformation leader, in contrast, operates in a world of bounded rationality and creatively shapes public perceptions of social conditions and designs responses to perceived problems and opportunities.

Conclusion

What this chapter demonstrates are the opportunities and limitations that presidents face in shaping and influencing the policy process. Presidents are generally in a strong position to set the nation's policy agenda. But a president's ability to determine the exact outcome of specific policies is problematic at best. President Clinton was successful in placing health care on the national policy agenda; he was less successful in determining outcome.

Presidents are constrained significantly in their role in the policy process by the constitutional and cultural setting within which they operate. There is no denying the fact that a presidential system of government characterized by separation of powers, checks and balances, and federalism, combined with the lack of a disciplined and ideologically cohesive political party system, makes the task of leadership much more difficult for a president than a parliamentary system does for a prime minister.

Presidents who have been successful in their role as a chief legislators have often had resources available to them that were not available to less successful presidents. One of the most important resources a president can have is if he can successfully claim a mandate for his policy agenda. A president who wins an election by a strong majority and an election in which he had clearly articulated his policy agenda can claim such an electoral mandate. This was the case with Lyndon Johnson in 1964 and Ronald Reagan in the 1980 presidential election. Such was not the case with President Clinton, who managed to win only 43.6 percent of the popular vote in the 1992 election.

Another resource a president can have is his popularity with the general public and his reputation as a skilled politician in the policy-making community. A president who enjoys strong popular support can turn this into an important resource in his dealings with Congress. It can give the president tremendous persuasive and bargaining power. A president can "go public" and successfully appeal directly to the public for support of policies. President Reagan had this resource at his disposal after the 1980 elections. President Clinton never enjoyed much popularity among the public. Even in the best of times his job approval rating among the general public never reached more than 53 percent during his first term in office.

Presidents who used strong rhetoric and were perceived as fighters were often able to win the sympathy of the people and use it to their political advantage. Despite the early failure of President Clinton in this regard, there is reason to believe that his strong rhetoric with respect to Republican initiatives on Medicare and Medicaid and his willingness to shut down the government over these issues may have helped him with the general public in this regard.

Some scholars have argued that overcoming the difficulty of presidential leadership in an antileadership system may require the president to mask a strong leadership role or to cast the leadership role in antihierarchical terms. This is the hidden-hand presidency characterized by the leadership of Thomas Jefferson, Andrew Jackson, and Dwight Eisenhower. But the style, character, and personality of President Clinton made such a leadership style impossible for him.

A president who fails to win a strong electoral mandate and does not enjoy high public support, as George C. Edward III (1989) has suggested, may be forced to operate on the margins of congressional decision making. Nevertheless, a skillful president can recognize and exploit opportunities in a changing environment and, even operating on the margin, can turn opportunities into notable accomplishments.

The main questions confronting a president in contemporary American society and politics are these: How can a pluralist society create a unity of purpose out of conflicting diversity of interests, institutions, and values? Can we, as a society, get our act together so we can develop habits of acting together?

4 CONGRESS AND HEALTH CARE

Congressional Structure and Process

Comparing the House and the Senate

In the opening chapter we saw that one of the explanations for the failure of health care reform was the structure of government. In this section we briefly look at some structural features of the House of Representatives and the Senate and how they have an impact on policy making.

An important difference between the House and the Senate is size. The Constitution requires that each state have two senators, so the Senate has 100 members. The size of the House has been fixed in law at 435. Size differences lead each house to develop rules and procedures that affect how they operate.

Because the House is much larger than the Senate, it has adopted rules to make it more orderly. Bills that come to the floor of the House must be accompanied by a rule stating what and how many amendments may be made to a bill and limiting the amount of debate. It is unlikely, therefore, that without leadership support, a nongermane amendment (one not directly related to the bill) could be added. This makes the Rules Committee important, and congressional leaders of both parties sit on that committee.

The Senate is smaller and more informal than the House. Bills that make it to the floor of the Senate have no rules attached to them. Senators can add amendments on the floor and debate is usually unlimited. This allows a small group of a bill's opponents to delay Senate consideration by holding on to the floor through a filibuster.

The Senate has a procedure to end debate, called cloture. Ending debate requires a positive vote by sixty senators. In the 103d Congress (1993–94), the Democrats did not have sixty votes. In the 104th Congress (1995–96), the Republicans did not have sixty votes.

Why is this significant? In the House, party leaders may have control over their members and over the floor. Certainly, Speaker of the House Newt Gingrich exercised control in a way that had not been seen for decades. The House passed most of the provisions of the Republican Contract with America. The Senate passed fewer of them because there were not enough Republicans to end debate (to say nothing about whether all Republicans agreed with the legislation). Without a sixty-plus vote, majority control in the Senate is limited.

A related aspect of how the Senate operates concerns unanimous consent procedures, which allow routine matters to go on in both houses without debate. In the Senate, unanimous consent performs the same functions as the House Rules Committee. By definition, unanimous consent requires no disagreement. One example of the use of this procedure is the naming of members to the conference committee to work out disagreements on legislation with the House. If just one member objects, the conference will be delayed. This was the case with the health insurance reform legislation in 1996.

The implications of these differences are profound. In the House, even a thin majority, if it is unified, can control what goes on. Majority rules. In the Senate, with its informal rules, limited controls on floor debate, and unanimous consent, minorities are protected and can create havoc with the agenda of the majority. In the Senate, therefore, small majorities must work with the opposition party. In the House, the opposition may have little say; this has been true under both Democratic and Republican control. The overall implication is that the many steps legislation needs to pass in each house and the features that effectively protect the opposition in the Senate make passage of legislation a difficult chore. Defending is easier than changing.

Another important distinction between the House and the Senate relates to differences in terms of office. The term of office for a member of the House is two years; the entire House, therefore, stands for reelection every two years. The term of office for the Senate is six years annually. Therefore, only one-third of the Senate stands for reelection every year.

Obviously, turnover in the House can come more rapidly than turnover in the Senate. Because of the 1980 elections, the Senate had a Republican majority. It would be six years until the Democrats regained control. While there was significant turnover in the House because of the 1994 elections and both houses of Congress saw Republicans elected to majority positions, the turnover in the Senate was much less. There were, relatively speaking, more moderate Republicans in the Senate and fewer conservative Republicans than in the House. So another explanation for the outcomes on budgets and Contract with America provisions is based on these different terms of office.

The Federal Budgeting Process

A critical factor in the outcome of health policy making in our two periods is the budgeting process, which affects the two periods in different ways. Because of its importance in both 1993–94 and 1995–96, we must spend some time describing the budgeting process.

The congressional budgeting structure divides the workload into four sets of committees. The most numerous are the authorization committees (also known as legislative or substantive committees). These committees create (and eliminate) agencies, establish their duties and powers, and set yearly ceilings or authorization on spending for each agency for each fiscal year. Essentially, these bills state the maximum level of spending for each agency or program. Examples of such committees include the Armed Services committees in each house, Finance in the Senate, Ways and Means in the House, and the Commerce committees.

The second important committees are the Appropriations committees, one in each house. Each Appropriation committee has thirteen subcommittees, and Congress must pass thirteen appropriations bills each year.

The third important set of committees are those that have jurisdiction over taxes, Ways and Means in the House and Finance in the Senate. Those two committees also have significant jurisdiction over programs such as Medicaid and Medicare.

The final significant committees are the budget committees, one in each house, designed to consider the budget as a whole. Through the budget committees, Congress adopts a budget resolution containing overall totals for spending and revenues. Because this is a resolution and not a law, it does not require a presidential signature. It is a planning document.

An important part of the congressional budget process is *reconciliation*. Reconciliation occurs when spending or revenue differs from the budget resolution. It is a law that requires the appropriate committees to make changes (usually budget cuts but could also include tax changes) to conform to the budget resolution. As we see below, reconciliation turns out to be an important component of our story.

The final element of the budget process is the Congressional Budget Office (CBO), the counterpart to the president's budget office, the Office of Management and Budget (OMB). The CBO's responsibilities include analyzing the impact of legislation (both authorization and appropriations) on the overall budget. It, too, has a critical role in health policy making.

Naturally, a major concern of the participants in the budgeting process is the problem of *budget deficits*. A budget deficit occurs when expenditures are higher than revenue. Because budgets have to passed every year, they are always on the policy agenda. Budget deficits became a major problem in the early 1980s, though concern was expressed about earlier budgets (Rushefsky 1996).

Faced with increasing deficits (eventually approaching nearly $300 billion), Congress and the Bush administration attempted to deal with the budget deficit in 1990. The administration was also pressured by the need for congressional support for the Persian Gulf intervention to repel Iraq's invasion of Kuwait in August 1990. The reconciliation process, in this case the Budget Enforcement Act of 1990, was used to cut spending and raise taxes by around $500 billion through FY 1995.

Two features of the act were of major importance. First, it placed limits on discretionary spending through FY 1995. The discretionary spending categories included defense, foreign aid, and domestic spending. It did not include the largest budget items, which do not require annual appropriations bills: Social Security, Medicare, Medicaid, and interest on the debt.

Second, the Budget Enforcement Act added a new element to the budget process, a pay-as-you-go feature (PAYGO). Under PAYGO, any changes in spending or tax laws would have to be revenue neutral; in other words, new or expanded programs or tax cuts could not contribute to an increased deficit. Any changes would have to be scored (called scorekeeping) by the CBO for their impact on the deficit.

The deficit-reduction package approved during the Clinton administration, the Omnibus Budget Reconciliation Act of 1993, produced a similar package of spending cuts and tax increases and extended the deficit-enforcement procedures of the 1990 legislation through 1998.

A major impact of deficit-reduction legislation, apart from its effect on the policy process, has been actual reductions in the federal budget deficit. In terms of actual dollars, the deficit peaked in FY 1992 at $290.4 billion. It declined to about $165.1 billion by FY 1995. For FY 1996, the deficit was about $108 billion, the lowest amount since FY 1981. In relative terms, the budget deficit peaked in FY 1983 at 6.3 percent of the gross domestic product (GDP). In FY 1992, it was 4.8 percent. Based on the estimate for FY 1996, the deficit was about 1.6 percent of GDP, the lowest since FY 1974 (Purdum 1996). Of course, the continued growth of the economy since the end of the recession in March 1991 contributed to deficit reduction. Despite this good news, deficit reduction and program cuts will haunt the policy agenda into the next century. Entitlement programs, such as Medicare and Medicaid (as well as Social Security), will continue to put pressure on the federal deficit (see Peterson 1995).

Committees

Perhaps the first political science work pointing out the importance of committees was *Congressional Government,* written in 1885 by Woodrow Wilson. Wilson observed that many of the decisions Congress made were done in committee and usually behind closed doors (Lazare 1996).

Congressional committees are important because they take on a significant portion of the workload from Congress. Smith (1993, 177) describes their roles:

> Most important legislation originates in a standing committee, most of the details of legislation are approved in committee, and standing committee members usually dominate floor and conference action.

The importance and autonomy of committees has diminished over the years as Congress has allowed more leadership control. Much of this has come about because of changes in the budget process, congressional reforms in the 1970s that weakened seniority and strengthened subcommittees, and changes made by the Republican leadership at the start of the 104th Congress (Smith 1993).

From our standpoint, committees played an important role in deciding the fate of health reform in 1994. A key issue is to which committee a bill is referred. A complex bill, such as the Clinton Health Security Act, affects so much of the economy that multiple committees can claim jurisdiction.

In the House of Representatives the major committees were the Ways and Means Committee and the Energy and Commerce Committee. Each committee had a key subcommittee: Health for Ways and Means and Health, and the Environment for Energy and Commerce (Rubin 1993). The Education and Labor Committee was also important. Congressional leaders in the House referred the bill to a total of ten committees, though the three named above were the most important (Evans 1995). In the Senate, the primary committees were Finance and Labor and Human Resources. Senate leadership did not resolve the jurisdictional question between these two committees and so made no referrals. Both committees considered the bill.

Evans (1995) points out that complex issues such as comprehensive health care reform tend to be dealt with by the House and Senate as a whole more than in committee. This fragmentation of jurisdiction served to confuse the public about health reform. The jurisdictional problem also showed one of the flaws of House Democratic leadership. Evans argues that the House Democratic leadership should have created an ad hoc committee to oversee the process, particularly given the priority placed on health care reform by the Clinton administration. The Republican House leadership in 1995 and 1996 often resorted to such ad hoc committees.

Another alternative institutional mechanism that the White House and congressional leadership could have chosen in 1993–94 was budget reconciliation. A major advantage of including health care reform within a budget reconciliation bill was that, unlike other legislation, it was not subject to a Senate filibuster. Only a simple majority in each house would be needed for passage. This was the tack that Republicans tried in 1995–96, especially concerning environmental legislation. The other advantage of the reconciliation strategy was time. Democratic congressional leaders agreed early in 1993 that if health care reform did not pass in 1993, it would be unlikely to pass in 1994 when a mid-year congressional election would loom (Johnson and Broder 1996).

The major difficulty with the strategy was that there was too much division within the Democratic Party to overcome opposition from the Republican Party. Further, Clinton was proposing budget-reduction plans, so there were the two big items that would be included in one bill.

Republican supporters of reform argued against the budget strategy, saying that they wanted a chance to modify any proposal. Further, Senate Minority Leader Bob Dole (R-Kans.) told the president in early 1993 that Republicans would "unanimously oppose his budget—no matter how the President framed it" (Johnson and Broder 1996, 125).

Robert Byrd (D-W.Va.), former Senate majority leader and the chairman of the Senate Appropriations Committee, cast the final blow against the reconciliation strategy. The Senate had adopted the "Byrd Rule" to keep only deficit-reduction items in the reconciliation bill. All it would take would be a point of order to keep health reform out of reconciliation (Johnson and Broder 1996). With the failure of the reconciliation strategy to get off the ground, the hard work would have to be done in committee.

Elections, Realignment, Divided Government, and Gridlock

The result of elections can have profound effects on congressional behavior within the structure and process described above. A major goal of elected officials is to be reelected. Apart from explaining the motivation and behavior of individual senators or representatives, elections can have an impact on public policy. Policies may be opposed or favored because of the imminence of elections, which, as we have seen, occur every two years for the House of Representatives. We argue that the Clinton health care plan or, more broadly, any health care reform plan in 1994 was doomed because of maneuverings around the 1994 elections. We also argue that the failure to cut the budgets for Medicare and Medicaid (and the overall failure to pass deficit-reduction legislation) and the passage of health insurance reform in 1996 were related to forthcoming elections.

Elections can also affect the balance of power in Congress. This process, known as *realignment,* may be defined as a change in the partisan makeup of the political parties. Realignment plays an important role in explaining policy outcomes and initiatives in our two periods, though in different ways. While there has been considerable discussion about whether a realignment has occurred since the 1930s, there does appear to have been a regional realignment beginning in the 1960s that eventually produced more ideologically coherent political parties (see Carmines and Stimson 1989; Edsall and Edsall 1991; Nardulli 1995). The Democrats became more liberal as southern conservative Democrats were replaced by southern conservative Republicans. Moderates became a smaller, though not insignificant, part of the Republican Party. Ideological distinctions reinforced partisan distinctions, leading to less bipartisanship and more unified party voting. Unified party voting occurs when a majority of one party votes against the majority of the other party. This practice increases the likelihood of gridlock.

Controlling Congress and Divided Government

In the first chapter we discussed the concept of divided government. To recall, *divided government* occurs when one party controls the presidency and the other party controls at least one branch of Congress. Divided government has characterized American politics at the national level for much of the post–World War II period. Some have argued that divided government leads to gridlock and the failure of the federal government to act on pressing issues. David Mayhew (1991) argues, instead, that the federal government has been able to accomplish much despite divided government. We would like to present a slightly different perspective on the issue of divided versus unified government.

Our perspective is that the real issue is whether a party has a working or effective, not just a numerical, majority in one or more houses of Congress. A working majority can take several forms. First, is the majority party unified on policy issues and ideology? If the majority party has a fairly wide ideological membership, there may not be a sufficient number of members of that party to enact the leadership's agenda. In general, the Democratic Party is more diverse (and less well organized) than the Republican Party. But there are divisions within the Republican Party as well, which affected the outcome of policy proposals in 1995–96. Minorities, whether of the opposite party or within the majority party, can often affect the course of events.

Second, is there a sufficiently large majority to override a presidential veto, especially if the president is of the other party? If the answer is no, as was true for the Republicans in both the House and the Senate in 1995–96, then the likelihood of enacting laws diminishes and the opportunities for compromise increases.

Third, is there a sufficiently large majority in the Senate to limit extended debate (i.e., filibusters)? If the answer is no, as was the case throughout the entire period, then controversial legislation is less likely to be acted upon.

Finally, can coalitions of like-minded legislators be crafted from both parties to enact legislation? If yes, then legislation can be passed even under conditions of divided government.

From our standpoint, then, we should ask whether there were working majorities in Congress for health issues. Overall, the answer is no, health insurance reform being the lone exception. Some legislation (other than health issues) was passed with little bipartisan support. Other legislation had large bipartisan support.

Gridlock

Obviously related to the above discussion is the issue of gridlock. As Mayhew (1991) points out, even during periods of divided control, significant legislation can be passed. Budget and tax-cutting legislation in 1981 is one example. To that we should add the 1986 tax reform bill, the 1990 Clean Air Act Amendments, the 1990 Americans with Disabilities Act, the Civil Rights Restoration Act of 1988, the Civil Rights Act of 1991, and health insurance reform, welfare reform, and increases in the minimum wage in 1996.

Yet the argument that we have experienced gridlock for a number of years should not be summarily dismissed. The two civil rights acts were passed after great difficulty. The Clean Air Act Amendments of 1990 should have been passed a decade earlier. In 1995–96, budget and policy disagreements between Congress and the president led to two shutdowns of government.

One of the best discussions of legislative gridlock is Kraft's analysis of policy making in the environmental policy area (Kraft 1996). Kraft argues that there are several reasons why legislative gridlock may occur. One, which we have already discussed, is separation of powers/checks and balances. A second is the increasing trend toward candidate-centered, rather than party-centered, elections. That is, candidates run independent campaigns, raising most of their own money. Republican victories in 1994 were a move back toward party-centered campaigns.

Kraft also notes that a lack of public consensus on a policy issue will also lead to gridlock. We address the role of public opinion in both of our periods explicitly in chapter 7. One more important reason for gridlock is the lack of effective leadership, either at the presidential level or within Congress or both. Such leadership can help craft the effective majorities discussed earlier. So Kraft points to several explanations for gridlock, and we can see how they play out in our two periods.

Presidential Agenda and Activist Government, 1993–94

Setting the Stage: The Electoral Connection

The president has an important role in setting the congressional agenda. To achieve that agenda, a president needs both public support for policy proposals and a working majority in Congress. The president should also be able to work with congressional leaders, employing all the tools of the presidency to persuade (see our discussion in chapter 3 and Neustadt 1990). Much of this ability is affected by elections. So what was the situation Bill Clinton faced in January 1993?

First, as discussed in chapters 2 and 3, Clinton had an ambitious, crowded agenda, including, in addition to health care reform, welfare reform, budget and trade issues, and a crime bill.

A second aspect is that a president's status with the public will affect his success with Congress. Clinton was a minority president, winning only a 43 percent plurality of the popular vote in a three-way race. Virtually all congressmen, Republican and Democratic alike, ran ahead of the president; there were no presidential coattails, and Democratic congressmen did not owe their election to him. Further, the president's popular support, as expressed in public opinion polls, was not much better than his electoral support during 1993–94 and sometimes lower, affected by early decisions (gays in the military and controversial appointments) and a continuing focus on scandals (e.g., Whitewater).

A third calculation is the electoral returns for Congress. It remained Democratic after the 1992 elections. But the Democrats gained only one seat in the Senate, for a total of fifty-eight senators, and lost seven seats in the House of Representatives. By our definition, a working majority did not exist in the Senate; there were not enough senators to end debate.

A fourth aspect has to do with partisanship in Congress. As the parties began to diverge ideologically and geographically, there was less tendency for bipartisanship or cross-party friendships (Broder 1996a). Compromise became more difficult.

Cohen and Schneider's (1995) analysis of the second session of the 103d Congress (1994) illustrates this polarization and change. Schick's (1995) analysis of party-line or partisan voting also demonstrates this tendency. Partisan voting on roll-call votes in 1966–84 averaged about 38.2 percent in the House and 41.6 percent in the Senate. The respective figures for 1985–94 were 57.9 percent in the House and 48.6 percent in the Senate. Partisanship within the major congressional committees with jurisdiction over health care (House Energy and Commerce and Ways and Means, and Senate Labor and Human Resources) increased from 1988 to 1994 (Talbert 1995). As Schick notes, partisanship is higher in the House than in the Senate because of the size and rules of the two houses, discussed above. But partisanship and party loyalty has increased in both houses. Schick attributes this polarization to the changing composition of the two parties and the long control of the House by the Democrats, resulting in a unified Republican Party. Talbert (1995) points out that Democratic committee leaders were also unwilling to look at proposals suggested by party moderates, especially in the House.

Schick also has an interesting view of unified versus divided control. Under conditions of unified control (same party controls the presidency and both houses of Congress), there is a greater tendency for partisan voting than under conditions of divided control.

Schick (1995, 255) summarizes the twin impacts of polarization (increased partisanship) and party control of Congress:

> If this pattern had prevailed with health care reform, legislation would have been reported by committee, Democrats and Republicans would have fought over floor amendments, and sufficient compromise would have been reached in conference to permit bipartisan passage. Health care legislation did not play out that way, but not simply because Clinton ignored the Republicans and went it alone with the Democrats. By the time health reform was on the congressional agenda, the parties had become so polarized that their differences could not be bridged by normal legislative interaction. Party behavior on legislation was markedly different during the 1993–94 (103d) Congress than it had been four years earlier. With the election of Bill Clinton, the Democrats controlled the government and Republicans were united in opposition. Party cohesion scores soared, and party lines were more staunchly defended than they had been during times of divided government.

Competing Proposals

A critical factor affecting the outcome of congressional deliberations in 1994 was that President Clinton's proposal, the Health Security Act, was one of a number of such proposals, some of which had more support than the president's. Alissa Rubin, who covered health care for *Congressional Quarterly Weekly Reports,* noted that "the emergence of competing plans in Congress signals the complexity of the political and policy battles ahead for the administration" (Rubin 1994a, 23).

This section briefly describes proposals that had been made by January 1994 (based partly on the analysis in the Kaiser Commission on the Future of Medicaid 1994). The Clinton Health Security Act was described in chapter 3.

Democratic Congressional Proposals

One competing proposal was a variation of the Health Security Act with some bipartisan support. This was the Managed Competition Act sponsored by Representatives Jim Cooper (D-Tenn.) and Fred Grandy (R-Iowa) and Senator John Breaux (D-La.), originally introduced in 1992. It was in many respects similar to the Clinton bill, but featured no employer mandate. For example, it required employers to offer a health insurance plan to its employees but did not order employers to pay for it. It called for insurance reforms and subsidies for low income people and the organization of voluntary purchasing cooperatives (Rubin 1994b). Because of the managed competition features and the lack of a mandate, it was often referred to as "Clinton lite" (Johnson and Broder 1996, 314).

A second Democratic alternative was more radical. This was the single-payer system embodied in the American Health Security Act, sponsored by Paul Wellstone (D-Minn.) in the Senate and Jim McDermott (D-Wash.) in the House. The bill would cover the entire population, tax employers, and be administered by the states. The program contained price controls over industry and substantial government involvement (Rubin 1994a). The virtues of the bill were its simplicity and savings. It was simple because it eliminated the multiple sources of payers replacing it with one administrative system. The savings came from price controls and the administrative simplicity. In December 1993, the Congressional Budget Office estimated that a single-payer system would save about 6 percent of national health expenditures (Rubin 1994a). The major criticism of the plan was political: it was opposed by those who were hostile to increasing government involvement; by the medical community, which is against government interference in the practice of medicine; and by insurance companies, which would see their health industry business disappear. Another criticism made of the single-payer plan was that it did not take into account the different needs of different parts of the population (Rubin 1994a).

Republican Congressional Proposals.

Republicans in Congress offered several proposals, at least in 1993. The oldest of the proposals was offered by House Minority Leader Bob Michel (R-Ill.) and Senator Trent Lott (R-Miss.), who would become Senate majority leader in 1996. Their Affordable Health Care Now Act was a voluntary program, requiring employers to offer but not pay for health insurance, expanding Medicaid to low-income people, and some insurance reforms.

A second Republican proposal was offered by Congressman Clifford Stearns (R-Fla.) and Senator Don Nickles (R-Okla.). The Consumer Choice Health Security Act employed an individual mandate in the sense that it provided financial penalties to those not purchasing insurance. Consumers would be responsible for their own payments, and there would no limit on how much they paid. The preference in the program was for catastrophic insurance.

The third Republican plan was the Health Equity and Access Reform Today Act, sponsored by Senator John Chafee (R-R.I.) and William Thomas (R-Calif.) and originally offered in a somewhat different form in 1991. Of the Republican bills, this was the only one that promised universal coverage of the population. Like the Stearns/Nickles bill, the Chafee/Thomas proposal was based on an individual mandate to purchase insurance. Again, employers had to offer insurance but did not have to pay for it. Like the Clinton and "Clinton lite" approaches, it would rely on health alliances or purchasing cooperatives and market reforms.

Another variant of Republican health insurance proposals, one that reappeared in 1995 and 1996, was offered by Senator Phil Gramm (R-Tex.). This was the medical savings account (MSA) proposal. The Gramm proposal was at the opposite end of the ideological stream from the single-payer plan. It would involve very little government intervention and sought to provide smaller insurance coverage on the grounds that comprehensive insurance shields consumers from the true costs of health care (Rubin 1994a). We return to medical savings accounts below. The Gramm proposal was not a major player in 1994; it does, however, illustrate the ideological range of health care proposals in this period.

Bipartisan Approaches

At least two bills crossed party lines, apart from the Managed Competition Act. One was a conservative bill proposed by Georgia Democratic Representative J. Roy Rowland and Florida Republican Representative Michael Bilirakis. Johnson and Broder (1996) described the bill as "minimalist." It included health reforms to help people with expensive health problems and allowed voluntary purchasing cooperatives for small employers. The bill did not include a way to pay for the reforms and did not cover the uninsured.

The other bipartisan bill emerged in the waning days of the health reform battle in 1994. It was a last-ditch effort crafted by a small group of senators on the Finance Committee, known as the *mainstream coalition*. We examine the mainstream coalition next.

Committee Action in 1994

Movement on health care reform in the various committees did not get off to a good start in 1994. One issue was whether to consider welfare prior to health care. Senate Finance Chairman Daniel P. Moynihan (D-N.Y.), a former academic with great experience with welfare policy, argued in January 1994 that he did not think there was a crisis in health care, though there were problems, and that welfare reform should come first. He was concerned that Republicans would make gains in the 1994 elections and would produce a welfare reform package more conservative than Democrats wanted (an accurate forecast). The importance of Moynihan's comment was that this was another example of the lack of unity within the Democratic Party for health care reform.

Additionally, in the period between the first and second sessions of the 103d Congress (Winter 1993–94), congressmen talked with their constituents about health care reform. They reported that constituents were ambivalent about health care reform: they wanted to change and to keep what they had; they wanted costs controlled, but were afraid of price controls (Katz 1994). This mixed message reinforced the hesitancy a number of representatives already had about health care reform.

In February 1994, the Congressional Budget Office (CBO) issued its report "scoring" the Clinton Health Security Act. It made several important points:

1. Individual and business premiums should be considered as part of the federal budget because they were mandated and an important part of plan.
2. Health care alliances should be considered federal entities.
3. Health expenditures would rise through 1999 and then decline; by 2004 they would be about 7 percent less than was projected under current law.
4. The Clinton plan would increase the deficit in the short term (by $74 billion from 1995 to 2000 and by $126 billion from 1995 to 2004) and then would reduce the federal deficit (Rubin 1994c).

The CBO report was critical in several ways. First, some of its rulings undermined the hopes of the Clinton administration. This was particularly true of the first point in the above paragraph. Essentially, CBO said that premiums should be considered taxes because they were mandated, even though that is not how premiums were or are treated. A similar statement was true about the alliances; because they were mandated and not voluntary, as in some of the other health care reform proposals, CBO ruled that they should be considered part of the federal government.

A second point concerning the budget deficit was the most devastating, even though the message was mixed. What the news media and opponents of the Clinton plan heard was that the Health Security Act would increase the budget deficit. This was true because of the subsidies for small businesses and low-income people; more of the population would be covered, and so the plan had to cost more. Yet the CBO also stated that in the long run, after 2004, the Clinton plan would reduce the deficit. Somehow, this last point was missed in the noise.

Finally, the CBO played an important role in the health debate because it was the referee or scorekeeper. It judged all health care reform proposals, and committees often waited for a CBO report until acting on a bill. Yet the knowledge base for CBO analysis was extremely limited. In an important article appearing in 1995, Robert Reischauer, who was CBO director at the time, and his coauthor confessed to how weak the knowledge base and therefore the estimates were. Yet what CBO reported was taken as gospel. The truth was, given the magnitude of the changes proposed, no one really knew what would happen (see Bilheimer and Reischauer 1995).

By the end of February 1995, key House subcommittees in Ways and Means and Energy and Commerce were missing their deadlines for marking up a health reform bill. One important impact of delay was that the time left in the legislative session was quickly diminishing, given Congress's work schedule. Delay continued to work against health care reform.

Further, Democrats on the committees were divided over a course of action to take. The chairman of the Ways and Means Health Subcommittee, Pete Stark (D-Calif.), noted that there was little support among Democrats for the mandatory alliances feature of the Health Security Act. At about the same time, Senate Majority Leader Tom Daschle (D-S.D.) and Senator John D. Rockefeller IV (D-W.Va.) said that the alliances were an important part of health care reform (Donovan 1994a).

While Democrats were divided about health care reform, so were Republicans, though they would eventually come to a consensus. In March 1994, some thirty-five Republican senators as well as some House Republicans met at a retreat to devise a position. The Republicans were split along three possibilities. One was to support the Chafee plan. A second was to support Phil Gramm's proposal for medical savings accounts. The third was support for Don Nickles's plan to use tax incentives. House Republican support was divided among Minority Leader Robert Michels's plan and the Cooper-Grandy bill (Rubin 1994d).

An intriguing proposal was developed by the chairman of the House Ways and Means health subcommittee, Pete Stark. One purpose of health care reform was to cover the uninsured. The simplest way to do this, Stark reasoned, was to expand on what we already had. Therefore, he proposed an addition to Medicare, a Part C, that would cover the uninsured. The Stark bill called for premiums of $2,400 per person, with the individual share at 20 percent and a $500 deductible. Employers would be required to pay 80 percent of premiums, and there would be national targets for public and private spending (Rubin 1994e).

By the middle of March, House subcommittees had taken some action. The House Ways and Means health subcommittee approved the Stark bill along strict party lines (i.e., no Republicans voted for it). The subcommittee also considered the other health care reform proposals, such as Clinton, Cooper-Grandy, Chafee and single-payer, and rejected all of them (Rubin 1994f).

Energy and Commerce Committee Chair John Dingell (D-Mich.) issued a proposed modification of the Clinton package. The modification would cut back the benefits package so as to reduce subsidies; retain universal coverage; keep the employer mandate with subsidies for small firms depending on size; drop mandatory alliances but allow voluntary alliances; institute a set of reforms that would require insurance companies to accept all applicants and prohibit them from rejecting applications with preexisting conditions; make states responsible for cost containment; and place caps on federal spending (Donovan and Rubin 1994a).

Through the spring, House and then Senate committees and subcommittees continued their agonizing consideration of health reform with little progress and virtually no consensus. The major roadblocks were the mandatory features: the employer mandates and the health care alliances.

A further blow to the health care reform case was the CBO analysis of the Cooper-Grandy bill. The CBO reported that Cooper-Grandy would reduce the number of uninsured by about 15 million people and would lower health care spending by 1 to 2 percent in 2004. That would still leave about 24 million Americans without coverage, and there would be about a $35 billion shortfall in subsidies for the poor. Additionally, the CBO estimated that the middle class would suffer a decline in benefits because incentives in Cooper-Grandy would push employers toward selecting low-cost plans (Rubin 1994g).

Three other issues had their impact on health care reform. One was whether abortion services should be included in a health benefits package. The issue was complex. Many private health insurance plans include such services. If it were part of a standard health care reform benefits package, then those opposed to abortion (right-to-life groups and the Catholic church) would oppose health care reform. If it were not included, not only would pro-choice groups be upset but a benefit currently offered would be eliminated.

The second issue was whether to tax employee health insurance premiums paid for by employers. Employer contributions are a major fringe benefit covering the bulk of the population. The tax code treats such contributions as a business expense and therefore exempt from tax liability. This encourages employers to offer health insurance benefits, often quite generous ones. The concern addressed in May 1994 was whether to tax such benefits as either a means to raise revenue, since virtually all health care reform proposals called for additional spending, or as a means of cost control, or both. The Clinton plan called for such a tax beginning in 2004 on plans more generous than the standard package. The Cooper-Grandy bill would impose a 34 percent tax on incremental costs for plans above the lowest cost plan. The Chafee proposal would allow deductions up to the average of lower-priced plans but then a tax on incremental costs for higher-cost plans (Donovan 1994c).

A third provision of health care reform proposals was intensely examined. This was the employer mandate, strongly opposed by small businesses and their organization, the National Federation of Independent Businesses (NFIB). Many of the proposals did not contain an employer mandate but instead contained *triggers,* deadlines by which action must be taken if a goal is missed. A trigger might call for employer mandates if a certain percentage of the population (say, 95 percent) were not covered by a certain date (say, 2002). This would be a hard trigger. A soft trigger would call for study of the issue (by a commission or Congress) if the target were missed. Democrats on the Finance Committee and part of the bipartisan Mainstream Coalition were divided over which direction to go (Rubin 1994i).

In May 1994, the Senate Labor and Resource Committee approved a bill combining the Chafee plan and an amendment proposed by committee chair Edward M. Kennedy (D-Mass.) that would exempt the smallest businesses from the mandate (though require a 2 percent payroll tax), allow businesses with over 1,000 employees to have their own insurance plans, and make alliances voluntary for businesses under 1,000 employees. It also expanded benefits but required higher out-of-pocket costs (Donovan 1994b; Donovan and Rubin 1994b).

There was yet another problem plaguing the Democratic effort in the House. Ways and Means Committee Chair Dan Rostenkowski (D-Ill.) came under federal indictment for post office fraud. He eventually gave up his chairmanship, then resigned from the House and pleaded guilty. Though his successor, Sam Gibbons (D-Fla.), proved more vigorous than expected in pursuit of health care reform, the time period between indictment and resignation delayed action in this important committee. Meanwhile the Ways and Means Committee continued to consider the Stark proposal and whether the health alliances should be mandatory (Rubin 1994h).

Finally, on June 9, a congressional committee reported a health care reform bill. This was the Senate Labor and Education Committee's approval of the Kennedy modification of the Health Security Act. The vote was 11–6, as all committee Democrats and one Republican, Jim Jeffords (R-Vt.), supported the bill. The bill contained an employer mandate, exempting only the smallest firms; state-established purchasing cooperatives, with exemptions for smaller businesses; caps on insurance premiums; and a more generous benefits package than contained in the president's proposal (Donovan 1994d).

By June 1994, while House and Senate committees continued to consider health care reform legislation, Senator Majority Leader George Mitchell (D-Maine) stated that he wanted a bill to the floor of the Senate by July. House Majority Leader Richard Gephardt (D-Mo.) became more involved in discussions.

In June 1994, House Minority Whip Newt Gingrich (R-Ga.) urged two courses of action on Ways and Means Republicans. The first action was to have as many votes on amendments as possible. The second was to defeat any amendments that would improve the Democratic bills, especially those aimed at meeting objections by small businesses (Rubin 1994i). Further, Fred Grandy, the Republican House cosponsor of the Cooper-Grandy bill, reported that Gingrich told House Republicans that he wanted Ways and Means Committee Chair Sam Gibbons's bill defeated (Cloud 1994a).

By the end of June, the Senate Finance Committee was deadlocked over health reform. Majority Leader Mitchell threatened to bring a bill up without Finance Committee approval at the same time that the House Ways and Means Committee was waiting for Finance Committee action. House committee Democrats were concerned that they might risk reporting a strong bill only to have the Finance Committee come up with a much weaker bill (as happened with the proposed energy tax; see Donovan 1994e; Woodward 1994).

By the middle of June, a bipartisan group of senators on the Finance Committee crafted a modest health care reform bill. The group, with slightly changing membership at times, became known as the *mainstream coalition* and included Democrats John Breaux of Louisiana, David Boren of Oklahoma, and Kent Conrad of North Dakota, and Republicans John Danforth of Missouri, John Chafee of Rhode Island, and David Durenberger of Minnesota. One moderate Democrat, Bill Bradley of New Jersey, quit the group because the plan lacked an employer mandate.

Features of the plan included the following: (1) insuring 95 percent of the population, reducing the ranks of the uninsured by about 20 million people; (2) a soft trigger, with a commission reporting to Congress every two years; (3) a managed competition approach; (4) allowing individuals and firms to join purchasing cooperatives; (5) taxing costly insurance plans to create incentives toward less costly plans; (6) a standardized benefits package; (7) partial subsidies on a sliding scale for the poor; (8) cuts in Medicare and Medicaid; (9) limits on federal health spending and automatic cuts (such as in subsidies) if limits were exceeded; and (10) a requirement that insurers cover all enrollees. This plan would become the major focus of Senate action (Rubin 1994j).

By the end of June, events began to move quickly. John Dingell, chairman of the House Energy and Commerce committees, told House leaders that he could not get a majority behind any bill and that his committee would not take any action. Republicans became somewhat more cooperative. Minority members of the Ways and Means Committee began voting for some of the amendments in Ways and Means.

Senate Minority Leader Bob Dole stated that he had forty members of his party supporting a proposal for insurance reform and low-income subsidies. The minority leader had originally supported the Clinton plan, then gradually moved away from it. By the end of June his position was "no employer mandates, no price controls and no taxes" (Rubin 1994k, 1799). His proposal reflected this stance. The features included: (1) universal access to insurance; (2) individuals and small businesses could buy into the Federal Employee Health Benefits Program (FEHBP); (3) a sliding scale of subsidies; (4) no standardized benefits package except for those who receive subsidies; and (5) allow the formation of purchasing cooperatives. In addition, the Dole plan offered several important insurance reforms: insurance companies had to accept all applicants and renew all plans; companies could require a six-month waiting period for new applicants; small companies would have to be given some form of community rating; and insurance would be portable (workers would not lose coverage when changing jobs) (Rubin 1994k).

By the middle of July, the White House and the Democratic National Committee (DNC) were preparing a major lobbying campaign and bus tour. At the same time, Democratic leaders were informing the Clinton administration that the employer mandate had to be phased in if included at all, and

House Democratic leaders were preparing to send a bill to the floor based on the Medicare C proposal with a possible option that would include FEHPB. House leaders were also considering delaying floor action until the Senate acted. Moderates in the House were preparing to bring the Cooper-Grandy bill to the floor (Rubin and Donovan 1994b).

On July 29, House Majority Leader Richard Gephardt unveiled a plan based on the Ways and Means Committee proposal. The provisions of the plan included a phased-in requirement that employers pay 80 percent of costs of premiums; that employers have to offer at least two plans (one unlimited and the other managed care); that smaller employers could enroll employees in either a private plan or Part C of Medicare; phased subsidies for low-income people; standardized benefits package with caps on out-of-pocket costs; some new taxes and tax credits; cost controls by limiting reimbursements under Part C; a commission to determine private sector costs; insurers could not experience rate; and states would be allowed construct a single-payer plan (Rubin 1994l).

At the same time that Democrats were trying to move forward on health care reform, Republicans were moving away. The not especially subtle signal of this was a memo by William Kristol of the Project for the Republican Future urging Republicans "to defeat any Democratic health care bill and 'send them to the voters empty-handed' " (Rubin 1994l, 2146). Additionally, Senate Minority Leader Bob Dole would not allow the Senate to move on health care.

Floor Action in 1994

Despite Republican threats of filibuster, debate on health care reform was set for August 9 in the Senate and August 15 in the House, with final voting in the House scheduled for August 15. Senate Majority Leader George Mitchell presented his compromise proposal, which would delay a possible employer mandate to 2002, contained mechanisms to avoid the mandate entirely, reductions in employer contributions, and exemptions for small businesses (Rubin and Donovan 1994). As August wore on, Mitchell compromised further, agreeing to cover 95 percent of the population by the year 2000 and lowering the amount of small employer contributions from 80 to 50 percent. The CBO review of the Mitchell plan was mixed. It would reduce the deficit, but parts were hard to implement (tax on high-cost insurance) and the sliding scale of subsidies might induce less work. Further, some 14 million people would remain without insurance (Rubin 1994m). Even with Mitchell's bill, there were not enough Democratic senators behind a single proposal to pass a bill, let alone stop a filibuster.

By mid-August, the House delayed debate on health care reform, largely because of a lack of consensus behind a single proposal. At the same time a bipartisan group of House moderates (J. Roy Rowland [D-Tenn.], Michael Bilirakis [R-Fla.] and Bill Thomas [R-Calif.]) crafted yet another proposal. The features of the plan included universal access to insurance with firms offering at least two plans, though they would not have to pay for them. The objective was to cover 90 percent of the population by 2004 (notice how the proposals become less and less ambitious). There would also be low-income subsidies on a sliding scale and insurance reform. There would be no set standard benefits package (Cloud 1994b).

As the acrimonious debate continued in August, Chafee and Breaux kept relaxing details of their plan in the hope of assembling a majority. The 95 percent goal was lowered to 92 or 93 percent. The employer mandate was replaced by a soft trigger. There would be insurance reform and a cap or limitation on insurance premiums. Medicaid and Medicare would be cut to pay for the program (Rubin 1994n).

In the meantime, the administration's crime bill was experiencing difficulties. It was originally defeated in the House on August 11. Two weeks later, it passed both houses of Congress, but took up valuable time from health care floor debate in the Senate. With the passage of the crime bill, Congress recessed in late August, and the prospects for even incremental change given the time left in the 103d Congress was small.

Mitchell tried one last time to come up with a compromise package, despite discouraging reports from the public and congressional Republicans. His last proposal, in late September, contained elements from the mainstream coalition's bill: health insurance reform; a standard benefits package to be set by a commission; a choice between a comprehensive and a less generous plan; workers could buy insurance through employers (though employers would not have to pay) or could also buy through a local FEHBP; voluntary purchasing cooperatives; sliding subsidies for low income; cuts in Medicare and Medicaid; tax cap on business insurance payments; and states could set up a single-payer system (Rubin 1994n).

On September 26, 1994, Senate Majority Leader Mitchell held a news conference in which he confirmed the obvious: health care reform was dead for the year. It would be up to the next Congress, if it chose, to reconsider the issue.

Explaining the Failure of Reform

Democratic Disunity. Clearly one of the problems facing the administration was that there was little unity behind a single health care reform proposal.

Instead some conservative Democrats were against the whole idea and other less conservative Democrats supported a modest proposal, with few if any mandatory features. In the middle was a group that supported a modified version of the Clinton plan (Cooper/Grandy). On the left were liberals who supported the single-payer plan. No one in either house was able to put together a bill that could produce a majority. This was most clearly seen in the House at two points. One was the failure of the Energy and Commerce committees to agree on a bill that could be reported to the floor. To the extent that any bill had a chance to be voted on by the entire House, it was the Ways and Means bill based on a new Medicare Part C program. A second indication of disunity among the Democrats in the House was that no floor debate ever occurred. The House leadership waited for the Senate to act, and the Senate never did. There was never a bill in either house that commanded a majority of the Democrats.

Republicans

The Republican position on health care reform was mixed. Some moderate Republicans, largely in the Senate (mainstream coalition) but also some in the House (e.g., Fred Grandy) supported the goal of modest reform. But most Republicans were against it. Further, the position of Republicans changed, eventually coming out against any reform. We can see this in the case of three important Republicans: Bob Dole, William Kristol, and Newt Gingrich.

Consider Dole, the Senate minority leader, first. On October 27, 1993, when the Health Security Act was finally sent to Congress, Dole said he supported comprehensive reform. Indeed, he was one of the cosponsors of the Chafee bill. In November he supported a more modest Senate bill that limited government involvement. By early January 1994 Dole was saying that he did not see a health care crisis and thus no urgency to act (Rubin 1994a). By the end of June 1994 he was proposing a modest bill that had support from forty Republican senators. He had enough votes to support a filibuster and his position was firmly against a strong government role. By July he was holding up debate in the Senate.

Dole had several motivations for his behavior. One was the genuine Republican conservative view against big government that was seen as embodied in the Health Security Act. But a second motivation was equally important. Dole was in the process of making his third run for the Republican nomination for the presidency (the other two were in 1980 and 1988). Winning the nomination meant that Dole had to capture the right wing of the Republican Party. Phil Gramm (R-Tex.) was also seeking the nomination and was carving out a position among conservative Republicans. Dole could not be seen as giving conservative ground to Gramm. Health care, even a modest program, was the ultimate liberal program (see Johnson and Broder 1996).

A second important figure among the Republicans was William Kristol. He had served as chief of staff to Vice-President Dan Quayle and then went to work for a conservative think tank, the Project for the Republican Future. From his position at the think tank, Kristol issued strategy memos to Republicans about how they were to deal with health care. His memos brought to the surface what would eventually become the posture of most congressional Republicans toward health care reform: opposition as a way to gain power (Johnson and Broder 1996; Skocpol 1996).

In one memo, published in the *Wall Street Journal* on January 11, 1994, Kristol wrote:

> But passage of the Clinton health care plan *in any form* would be disastrous. It would guarantee an unprecedented federal intrusion into the American economy. Its success would signal a rebirth of centralized welfare-state policy at the very moment that such policy is being perceived as a failure in other areas. And, not least, it would destroy the present breadth and quality of the American health care system, the world's finest.

Kristol's memo included a number of incremental, conservative changes, some of which became part of the 1995–96 debates (such as insurance reform and medical savings accounts).

In July 1994, when the Clinton plan was no longer a major factor and modifications were on the table, Kristol wrote another memorandum urging Republicans to oppose all compromises "sight unseen" (Quoted in Skocpol 1996, 146).

Newt Gingrich's role in his years in Congress was primarily that of a strategist, with the objective of achieving majority rule for Republicans in the House of Representatives and end decades of Democratic rule (Sabato and Simpson 1996). He did this in several ways.

One was to help develop a group of young conservative Republican candidates who would get elected to the House. Using his "leadership" political action committee (GOPAC), he provided campaign funds to candidates throughout the country. He also provided them with campaign material. And he joined with other young conservative Republicans in Congress to form the Conservative Opportunity Society, to consider various strategies and tactics for gaining control of the House.

Another strategy was to bring down the Democrats by delegitimizing them. This included speeches at the end of the day on the floor of the House denouncing the Democrats. Most of the time, the House chamber was empty, but Gingrich's speeches were carried on the cable network C-SPAN, much to the dismay of Democrats (Balz and Brownstein 1996). Similarly, Gingrich (and other Republicans) pushed scandals, such as the banking and post office scandals.

The most ambitious effort along these lines came when Gingrich pressed ethics charges against House Speaker Jim Wright (D-Tex.). While Gingrich was warned off the effort to take on the powerful speaker by members of his own party, Gingrich continued the assault, ultimately leading to Wright's resignation.

Another path to Gingrich's ultimate goal involved health care. As early as 1991, Gingrich saw health care reform as a barrier to his long-sought goal of a Republican House majority. A national health insurance system would be the final piece of the welfare state created by Franklin Roosevelt and his New Deal. Such a system might cement the loyalty of a large portion of the population to the Democratic Party well into the next century. His objective became, then, to defeat any kind of health care reform from succeeding (Johnson and Broder 1996). It should also be pointed out that Gingrich's opposition to health care reform was as much policy/ideologically oriented as politically strategic. As a conservative, Gingrich naturally opposed what he saw as a massive extension of government programs. The ideology and politics combined, and there would be no room for compromise.

His opposition showed at several places. Recall Fred Grandy's comment that Gingrich advised House Republicans on the Ways and Means Committee against voting for any amendment that would improve the chances of a health care reform bill's passage. In September 1994 Gingrich called for an end to the health reform effort and warned that if Democrats continued to push for it, Republicans would not support the General Agreement on Tariffs and Trade (GATT), an agreement Republicans overwhelmingly supported (Cloud 1994c; Johnson and Broder 1996). In July 1994 Senate Finance Committee Republicans issued a similar warning (Johnson and Broder 1996). Gingrich also held up the voting on GATT until after the November 1994 elections so that the Democrats would not get credit for its passage.

The Democratic response to Republican obstructionism on health care reform was to dismiss all Republican proposals. When moderate Democrats sought to forge a bipartisan plan with moderate Republicans, the Democratic leadership challenged the loyalty of the moderate Democrats and disregarded the proposals (Talbert 1995).

The 1994 Elections

In chapter 2, we pointed out that an important element in agenda building is the political stream, which includes public opinion, interest-group activity, and elections. While we consider interest groups and public opinion in subsequent chapters, our focus turns now to the 1994 midterm elections.

Those elections were both affected by and profoundly affected the debates over health care reform policy. We have seen that Republicans, especially in the House of Representatives, saw the defeat of the Clinton Health Security Act as a means toward victory in November. Certainly one of the reasons for the results of the 1994 elections was dismay over the failure of some kind of health care reform.

A major event of the 1994 elections was the development of the Contract with America. The Contract, a strategic step by Newt Gingrich, had its origins as early as 1980 when Republican presidential candidate Ronald Reagan and other Republican candidates pledged at a campaign event on the steps of the Capitol to increase the defense budget and cut taxes. Gingrich had participated in planning the event and sought to re-create it. Three years later, a member of the Conservative Opportunity Society (COS), Judd Gregg, wrote a memo suggesting issues that COS should consider; many of those issues were eventually incorporated into the Contract (Balz and Brownstein 1996).

In early 1994, Gingrich asked Dick Armey (R-Tex.) to work on the substance of the Contract, within certain guidelines, such as having ten provisions and sufficient support. This reaffirms the notion of Gingrich as primarily a strategist. Republican candidates were polled to see what they wanted in the Contract, and a series of focus groups were held to see how ideas within the document would play among the public (though no survey research was conducted on this). On September 27, some 300 Republican House candidates signed the Contract on the Capitol steps. The Contract was also publicly marketed, particularly a brief version of it in *TV Guide* (Balz and Brownstein 1996). The Contract was not unique. Bader (1996) found that congressional majority party leadership issued policy agenda under conditions of divided government.

The Contract with America is not important for its impact on voting; there is considerable evidence that it had little effect on voters' decisions. According to a *New York Times*/CBS News poll just before the elections, most voters (about 71 percent) had not heard of it and even among the small minority who had heard of it, most said that it would not have affected their decision to vote (Jacobson 1996).

But the Contract is important because of its substance. It was, in effect, a campaign platform, similar to what parties adopt during their presidential nominating conventions. It was a pledge to vote on certain legislation, some on the first day of the new Congress and the rest within 100 days.

Two aspects related to health care were not in the Contract. First, the

Contract called for a balanced budget amendment. But the Contract did not say how the budget was to be balanced; as a constitutional amendment, the details would be left up to future Congresses. Second, the Contract made no mention of Medicare, Medicaid, or any other health policy proposals. Given its lack of public support (largely out of ignorance of its provisions) and the two missing elements, one could not argue that there was a mandate for addressing health care issues. Yet, as we see below, Congress turned precisely to those policy concerns.

The elections themselves were a tremendous victory for the Republicans. They regained control of the Senate for the first time since 1986 and control of the House for the first time since 1954. The Senate went from a 56–44 Democratic majority to a 53–47 Republican majority. The House went from a 256–178 Democratic majority to a 230–204 Republican majority. Seventy-three freshman Republicans were elected, most of them loyal to Newt Gingrich for his help in their victories. Furthermore, no Republican incumbent lost in either the Senate, the House, or gubernatorial elections. The Republicans also made substantial gains in state legislatures. The question to be asked is why the massive change just two years after the Clinton victory in 1992.

Schneider (1994) suggests two reasons: the desire for change and conservative ideology. Voters in 1992 wanted government that would work, but became dismayed by what they saw as big government: "an economic stimulus program, a broad-based energy tax, expensive new crime prevention programs, a massive health care reform plan" (Schneider 1996, 2632). These and other actions by the administration alienated conservatives and when some did not pass, such as the economic stimulus program and health care reform, upset voters who wanted change. Clinton's popular approval rating was also low. Many of those who voted for Republicans voted in protest against Clinton policies (see also Balz and Brownstein 1996) and wanted less government. Schneider (1994) pointed out that the lack of trust in government was associated with voting Republican.

Jacobson (1996b, 204) offers the following explanation for Republican victories in the House:

> In 1994, the Republicans won the House by fielding (modestly) superior candidates who were on the right side of the issues that were important to voters in House elections and by persuading voters to blame a unified Democratic government for government's failure.

Balz and Brownstein (1996) have a slightly different view of the Republican victories. They see three broad trends coming together in 1994. The first is economic stagnation, essentially the decline of economic progress for the middle class (and lower classes) since about 1973 (see Krugman 1994; Madrick 1995; *New York Times* 1996; Phillips 1990). The second trend was cultural fragmentation. This included racial polarization, immigration issues, and the breakup of the traditional two-parent family. Balz and Brownstein's third trend was political alienation, "collapse of faith in government and political system itself, partly for its failure to reverse these other worrisome trends" (Balz and Brownstein 1996, 12). The Contract with America reflected many of these concerns, calling for smaller government.

So the reasons for the Republican victories were many. But in the aftermath of their victory could also be seen the seeds of Republican destruction. The elections, Schneider (1994) warned, should not be seen as an ideological mandate. Schneider said the real mandate, looking at both the 1992 and 1994 elections, was for change and for bipartisanship. Failure to understand the voters' genuine desires could lead to policy and political failure.

The Republicans Take Control

Newt Gingrich, now Speaker of the House, sought to assert control of the institution from the beginning. First, he picked the committee chairmen who would be responsive to the leadership's desires, bypassing seniority in three committees. The leadership also became responsible for committee assignments. He assigned the day-to-day control to the number-two Republican, House Majority Leader Dick Armey (R-Tex.), though he kept monitoring the course of legislation, especially those called for in the Contract with America. Some committee jurisdictions were changed and committee staff was significantly reduced. At least for a while, the Republican majority in the House acted in a disciplinary fashion, somewhat reminiscent of the British Parliament (the Westminster system):

> The party had a program, the "Contract with America." The Speaker chose the committee chairmen and the Majority Leader told them when to get which bills done. It was clear when dissenting votes would be tolerated, or treated as "free votes" on the British model, and when they would not. (Clymer 1995d)

Gingrich and the Republican House leadership also made use of ad hoc groups and task forces to develop consider issues and write legislation (Peters 1996; Strahan 1996). One example of this was the Speaker's Advisory Group (SAG), made up of top party leaders who oversee committee activities (Peters 1996).

The House succeeded in fulfilling its promise in the Contract. It voted on a number of bills on the first day of the new 104th Congress and voted on all the Contract provisions within the 100-day time limit. All but term limitations passed. Strahan (1996) writes that the Contract was important, not just for its substantive features, but also because it provided an agenda, at least for the first few months of the new Congress, and an opportunity for the new leadership to exercise its power. The result was that those first few months "acclimated Republican members to a party-centered, leadership-directed mode of operation" (Strahan 1996, 5).

There was less change in the Senate. Though it had a Republican majority, the "Long March of Newt Gingrich" (Peters 1996, 3) was not necessary. Republicans controlled the Senate from 1981 to 1986 and so had had experience with majority rule. Further, the smaller size of the Senate did not lend itself to the tight discipline imposed upon the House. Finally, the new Senate Majority Leader, Bob Dole (R-Kans.), was, by personality and experience, more of a compromiser than a strategist. Seniority was still the key to chairing committees.

The Senate, though Republican controlled, was a moderating influence on the more radical House. No senator signed the Contract with America, and some of the Contract's provisions would die in the Senate. The major example was the balanced budget amendment, which failed by one vote to reach the two-thirds majority necessary to propose a constitutional amendment. One Republican, Mark Hatfield (R-Ore.), voted against the amendment. Hatfield was also the chairman of the Senate Appropriations Committee. Though some Republican senators wanted Hatfield chastised and removed from his chairmanship, something that likely would have happened in the House, Hatfield retained his position (Cassata 1995).

Addressing Health Care in the 104th Congress

As we have seen, comprehensive health care reform failed in Congress in 1993–94. Most Republicans were against such a program, and some (Gingrich, Krystol) saw its defeat as the path to victory in the November 1994 elections. That does not mean that health care would not be an important agenda item in the 104th Congress.

Those who supported comprehensive reform turned to incremental changes as the road to reform. One possible target for reform were children. This approach was reminiscent of what happened after national health insurance was defeated during the Truman administration. Supporters of change then focused on health care for the elderly, a group that was felt would be generally viewed as deserving. The result, eventually, was the passage of Medicare (and Medicaid) in 1965 (Marmor 1973; Starr 1982). The kinds of changes addressed in 1995–96 were incremental and something more (see Families USA 1996a).

The more than incremental changes concerned the two major government health care programs, Medicare and Medicaid. The House proposed major changes in the program combined with significant reductions in spending. The smaller changes concerned insurance reform. While Congress passed legislation affecting all these programs, only the insurance reforms became law. We consider the Medicare and Medicaid changes first.

Medicare

To understand the proposed changes in Medicare (and Medicaid), it is necessary to place them in context. For both programs, the context was the attempt to balance the budget, largely through spending reductions. In the case of Medicare, questions about the viability of the hospital trust fund also played a role.

Balancing the Budget

The Contract with America called for a balanced budget amendment that would produce a zero deficit by the year 2002. The defeat of the proposed amendment in the Senate meant that Congress would have to take the legislative route to a balanced budget.

The first step in the process, as discussed earlier in this chapter, is the passage of a budget resolution. The House moved first. Its budget resolution called for $1.04 trillion in spending reductions for fiscal years 1996–2002. The reductions included $288 billion in savings in Medicare; $187 billion in Medicaid savings; $219 billion in savings from mandatory programs other than Social Security (which was untouched by the balanced budget plan), Medicare, and Medicaid; and $192 billion in discretionary spending. Defense spending would be increased. The budget resolution also called for $353 billion in tax cuts.

The Senate budget resolution called for $958 billion in total reductions. This included $256 billion from Medicare, $176 billion from Medicaid, $209 billion from other mandatory spending, and $190 billion in discretionary spending. The Senate said that a tax cut of as much as $170 billion could be enacted only if the Congressional Budget Office certified that the congressional plan would actually produce a balanced budget by 2002.

In June 1996 the House and the Senate agreed on a compromise budget resolution with the following features: $983 billion in total reductions, $270 billion from Medicare, $180 billion from Medicaid, $174 billion in other mandatory spending, $190 billion from discretionary spending and a $33.7 billion increase in defense spending over the Clinton administration defense proposal. The tax cut would be up to $245 billion with CBO certification (Hager and Rubin 1995). Between the Contract provisions and the budget resolutions, the new majority was on a roll. The hard work of the budget process was yet to come: a reconciliation bill and the thirteen appropriations bills.

Addressing Medicare

Medicare is one of the federal government's largest programs. By 1994 its costs were increasing by almost 11 percent a year and had grown into a $166.1 billion program (Levit et al. 1996). Its size made it an attractive target for budget cutters. The Clinton budget cut in 1993 called for $56 billion in Medicare cuts (Shear 1995). The congressional budget resolution in 1995 called for slowing the growth in Medicare to about 6.5 percent. Because Medicare was so important to the balanced budget goal, Gingrich set up several overarching committees to oversee the work of the House Ways and Means and Commerce committees (Balz and Brownstein 1996).

The large cuts called for in the budget resolutions set up an opportunity for the Democrats (and President Clinton) to put the Republicans on the defensive. Democrats charged that Republicans were trying to cut Medicare, a popular program especially among its chief beneficiaries, the elderly. Campaign ads charged Republican congressmen with voting with Speaker Gingrich to cut the program.

Republicans argued otherwise. They noted that spending on Medicare in 2002 under the Republican plan would be greater than in 1995, a correct statement. So how could a spending increase be seen as a cut?

The Democratic response was to argue that proposed spending in 2002 (and in the years between 1996 and 2002) would be less than under current law. Under current law, entitlement programs such as Medicare are adjusted for changes in the number of recipients (an increase in the case of Medicare) and for cost of living. This is known as *baseline spending*. Republican proposals would cut Medicare spending below the baseline (Shear 1995). Shear points out what this argument looks like if defense spending were being considered:

> While true, the [Republican] argument sidesteps the effects of reducing the rate of growth on the baseline. And when defense spending is restrained in a similar manner, Republicans refer to "cuts." Defense spending went from

> $287 billion in 1987 to $295 billion in 1992. While it grew and was not cut, it might as well have been slashed: $295 billion in 1992 bought far less defense—fewer active divisions, air wings and naval forces—than $287 billion bought in 1987. (Shear 1995, 736)

There were a number of options for achieving these reductions in Medicare spending but the specific plan to achieve such reductions was not immediately produced. Such options included converting Medicare into a voucher system, whereby Medicare recipients would be given a piece of paper worth the average amount of Medicare payments and then could use the voucher to purchase health insurance. Other options included increasing cost sharing on the part of Medicare recipients through higher premiums, deductibles, and co-payments and cutting payments to providers (Vobejda and Rich 1995).

In September 1995 House Republicans unveiled the specifics of their Medicare proposal, drafted by an eight-person task force. The plan, the Medicare Preservation Act of 1995, contained four major provisions: (1) slight increases in Medicare premiums in Part B (doctor bills) rather than the relative decreases that would take effect under current law (keep premiums at 31.5 percent of Part B, rather than 25 percent); (2) wealthier Medicare beneficiaries would pay considerably more than under current law, as much as triple current premiums; (3) beneficiaries could choose to join private plans, such as a health maintenance organization, in return for which they would receive some added benefits; and (4) Medicare recipients could decide to set up a catastrophic or high-deductible policy and a medical savings account that could be used to cover medical expenses (Pear 1995e). An earlier draft of the Republican proposal included financial incentives for joining HMOs, but it was dropped because of fears of commercialism (Pear 1995f).

The proposal was about $80 billion short of the target of $270 billion in savings. A vaguely described "fail-safe" mechanism was included in the proposal in case yearly savings were not met because of movement into alternative plans (HMOs and catastrophic/medical savings accounts). Unspecified steps would be taken to make up for the shortfall (Rosenbaum 1995b).

Further elaborations of the House Medicare proposals suggested that the premiums Medicare recipients paid would double and that antitrust laws would be relaxed to make it easier for providers to form networks to offer plans. In any event, by the end of September 1995, no bill had been submitted (Pear 1995f). The Senate Republican proposal to save on Medicare expenditures focused on reductions in payments to providers and cuts in benefits (Pear 1995h).

Republicans looked to cut the growth in Medicare spending for various reasons. First, the balanced budget goal was important in and of itself to them. Second, the balanced budget goal was a means to an end, the end being the shrinking of the size of the federal government (Balz and Brownstein 1996; Schneider 1995). Third, Medicare was one of the largest federal programs and, as we have seen, was growing at a rapid rate. With Social Security, interest on the debt, and defense spending (which was slated to increase) not targeted for cuts, Medicare was the next logical place to look.

Another element seemed to reinforce the Republican view that Medicare needs to be examined. In April 1995, the trustees of the Medicare and Social Security trust funds issued a report that said the Medicare Part A (hospital) trust fund would go bankrupt by the year 2002 (coincidentally the year Republicans picked to balance the budget). Republicans jumped on the report, asserting that changes needed to be made in Medicare and that President Clinton's budget did not address this issue (Pear 1995a). This provided Republicans with a different kind of justification for its Medicare proposals: it was not just cutting the program but protecting or saving it. As a result of polls and focus groups conducted by Republicans, the words "preserve," "protect," and "improve" were used to describe Republican proposals. The word "cuts" was forbidden; the word "strengthen" was also eliminated because it had the connotation of increasing coverage (Maraniss and Weisskopf 1996).

One interesting point about the Medicare proposal was that in some ways it was similar to what the Clinton administration had proposed as part of its Health Security Act. The Clinton plan called for limits on annual increases in insurance premiums as a last resort in the event that managed competition did not control health care spending. The belief was that the limits would be reflected in changes in payments to providers. The Republican plan called for a "benefit budget" that limited the amount of money to be spent on Medicare in a given year. To achieve that limit, government could reduce payments to providers and insurance plans. Both plans also envisaged a greater role for managed care as a means of controlling costs (Pear 1995g).

Republicans argued that there were differences as well. The Health Security Act would have covered the entire population and therefore would expand government's role. Their proposal was designed to increase the private sector's role in caring for the elderly, thereby reducing government's role. Medicare is such a large program, however, that its practices are often adopted in the private sector (Pear 1995g).

The Medicare proposals were criticized. One observer described the process of how the $270 billion reductions figure was arrived at:

> The Republicans decided that they wanted to balance the Federal budget by 2002. Then they agreed on a tax cut of $245 billion. Then they determined how much they could squeeze out of other Government programs. And $270 billion was what was left—what was needed from Medicare to make the ledger balance. (Rosenbaum 1995a)

Another charge was that the $270 billion was not necessary to protect Medicare from the impending emergency. Only $90 billion of the $270 billion in proposed cuts would come from Part A, where the trust fund is an issue. The other $180 billion would come from Part B. The changes proposed by the Republicans would forestall Part A trust-fund bankruptcy by only a few years. The trustees have been issuing reports of impending doom as far back as 1980, when they predicted bankruptcy in 1994. Each time changes were made, bankruptcy was averted. Given the above analysis about the relationship between Medicare and tax cuts, Democrats argued that Medicare recipients were being asked to bear the burden of the reductions so that tax cuts for the wealthy could be given. The reality is that given the size of the proposed budget cuts, even in the absence of tax cuts, Medicare would have remained an irresistible target (Rosenbaum 1995a).

The proposed Medicare cuts quickly became embroiled in partisan bickering. Democrats were opposed to the balanced budget goal and saw Medicare as a perfect vehicle for a counterattack. They also argued that the proposals were being hastily drawn up and pushed too quickly (Apple 1995).

Democrats in both the House and the Senate offered alternatives to the Republican plans. The Democratic proposals would reduce spending by $90 billion over the same seven-year period, primarily through reductions in payments to providers. The smaller figure, they argued, was more targeted to financial solvency then the broader Republican proposals. Democrats also noted that their plan would keep the Part A trust fund solvent through the year 2006 (Pear 1995h).

The Clinton administration, apart from attacking the Republican proposals as extreme, provided its own set of Medicare cuts. In June 1995, as Congress was finalizing its budget resolution, the administration offered its proposal as part of a ten-year balanced budget plan. Medicare spending would be reduced by a net of $124 billion over that time period. Cuts would come primarily from reductions in provider payments, rather than from benefits. The proposal also looked toward managed care and other alternative provider arrangements to achieve savings (Toner 1995).

In December 1995, as budget talks between the administration and Congress continued (following), the administration offered a revised plan. The goal was the same reductions as in June, $124 billion, but the time period was reduced to seven years, to 2002. The proposal would, the administration said, extend solvency of the Part A trust fund to 2011. Unlike the Republican plan, medical savings accounts were not included (Wines 1995).

Democrats labeled the cuts extreme and were able to use Republican leaders' own words against them. A flyer from the Democratic National Committee (1996) quoted three of them. Senate Majority Leader Bob Dole was quoted as saying, "I was there, fighting the fight, one of twelve, voting against Medicare, because we knew it wouldn't work, in 1965." House Republican Majority Leader Armey said that Medicare did not belong in a free world. Newt Gingrich said that "now we didn't get rid of it in round one because we don't think it's politically smart. . . . But we believe [Medicare is] going to wither on the vine." In fairness to Gingrich, he argued that the quote was that the Health Care Financing Administration, the agency that administers Medicare, was what he wanted to wither on the vine. A reading of the entire paragraph suggests, however, that he did indeed mean Medicare and not just the agency (Clymer 1996b).

Democrats had been reeling from the onslaught of the disciplined Republican troops; Medicare was the first real opportunity to regain ground. Indeed, it is not too much to say that Medicare proved to be the means of derailing the Republican budget proposals. Public opinion polls showed that the Democratic attacks were effective. The combined arguments that the proposed Republican cuts were too severe and were necessitated by the desire to extend tax cuts to the wealthy resonated with the public (Schneider 1995b).

In a sense, there was much less difference between the Clinton proposal and the Republican proposal than met the eye. The Congressional Budget Office issued an analysis noting that Medicare spending over the seven-year period under the administration proposal differed by only about 2 percent from the Republican proposal ($1.68 billion versus $1.65 billion). There was a difference between the two proposals in terms of how much spending would take place under current law. The administration used spending estimates provided by the Office of Management and Budget, which projected, for example, Medicare spending in 2002 at a little over $325 billion. The Republican proposal relied on Congressional Budget Office estimates, which projected Medicare spending of about $340 billion in 2002. The difference in projections provides the difference in proposed spending reductions, $124 billion in the administration plan and $270 billion in the Republican plan (Pear 1995n).

As the time came closer for voting on the Medicare changes, Republicans sought to maintain their majority support by making changes or tinkering with the bill. The problem for the Republicans in the House was that if no Democrats voted for the Republican measure, a loss of more than sixteen Republicans would defeat the measure. So began what the *New York Times* called a "frantic vote-trading bazaar. For example, representatives from New York and New Jersey sought changes that would maintain payments to foreign-born doctors in training. Rural areas sought higher monthly payments per beneficiaries" (Clymer 1995f).

On October 19, 1995, the House voted 231–201 for the Medicare reductions. The debate was heated. Consider the following two quotes ("Excerpts from House Debate on G.O.P. Plan to Overhaul Medicare System," October 20, 1995):

Charles Rangel (D-N.Y.): No one knows better than I how important a campaign promise is, and I recognize when you promise $245 billion to those who support the goals and aims of the Republican Party that you must keep that promise.

The questions is, Have you no shame in how far you can go to raise the money? Student loans, school lunches, housing for the poor and now we're talking about the crown jewel. The crown jewel isn't a $245 billion tax cut, the crown jewel are aged Americans. . . .

Oh, I know that Republicans have fought Medicare from the inception. Every time it comes up you've always been there. Always been there to vote it down and here you come again where hospitals that service the poorest of the poor, in the rural areas, in the inner cities, when they have no support system, there you are reducing the benefits.

People get up here time and time again saying that's just not so. Well why don't you go to the hospital people and ask them why they believe that you're destroying them. Why don't you go to those that are in nursing homes and ask why they are so frightened.

Dave Camp (R-Mich.): Some who oppose our program call it extreme. What is extreme is that year after year the Democrats' answer to Medicare has been to raise taxes. Almost every year Democrats dug deeper into the pockets of working Americans just to get through the next election. . . .

Could we put the Medicare crisis off a few years if we raise taxes again? Sure we could. Could we avoid the vicious attacks by special interest groups if we didn't reform the system? Sure, but we're not going to do that. We're going to preserve, protect and strengthen Medicare, not to get through the next election but for the next generation.

The president promised he would veto the budget reconciliation bill that would contain the Medicare proposals (Clymer 1995g).

Medicaid

Medicaid was also an important part of the budget story in 1995–96, though its dynamics were a bit different. Unlike Medicare, Medicaid is a joint federal-state program. The federal government sets overall eligibility and program standards and contributes between 50 and 80 percent of total costs. States set specific eligibility requirements, benefits packages, and administers the program. The costs of the program were increasing for both the states and the federal government. This meant that governors would be interested in changes that affected their budgets and their states. Medicaid is a smaller program than Medicare, both in the number of people covered and costs.

Medicaid is a means-tested program. That means that income eligibility requirements must be met before an applicant can be accepted. Medicare covers the entire eligible population (the elderly, the disabled, and those with kidney failure); Medicaid covers a little more than 40 percent of those living under the poverty level. Additionally, Medicaid is really two programs. One covers the poor, and the other covers the elderly poor who need long-term care (White 1995b). While most Medicaid recipients are in families with children, much of the money is actually spent on the elderly. By contrast, Medicare spends a very small amount of its funds on nursing home care.

There was one other difference between the two programs: at least at the outset of the 104th Congress, Medicaid's fate would be tied up with welfare reform.

Republican Proposals

The Republican proposals for Medicaid are fairly simple to explain. First, they wanted to cut the federal share of Medicaid spending by about $175 billion over the seven years ending in 2002. For the most recent two years, 1992–94, the federal share of Medicaid increased by a little over 9 percent, the state share by over 10 percent (calculated from tables in Levit et al. 1996). The Republican plan proposed reducing Medicaid spending to an annual growth of 4 percent.

The proposed cuts were deeper than for Medicare. First, the growth rate that Congress sought to achieve for Medicare was 6.4 percent, more than 50 percent higher than for Medicaid. Second, though the proposed cuts in dollar figures is larger for Medicare (15 percent in the House plan), Medicare is a bigger program than Medicaid; the proposed cuts in the House plan was almost 20 percent (Pear 1995b).

A second feature of the Medicaid proposals was revolutionary. The Republicans wanted to convert Medicaid into a block grant. Under current law, the amount of money spent on Medicaid is a function of state eligibility and benefits provisions and the number of Medicaid recipients. Under these conditions, Medicaid is both an entitlement and an uncontrollable expense. It is an entitlement because people who meet state and federal eligibility requirements join the program; it is uncontrollable because the federal government does not appropriate a specific amount of money for the program. A block grant would change all this.

Under a block grant, the federal government would give the states a specified amount of money each year (according to a distributional formula), and they would get no more funds. The Republican proposal, given the numbers discussed earlier, would result in a cut in the amount states received. Medicaid would now become a controllable and easily budgetable expense for the federal government. In return for the cuts, states would be given considerable flexibility in designing the program. Rules that normally accompany federal funds would be considerably reduced. States liked the flexibility and were willing to take some cuts in the grants to get that flexibility (Serafini 1995b). Governors, especially Republican governors, were supportive of the change, but concerned about the distribution formula.

The block grant, the controllable expenses, and the flexibility all pointed to the revolutionary nature of the proposed changes. In the early days of the Reagan administration, when cuts in social spending were being made, there was discussion of *safety net* programs. Medicaid was one of those safety nets. The block grant proposal changed the metaphor from safety net to *lifeboat*. The difference between the two is that a safety net is designed to catch all who fall (though Medicaid covers less than half the poverty population); a lifeboat has limited seating. Only those who can get in will be saved. Medicaid would no longer be a federal entitlement program. Under the Republican proposals, if the number of poor people rose unexpectedly, say, because of a recession, the size of the block grant would not be increased. Inflation would not necessarily be taken into consideration, nor would demographic changes be accounted for. The absolute and relative size of the elderly population will continue to increase into the twenty-first century and with Medicaid paying a sizable portion of long-term care expenses, the pressures on Medicaid would mount (Havemann 1995). On the average, Medicaid pays $955 per child per year under the age of twenty-one, $1,717 for adults twenty-one to sixty-four years of age, $7,216 for disabled recipients, and $8,704 for the elderly (Fraley 1995a). It would be up to the states to take action to meet the new needs, if they were so inclined. It could also set up competition between different groups of beneficiaries if cuts had to be made; the elderly, a potent political force, would likely fare better in such a competition than children (Fraley 1995a).

So the Medicaid proposal had four areas that would create controversy:

the formula for distributing the block grants to the states, the size of the proposed cuts, the end of the entitlement status, and the linkage between Medicaid and welfare reform.

The nation's governors, who were interested in change, particularly with regard to Medicaid (a much bigger program than welfare), had difficulty agreeing on a distribution formula. Part of the problem were differences between Republican and Democratic governors, the former approving of the changes (though not necessarily the formulas) and the latter fearing the cuts were too deep (Clymer 1995c). The budget resolution adopted in June 1995 did not include the term "block grants," and Republicans from some areas (especially in the Northeast, e.g., New Jersey) were opposed to the distribution formula.

Republicans in the Senate, though generally agreeing with the House proposal, had some difficulties with other parts of the Medicaid proposals, particularly those concerning nursing homes. The Senate Finance Committee voted to retain provisions of the current Medicaid law that prevented spouses from impoverishing themselves in order to qualify their spouses for nursing homes. Attempts to maintain federal nursing homes standards, however, failed (Fraley 1995c).

Like Medicaid, the Republican plan was included in the massive reconciliation bill. Clinton, in his June 1995 balanced budget plan, proposed cutting Medicaid by only $54 billion. This would be achieved by imposing a cap on spending per recipient (rather than on the program as a whole), allowing states to move Medicaid patients into managed care organizations, and reducing hospital payments without the benefit of a federal waiver (Hager 1995). He argued, as he did with Medicare, that the Republican cuts were too deep and that the entitlement status of Medicaid should be maintained.

The Train Wreck: Budget Battle

The huge budget battle between President Clinton and the Republican-controlled Congress reached its peak in the fall and winter of 1995. The battle, described as a head-on train wreck between Congress and the White House, took place over three sets of budget issues. First was the reconciliation bill that contained the cuts called for in the June budget resolution. This legislation included the Medicare and Medicaid changes discussed above. Enacting the reconciliation bill was necessary to achieve a balanced budget by 2002.

The second vehicle for disagreement was the debt-ceiling bill that would come due in November 1995. The federal government cannot borrow money past a ceiling established by law. Failure to enact such legislation could result in shutting down government and potentially defaulting on federal debts. The debt ceiling of $4.9 trillion would likely be reached by October 1995.

The third vehicle was the appropriations bills. By October 1, 1995, fiscal year 1996 began, but only two of the thirteen appropriations bills had been signed into law. A number of appropriations bills had not been voted on by the Senate.

Apart from disagreements about the actual dollar amounts in the appropriations bills, there was another issue. Some of the bills in the House, especially those concerning environmental programs, contained riders (amendments) not directly relevant to the bill. The inclusion of the riders and the controversy over them slowed the appropriations process.

Both the president and Congress had tools to use against the other. The budget legislation, both reconciliation and appropriations, could not be enacted without Clinton's approval, and Republicans lacked the majorities needed to override a veto. On the other hand, Congress did not have to pass a new debt-ceiling bill. Thus the stage was set for the train wreck.

The wreck came November 14, 1995, when the federal government shut down for six days. It reopened, as a result of a continuing resolution, which provided operating funds for a limited period, though the period could encompass the remainder of the fiscal year. On December 15, with still no agreement between the president and Congress, the federal government shut down for another twenty-one days.

On November 16, Congress passed the reconciliation bill, and on December 5 President Clinton vetoed it. In June the president had agreed on the balanced budget goal, but over ten years. In December he agreed to the 2002 goal, though with smaller tax and Medicare cuts than envisioned in the reconciliation bill.

Clinton's decision to agree to the 2002 balanced budget goal (and his earlier 2005 balanced budget goal) was based on the calculation that unless he was committed to balancing the budget, he would not be effective in negotiating with Congress or challenging them on specific actions such as Medicare, Medicaid, and tax cuts. The Republican gamble was that Clinton, who was seen by them as a weak president, would cave in to pressure. His acceptance of the balanced budget goal reinforced the view. Closing the government would force him to make concessions on budget and appropriations bills.

The Republican high-stakes gamble was a mistake. Emboldened by public opinion polls that showed the public blamed Congress more than the president, Clinton held firm, and the Republicans retreated. In negotiations with the president, Speaker Newt Gingrich became vulnerable to the president's charm (Weisskopf and Maraniss 1996). At one point, House Majority Leader Dick Armey was assigned to accompany Gingrich to the White House to prevent the Speaker from giving away too much.

An important impact of the budget gridlock was felt by Gingrich. Because of his tendency to say outrageous things, he became the embodiment of the Republican revolution, and his public approval ratings plunged. Though the Speaker, in private, was against closing the government (other leadership members were in favor of it), Gingrich took much of the blame. The most striking incident came in November 1995. Gingrich, along with President Clinton and other leaders, attended the funeral of slain Israeli Prime Minister Yitzhak Rabin. On the return to the United States, the Speaker complained about being snubbed by the president. The president did not ask him to talk about the budget negotiations and then the Speaker had to exit Air Force One from the back rather than the regular exit Clinton used. Gingrich said that this was one reason why a continuing resolution was loaded with items that the president disliked and thus vetoed it. Gingrich was seen by the public and the press as petulant (Maraniss and Weisskopf 1996).

Senate Majority Leader Bob Dole was in an ambivalent position. He needed to walk the line between Gingrich and Clinton. He was likely closer to the president in views toward the budget. He also wanted to end the stalemate so that he could get on with his presidential campaign. On the other hand, he wanted to maintain his relationship with Gingrich (Maraniss and Weisskopf 1996).

Though the budget battle, especially Clinton's public role in protecting Medicare, Medicaid, education, and environment programs, was very helpful to the president (his approval ratings went up), in the end Congress gained much of what it wanted. They got the president to agree to the 2002 balanced budget goal, though the president's plan left much of the budget cutting to the final years of the period. Further, the continuing resolutions that did pass contained cuts from the previous year's appropriations (Pear 1996a). The Republicans also played loose with the budget rules. The CBO scoring was that the budget had to be balanced in 2002; it did not have to be balanced after (or before that period). The Republican tax provisions would have resulted in revenue losses of some $55 billion after 2005 (up from $33 billion in 2002) (Allen 1996). Further, the two sides were not that far apart in the budget negotiations, a phenomenon similar to what occurred with Medicare cuts (Weisskopf and Maraniss 1996). Indeed, the Medicare portion of the Republican balanced budget deal was paralleling what was contained in the Health Security Act: "enticing seniors into private plans that accept a flat fee to provide basic benefits, reducing the inflation the government uses to pay doctors and hospitals to a rate closer to actual inflation and increasing out-of-pocket payments for the wealthiest Medicare recipients" (Pearlstein and Chandler 1995, 14). The total difference in spending between the president and Congress was less than $10 billion over the seven years; given the size of the economy over that time (more than $7 trillion a year), that was a small amount that was easily negotiable. Differences in economic assumptions could also have been ironed out to make agreement easier (Pearlstein and Chandler 1995).

Finally, in April 1996, seven months into fiscal year 1996, the president and Congress agreed on a budget. In total, some thirteen continuing resolutions were passed on the way to the agreement (Gray 1996).

Fiscal 1997 Budget Proposals

In March 1996 President Clinton sent his fiscal 1997 proposals to Congress. It called for reductions in spending for Medicare of $116 billion and $54 billion in Medicaid. In May 1996 Congress passed its FY 1997 budget proposal. It called for Medicare spending reductions of $168 billion and $72 billion for Medicaid (Hager and Rubin 1996; Wines 1996b). The balanced budget goal remained 2002, so both proposals were now over a six-year period, rather than seven years.

The Republican proposal moved a bit closer to Clinton in Medicare and Medicaid spending from the original 1995 budget resolution. It sought to end the entitlement status of Medicaid. For Medicare, the Republican plan called for moving recipients into private plans and employing medical savings accounts (Wines 1996a). The Medicare portion, described as "kinder" than the previous proposal, dropped the increase in Part B premiums (Rubin 1996). Not all agreed with the description. The Center on Budget and Priorities found that the proposed cuts in Medicare in May 1996 were not much different from the January 1996 proposals in the midst of the budget stalemate. For Medicaid, the proposed reductions were not significantly smaller than in 1995 (Greenstein and Kogan 1996).

Congress was still considering changes in Medicaid legislation. A bill approved in June 1996 by the House Commerce Committee would change Medicaid into a block grant, though there would be a small pool of federal funds, an "umbrella fund," in the event of a recession. But the amount of these reserve funds was equal to only 3 percent of total federal Medicaid funds under the proposal and could only be used on a one-time basis. The bill called for the $72 billion, six-year reductions contained in the budget resolution and would also lower the state matching share from 50 to 40 percent. This could mean that states would spend almost $180 billion less in Medicaid over the six years than under current law.

The bill removed the requirement that states provide services under Medicaid that were of sufficient scope, large enough and long enough to meet the goals of Medicaid. The proposal also allowed states to treat people with different diseases differently. For example, a state could offer extensive treatments for someone suffering from cancer but little services for someone suffering from AIDS. States could also impose high co-payments on Medicaid recipients. These and other provisions of the bill gave great flexibility to the states, as the governors wanted, but represented a major restructuring of the program (Families USA 1996b).

One last piece of legislation from 1996 should be mentioned. In August, President Clinton signed the Personal Responsibility and Work Opportunity Reconciliation Act of 1996. The act ended the sixty-year welfare entitlement program, Aid to Families with Dependent Children (AFDC), and replaced it with the Temporary Assistance for Needy Families (TANF) block grant. Much of the act was based on portions of the Contract with America. From our standpoint, the question is what impact the new legislation had on Medicaid. Under the now deceased AFDC program, welfare recipients were automatically eligible for Medicaid.

The new legislation stated that recipients of TANF were not automatically eligible for Medicaid. TANF created a "pre-welfare reform eligibility criteria" to determine Medicaid eligibility. The eligibility criteria are summarized as follows:

1. The individual meets the income and resource standards for determining eligibility under the State AFDC Plan in effect on July 16, 1996, using the income and resource methodologies under that plan; and
2. Based on the AFDC State plan in effect on July 16, 1996, the individual
   a. meets the AFDC definition of "dependent child" (i.e., meets AFDC age requirements, is a needy child, is living with one of the list of specified relatives and is "deprived of parental support or care" due to death, absence, incapacity or unemployment of a parent);
   b. is a relative of and living with a dependent child; or
   c. is pregnant and expects to give birth in the month or the following three months, and the child (when born) would qualify as an AFDC dependent child. (Greenberg and Savner 1996, 15).

States could make some minor adjustments to the standards by lowering their income standards slightly and by providing for some transitional Medicaid benefits under certain conditions (Greenberg and Savner 1996).

Insurance Reform

Republican proposals to cut spending for Medicare and Medicaid passed Congress but were vetoed by President Clinton. While the battle over the two large federal health care programs and the federal budget were occurring, other smaller health care reform changes were being considered and would ultimately be successful. The changes involved health insurance policies. One of the bills focused on issues concerning job transition and preexisting conditions. The other concentrated on an issue involving managed care organizations. We begin with the job transition issue.

Health Insurance Reform and "Job Lock"

The issue can be seen clearly in an August 1991 poll conducted by the *New York Times*/CBS News. The poll asked, among other questions: "Have you or anyone else in your household ever decided to stay in a job you wanted to leave mainly because you don't want to lose health coverage?" (Eckholm 1996). Thirty percent of the national sample said that either they or a member of their household did in fact stay in their job for that reason. This problem has been called *job lock*. The fear is that if a wage earner in a job offering health insurance changes jobs, either the new job would not offer health insurance or (more directly to our point) the wage earner or a member of his/her family might be denied coverage because of a preexisting condition. *Portability* was another term to describe the problem: to what extent a worker could carry health insurance into a new job.

Under federal law (COBRA), employers who offered health insurance as a benefit had to continue coverage for an employee who lost his or her job for a minimum of eighteen months, though employers did not have to pay for the premiums. Paying for the premiums would be difficult for unemployed people, and the coverage would end when they found new jobs.

Health insurance reform seemed like a natural winner. The president was in favor of it, congressional Republicans and Democrats were in favor of it, the health insurance industry was in favor of it. Yet it still took over a year for a bill to pass, and for a while it looked as though it might not pass at all. As usual, elections played a role in both the delay and the final passage.

Health insurance reform was a quiet part of the 1993–94 debate. President Clinton's Health Security Act addressed the job-lock issue by requiring individuals to enroll in a health plan and employers to join or form one. Bob Dole, as Senate minority leader, offered a plan in June 1994 that addressed the portability issue. The mainstream coalition proposal in late summer 1994 also contained health insurance reform.

In June 1995 President Clinton outlined, as part of his ten-year plan to balance the budget, a series of modest changes in Medicaid payments and health insurance reforms. The administration proposed federal regulation of the health insurance industry. Before this, the states were the primary regulators of the industry. Because the portability issue involves workers who cross state lines, however, it was an issue that only the federal government could address.

The proposal prohibited insurers from refusing to provide coverage to individuals with preexisting medical conditions, nor would they be able to deny renewal of health insurance policies. The measure also required insurers to cover small businesses and limit experience rating. Finally, the proposal would provide federal subsidies to enable former employees to afford premiums under COBRA (Pear 1995c).

In July 1995 a bipartisan health insurance bill was introduced in the Senate. The sponsors were Nancy Landon Kassebaum (R-Kans.), the chair of the Senate Labor and Human Resource Committee, and Edward M. Kennedy (D-Mass.). The bill, known as Kennedy-Kassebaum, contained the preexisting conditions provisions, though with some added wrinkles to make it more palatable to the insurance industry. For example, the bill allowed higher premiums for one year to those who had treatment for a chronic disease such as cancer or diabetes in the six months prior to obtaining the new policy (Clymer 1995a).

Another added touch to the bill was that it covered employers who were self-insured, that is, did not buy coverage from an insurance company. This was an important consideration. Some 60 percent of all workers are covered by employer self-insurance and, under the provisions of the Employee Retirement Income Security Act of 1974 (ERISA), such insurance cannot be regulated by the states (see Patel and Rushefsky 1995). The bill required employers who provide insurance to provide insurance to all workers who ask for it and prohibited workers from being excluded from insurance coverage because of previous conditions. Further, the proposal would prohibit employers from canceling insurance in the event a worker came down with an expensive illness, such as cancer or AIDS (Clymer 1995a).

The politics of the proposal were illuminating. The Kennedy-Kassebaum bill did not contain any tax features, such as medical savings accounts (to follow). This was designed to prevent the bill from going to the Finance Committee (a more conservative committee than Labor and Human Resources), which already had a large agenda. Thus the bill stayed with Labor and Human Resources (Clymer 1995a). As we see a bit later on, presidential politics also played a role in the deliberations.

In August 1995 the Senate Labor and Human Resources Committee unanimously reported the bill. The provisions of the bill called for a twelve-month limit on how long insurance companies might refuse to pay for preexisting conditions, eliminated any waiting period if the enrollee had not let his or her insurance coverage lapse for more than thirty days, and required insurers to renew policies. The General Accounting Office said the legislation could help as many as 21 million Americans ("Senate Panel Passes Health Insurance Bill" 1995). The bipartisan nature of the vote suggested the depth of the support for this kind of insurance reform.

The fate of insurance reform in the House was not so simple. No action was taken until early 1996. President Clinton, in his State of the Union message in January, called for congressional action on insurance reform.

One set of problems, ultimately the least important, was jurisdictional. Four committees could potentially claim jurisdiction over the House bill. The dominant committees were Commerce, Ways and Means, and Economic and Educational Opportunities. The Judiciary Committee could also stake a claim. To deal with the jurisdictional issues, a health task force was created, headed by J. Dennis Hastert (R-Ill.) (Pear 1996b; Serafini 1996a).

House Republicans added provisions to the basic Senate bill that would make it less likely that insurance reform would pass. The added provisions included "medical malpractice, antitrust law, special savings accounts for medical expenses and tax deductions for the health insurance costs of people who are self-employed" (Pear 1996b). The provisions were attached to the bill to please conservative Republicans and some committee chairs. Democrats argued that the underlying purpose of the bill was to kill the legislation because some of the provisions, such as medical savings accounts, might prove unacceptable to Democrats. The Republicans denied the accusation (Pear 1996b).

On March 19, 1996, the House Ways and Means Committee approved the insurance reform bill. It included the provisions that Democrats found objectionable, but the bill passed by a 25–11 vote, although most Democrats opposed it. Indeed, the Democrats proposed the Kennedy-Kassebaum bill in committee, and it was rejected 21–15, with Republicans voting against and Democrats voting for it (Pear 1996c). In any event, passage of the bill in committee meant it could go to the floor of the House.

A day later, March 20, the House Commerce Committee passed the bill 38–0. The difference in vote was that the Commerce Committee did not have authority over the tax provisions and so that portion of the bill was moot as far as Commerce was concerned (Pear 1996d).

When debate began in the House and the Senate, a major issue came up. As we have seen, the House bill contained a provision allowing for medical savings accounts. The Senate bill, emerging from the Labor and Human Resources Committee, did not contain the provision; a vote on MSAs in committee was defeated. What was so controversial about medical savings accounts?

A medical savings account program would work as follows: A worker and/or employer would deposit money each year into a savings account. The amount contributed to the accounts would be tax deductible. Then, when a medical expense was incurred, money would be withdrawn, tax free, from the account. To cover very costly medical expenses, workers would purchase insurance policies that had high deductibles (a catastrophic policy). A high-deductible insurance policy is one that would not pay until, say, the first $1,000 or $3,000 of medical expenses were paid. Catastrophic insurance policies are cheaper than either traditional or managed care insurance plans. Such a plan was proposed by House Ways and Means Chairman Bill Archer (R-Tex.) in August 1995 (Clymer 1996e; Freudenheim 1995), and it was included in the vetoed budget reconciliation bills. It was also strongly supported by Senate Minority Leader Bob Dole and House Speaker Newt Gingrich. A major backer of medical savings accounts was Golden Rule Insurance, which contributed to a number of Gingrich causes (Dreyfuss and Stone 1996; Serafini 1995a).

A problem associated with medical savings accounts is that people who anticipate little or no medical expenses are likely to choose such a plan. On the other hand, those anticipating considerable medical expenses, such as those with chronic medical problems, would be more likely to choose a traditional fee-for-service or managed care plan. The Medicare market can be segmented in just such a way. MSAs were included in congressional Medicare proposals as well as the House version of the Kennedy-Kassebaum bill.

Democrats challenged the inclusion of the extra provisions, arguing that the tax incentives for the medical savings accounts would benefit the healthy and wealthy and might lead to increases in premiums for other consumers. The argument was that if the healthy went to medical savings accounts plans, the less healthy would be left with conventional insurance. Because the conventional insurance population would be sicker and more likely to use health services than before, health insurance premiums would rise. This might price some elements of the population out of the insurance market. The ironic result of such a change, Democrats and others argued, was that fewer people might be covered as a result of a bill originally designed to extend insurance coverage (see Lav 1996; Pear 1996f).

Election-year politics stalled work on the bill. House Republicans were concerned that the president would get credit for the bill. By the end of March, Kennedy and Kassebaum promised to fight off amendments. House Republicans wanted their added provisions to gain support from the conservative Republican freshman class as well as put their stamp on the legislation. They also saw the revised bill as one able to control health care costs. Democrats wanted the measure to include a requirement for equal coverage of physical and mental health, to require coverage of at least a forty-eight-hour stay for postpartum care (normal deliveries), and to forbid lifetime limits for people in an employee health insurance plan. As *New York Times* health policy reporter Robert Pear wrote: "the chances for adoption of a health insurance plan decline sharply as the legislation becomes more intricate and convoluted" (Pear 1996e). One Democratic member of the House asked: "When there is something we all agree on, why can't we do what's doable?" (quoted in Pear 1996e).

On March 28, 1996, the House passed the bill 267–151 with the three provisions Democrats found objectionable. Gingrich said during the debate on the House floor that those provisions might be removed if the president threatened to veto it (Pear 1996g).

The Senate debated the Kennedy-Kassebaum bill in April 1996. Bob Dole offered an amendment to include medical savings accounts, which was defeated 52–46. Five Republicans joined the unified Democrats in defeating the amendment (Clymer 1996a). On April 23, the Senate unanimously passed the bill. It would still need to go to a House-Senate conference committee to iron out the differences.

Apart from the inclusion of the House provisions on medical malpractice and medical savings accounts, the Senate bill required insurers to cover mental illnesses. It should also be pointed out again that even the most modest version of Kennedy-Kassebaum extended federal control over health insurance in what had previously been a state-regulated industry (Clymer 1996b).

Presidential politics played a role in delaying the bill. Although the Senate rejected Senate Majority Leader Dole's amendment to Kennedy-Kassebaum that would include medical savings accounts, Dole still wanted the provision included in the bill. Clinton was against the provision and Dole was emerging as the Republican presidential nominee in 1996 against Clinton. Dole's strategy was to name to the Senate-House conference committee senators supportive of MSAs. Republicans thought Clinton would have to accept the bill with the MSA provisions or take the blame for failure of health insurance reform. Democrats, for their part, thought that Republicans would be seen as obstructionist, similar to what occurred with the budget battles (Clymer 1996c).

The battle of the conferees tied up the legislation for weeks. Trent Lott (R-Miss.), the Senate majority whip, proposed the list of conferees. Kennedy objected and offered his own list. Lott then objected to Kennedy's list, and no one was named. Dole did not participate in the debate, but did approach Kennedy during a quorum call and said, according to Kennedy, that he needed the MSAs politically, though he was not deeply committed to them. Kennedy, denied the opportunity of making complaints on the Senate floor, held a news conference in the Senate gallery (Clymer 1996d).

By June 1996 it appeared that health insurance, despite widespread support, was doomed. Democrats proposed trying medical savings accounts on a trial basis, but Republicans rejected the offer (Clymer 1996e). Democrats, on the other hand, wanted a vote on minimum-wage legislation, and Republicans were blocking that (Wines 1996c).

One interesting aspect of the deadlock was the resignation of Bob Dole from the Senate in June 1996 to concentrate on his presidential campaign. His successor, Trent Lott, was dedicated to getting legislation through Congress, though he expressed some frustration with the lack of movement and obstruction in general. By the end of June 1996 the conference committee had been unable to meet because of Senate Democratic opposition (Wines 1996c). Wines describes the problems in the Senate as follows:

> Twenty years ago, the proper way to block legislation in the Senate was to filibuster it, and that was considered a tactical weapon to be used only rarely. Today senators filibuster so often that the mere threat of extended debate suffices for the actual all-night session, and both sides assume that nothing will get passed unless a filibuster-proof 60 votes are on its side.
>
> Senators routinely block action by raising objections to debate, by placing "holds" on nominations and by threatening to offer amendments that they know will tie the chamber in oratorical knots. (Wines 1996c)

Eventually, the conferees met in July 1996 and a compromise was reached on Kennedy-Kassebaum. Medical savings accounts would be tried on an experimental basis, limited to 750,000 people, allowing long-term care expenses, including insurance, as a tax deduction and increasing the tax deduction on health insurance for self-employed people. Provisions requiring coverage of mental health were dropped in conference. On August 21, 1996, Clinton signed the bill (Havemann 1996).

One last law addressing health insurance issues was passed by Congress and signed in September 1996. One provision restored mental health coverage, deleted in the conference committee over the Kennedy-Kassebaum bill. The other, more publicized portion, mandated that insurers, especially managed care plans, cover a two-day hospital stay for mothers for normal deliveries and four days for cesarian births. The problem with postpartum care was that managed care plans were limiting such stays to one day to control costs (Pear 1996h).

The 1996 Elections

The 1996 elections produced mixed results. President Clinton won reelection with 379 electoral votes to Bob Dole's 159. The popular vote was considerably closer, with Clinton gaining just a bit less than 50 percent of the vote (49.2 percent); Dole received 40.8 percent of the popular vote, and third-party candidates divided up the rest. Voter turnout (about 48.8 percent) was one of the lowest in the twentieth century.

The congressional elections showed mixed results. Republicans gained in the Senate, extending their margin from 53–47 to 55–45. In the House, Republicans maintained their majority but saw their margin shrink from 236–198 to 227–207 (with one independent). In neither house were there enough Republicans to overturn a presidential veto, and the Senate majority remained short of what is needed to end a filibuster.

Health care played a role in the elections. More than a year before the elections, the Democrats opened fire on the Republicans for their proposed changes in Medicare and Medicaid. Clinton and Vice-President Al Gore constantly repeated the refrain of protecting Medicare, Medicaid, education, and the environment. The Democratic National Committee ran an ad in August 1995 accusing the Republicans of wanting to cut Medicare. The AFL-CIO spent $35 million to unseat House Republicans, again using the health programs as a hammer. The effort was partly successful; the House remained in Republican hands, though with a smaller majority. Fewer incumbents lost reelection than in previous elections.

Sixty-seven percent of those who thought Medicare and Social Security were important issues voted for Clinton, but they constituted only 15 percent of the electorate. More important were political ideology and the state of the economy. Fifty-six percent of the electorate thought that the state of the economy was good, and 63 percent of them voted for Clinton. The Clinton campaign and House Democrats won majorities among voters identifying themselves as liberal or moderate (Baker 1996).

Equally as important were two other considerations: divided government and region. Exit pollsters asked voters whether they would vote for a Republican or Democratic Congress if Clinton were reelected. Respondents were split and divided government was continued (Baker 1996). Broder (1996b) argues that in the short run, voters were putting both parties on probation: "For the longer haul, the Republicans still have to convince voters that they have a social conscience, and Democrats must prove that they have the fiscal discipline that voters clearly want" (Broder 1996b, 7).

The other issue was the regional realignment discussed earlier. Clinton won at least a plurality in all regions of the country except the South, where he tied with Dole. The South was the one region where Republicans carried a majority (Baker 1996). This produced what Schneider (1996, 2723) called "two different elections." This sectionalism reinforced the ideological and cultural differences between the two parties.

Conclusion

At the beginning of this chapter we examined a number of factors that affect policy making in Congress. These factors were structure and process, and elections. How well do they explain health policy outcomes in the 103d and 104th Congresses?

Start with structure. We noted differences between the House and the Senate. The House, the larger body, was characterized by more frequent elections and reliance on rules to guide the process. The Senate was more informal, with fewer limits on debate and amendment and more freedom to individual members.

We also looked at the impact of the budgeting process and the budget deficit on policy making. Two important points were made here. First, there was a mechanism, reconciliation, for making significant budget cuts. Second, the PAYGO rule prohibited new programs unless they were budget-deficit neutral, meaning new revenues or other program cuts had to be found. This budget-deficit politics would work against new programs (such as national health insurance) and in favor of program cuts (e.g., Medicare and Medicaid).

The third element of structure involved committees. Committees are where much of the detail work of Congress is done. But the fragmentation of power and authority in Congress meant that complex plans, such as comprehensive health care reform, would be the subject of multiple jurisdictions. For cutbacks in a single program, such as Medicare, multiple jurisdictions were less important.

The other major area discussed focused on elections and related factors such as divided government, gridlock, and realignment. Members of Congress react to the imminence of elections because of their desire to be reelected and to maintain or gain control of the House or Senate. Much of the electoral history of the United States in the post–World War II era has produced divided government, where one party controls the presidency and the other controls one or more houses of Congress. Divided government exacerbates the institutional jealousies created by the constitutional system of separation of powers/checks and balances. The result can be, though it is not always true, gridlock, an inability to make policy. We suggested that the real issue was whether a working majority existed in a particular legislative body. Finally, realignment appeared to increase the ideological coherence of the political parties, making compromise more difficult.

All these factors were important in explaining health care outcomes. While Democrats had a numerical majority in the House and the Senate during the 103d Congress, they did not have a working majority. There was little party unity on comprehensive health care reform; the Democrats did not present the public or the Republicans with a unified stance. Most Republicans were against reform and could use House and Senate rules to impede the process by voting against amendments to improve the chances that a bill would pass or by threatening to filibuster other needed legislation (e.g., GATT). Republicans saw the defeat of health care as an opportunity to achieve a historic electoral victory in 1994. The multiple committees that considered health reform legislation also made it more difficult for House and Senate Democratic leadership to produce a bill around which the party could unite. The complexity of the Health Security Act and its potential impact on the budget deficit also played havoc with its chances for success.

With their victories in November 1994, Republicans had the opportunity to enact significant policy changes, many of them found in the Contract with America. The Republican record in the 104th Congress was mixed. Republican leadership, committed to the Contract and ideologically cohesive, brought structural change to the House. Committee chairs were appointed by the Speaker based on support for the program. Ad hoc task forces produced uniform policy positions and moved committees to proceed quickly. But not all Republicans in the House agreed with the agenda, and the Senate, though controlled by Republicans, was less affected by new leadership. It did not agree with all the Contract items. A working majority was not present in the 104th Congress any more than it was in the 103d.

Some of the Republican agenda passed, but those parts related to the budget did not. Indeed, the most critical mistake Republicans made in 1995–96 was to challenge President Clinton by allowing the federal government to shut down twice. Clinton did not back down, as Republicans hoped he would, and the public blamed Congress for the shutdowns. Medicare and Medicaid were integral parts of this.

Elections played an important role in health policy outcomes. The 1992 elections helped put national health insurance on the policy agenda. The 1994 elections were seen as an opportunity to defeat that agenda and its defeat helped Republican victories. The 1996 elections provided an incentive for Republicans and Democrats (though mostly Republicans) to compromise and allow passage of legislation that might not have been enacted otherwise: welfare reform, minimum wage increases, health insurance reform, a telecommunications bill, and the Safe Drinking Water Act. Republicans, especially, wanted a successful record to run on. Note that Medicaid was taken out of the welfare-reform bill.

Mr. Clinton and the Republicans did not work together in the ordinary sense. But they used each other's desire to prosper in the November election, and the strength they had honed in opposition—the Republicans in 1994, Mr. Clinton in late 1995 and early 1996—to force the other side to give way sufficiently that both could swallow the results.

The 103d Congress also had its share of accomplishments: the Brady bill, the national service corps, the 1993 budget-deficit agreement, ratification of two trade bills (GATT and NAFTA), and a crime bill, among others. Its major failure was in health care.

The accomplishments of Congress in these two periods were marked by many successes and some major failures. But while changes made were not pathbreaking in the sense that New Deal legislation was, the legislative accomplishments were important. And while it may be argued, as we argue in the final chapter, that the health legislation eventually enacted has some important flaws, the system did work as intended.

5 INTEREST GROUPS

An interest group is an organized collection of people with common goals and concerns who seek to influence government policy (Berry 1997). Truman (1951, 33) defines an interest group as "any group that, on the basis of one or more shared attitudes, makes certain claims upon other groups in the society for the establishment, maintenance, or enhancement of forms of behavior that are implied by the shared attitudes." The basic elements of the two definitions are a group of people, some common interests, organized, seeking to influence others (the public, other groups, government).

Interest Groups and the Constitution

As in areas such as political parties, the U.S. Constitution is silent about interest groups. The First Amendment to the Constitution nevertheless provides protections for the formation and activities of interest groups. The rights granted by the First Amendment include free speech and press, assembly, and petitioning government.

The first two rights, speech and press, have become subsumed under the term *freedom of expression.* While freedom of expression has been expanded in controversial areas such as obscenity, there is little doubt that freedom of speech and of the press were meant to defend political expression. These two freedoms provide protection for the utterance of ideas necessary in a democratic society. In the context of interest groups, this means that interest groups can advocate policies or changes in policies and try to influence other members of society (without the use of coercion).

The last two freedoms, assembly and petition, are at the heart of protections affecting interest groups. The right to assembly means to gather together. It allows groups to meet and make decisions, plans, and so forth without government interference. The right to petition refers to the right to complain to or lobby government about its policies. Given our definition of interest groups, which emphasizes organized, collective, and influencing government, one can see how these two rights are vital to interest groups.

Having said that, we should point out that the Founding Fathers, those who wrote the Constitution and the Bill of Rights, were neither familiar with nor pleased about interest groups. The term had not come into general use, and to the extent that there were interest groups in society the Framers did not like them (see below). Further, as Lindblom and Woodhouse (1993) point out, the Bill of Rights freedoms were designed for individuals, not for groups: "Whether business corporations and other large institutions necessarily should enjoy all of the same liberties originally intended for individual citizens is one of the major issues unsatisfactorily addressed to date in democratic theory and practice" (p. 75).

It should also be pointed out that there is judicial precedent for giving protection to organizations. The Fourteenth Amendment to the Constitution, originally designed to give Bill of Rights protections to the freed slaves from state action after the Civil War, was interpreted by the courts instead to grant freedom to corporations from state regulation.

The Mischiefs of Faction

The view of the Founding Fathers toward interest groups was captured most succinctly by James Madison in the *Federalist Papers* (#10). This series of essays argued for the adoption of the proposed constitution and was published in newspapers around the time of the New York State ratification convention. Madison began his essay by writing that perhaps the most important advantage of the new government would be its ability to "break and control the violence of faction" (Hamilton, Madison, and Jay 1961, 77). He then provided us with a definition of a faction, one that shows Madison's disdain for them:

> By a faction, I understand a number of citizens, whether amounting to a majority or minority of the whole, who are united and actuated by some common impulse of passion, or of interest, adverse to the rights of other citizens, or to the permanent and aggregate interests of the community. (Hamilton, Madison, and Jay 1961, 78)

Note that Madison's definition can apply equally as well to political parties, which, like interest groups, were unknown at the time.

Madison wrote that the tendency to form factions was inherent in mankind. Some of the differences he saw as important, such as disagreements concerning religion or government. Others he saw as trivial or frivolous, just another part of the inherent frailties of people. The most important source of factions, however, was economic:

> But the most common and durable source of factions has been the various and unequal distribution of property. Those who hold and those who are without property have ever formed distinct interests in society. Those who are creditors, and those who are debtors, fall under a like discrimination. A landed interest, a manufacturing interest, a mercantile interest, a moneyed interest, with many lesser interests, grow up of necessity in civilized nations, and divide them into different classes, actuated by different sentiments and views. (Hamilton, Madison, and Jay 1961, 79)

The dilemma, as described by Berry (1997), is that we do not want to take away people's freedom, including the freedom to pursue their self-interest. On the other hand, pursuing one's self-interest may not be in the interest of society as a whole.

This problem, curing the mischiefs of faction, as Madison saw it, was at the heart of what government should be doing. Madison wrote that we could either forbid factions or allow them free rein. Typically, Madison saw both alternatives as unacceptable and chose instead to regulate their behavior. In *Federalist* #10, he said that a large republic was more likely to withstand factions than a smaller country, especially one that was characterized by a pure democracy. A representative government combined with separation of powers and checks and balances would suffice to prevent even a majority from rolling over its opposition.

Growth of Interest Groups

Much political science literature has focused on interest groups in American society. The decentralized and fragmented nature of American government provides access points for interest groups to petition and monitor government. Congressional reforms of the 1970s opened up committee proceedings so that not just hearings, most of which were public, but the all-important markup sessions in committees and conference committee proceedings were opened to the public (Loomis and Cigler 1991).

What is also important is the growth in the number of interest groups and in organizations with representation in Washington. Rauch (1994) reports that just before 1930 there were about 400 lobbies in Washington; by 1950, that number had increased to over 2,000. Rauch also examined the number of groups listed in the *Encyclopedia of Associations*. In 1956, the number was about 5,000; by 1993, the number climbed to more than 23,000 groups.

This same proliferation of groups can be found in the health care area. In

1979, the number of health groups in Washington was a little over 100. In 1991, the number was approximately 740 (Rauch 1994). Baumgartner and Talbert's (1995) calculations show a similar trend. They found that the number of health and social interest groups increased from 674 in 1960 to 3,971 in 1992 (calculated from the *Encyclopedia of Associations*). Equally important, Baumgartner and Talbert note that while interest groups in all areas increased in number over this time (their article compared groups in trade, agriculture, education and culture, and health and social), the increase was greatest in the health and social area.

Why this massive increase? A number of explanations have been offered (Rauch 1994; Loomis and Cigler 1991). Of the possible explanations (weakness of the party system, movement toward a postindustrial society, government's sponsorship of new interest groups, etc.), one that seems most appropriate to our topic is the expansion in government. Loomis and Cigler (1991) point out that growth occurs in spurts (see also Baumgartner and Jones 1993). One spurt came with the New Deal programs of the 1930s. A second one came with the beginning of the Great Society programs in the 1960s and continued into the 1970s.

This expansion of government went in two somewhat related directions. First, government expanded services provided. Examples of these include Social Security and welfare programs in 1935 and Medicare and Medicaid in 1965. More people were affected by what the federal government did, and, of course, taxes increased to pay for the new programs.

The second direction of government growth was in the area of regulation. While federal regulation dates back to the founding of the Interstate Commerce Commission in 1887, the nature of government regulation began to change, especially in the 1960s and 1970s. The older regulation, over things such as surface and air transportation, was known as economic regulation. It focused on specific industries and concentrated on prices and entry/exit. Social regulation ran across a broad array of industries and activities. For example, occupational health and safety affected virtually any kind of activity, as did environmental and consumer protection, civil rights, and so forth.

The basic point is that given the growth in what government did, those affected by government activities formed groups to engage in a variety of interest-group activities (see following). Beneficiaries of services formed groups to defend those services. Those who were affected by regulations also sought to affect government policy. The result of this growth is captured by Heinz et al. (1993, 385):

> By the late seventies, policy domains had become complex environments populated by substantially increased numbers of private interest representa-

tives and multitudes of executive branch agencies, independent regulatory bodies, the courts, and a greatly expanded congressional staff, all of which were processing a daunting volume of legislation, regulation, and litigation. Policy making had become more significant for more groups, but less controlled by the groups it affected.

Another way of looking at the growth of interest groups and their concern about government activity is through the theory of regulation developed by James Q. Wilson (1980). Wilson argued that policy proposals can be distinguished on the basis of perceived costs and benefits to affected groups. The distribution and magnitude of the costs and benefits are what give proposals their political significance.

From this insight, Wilson developed a typology based on distribution of costs and benefits. The distribution factor focuses on whether costs and benefits are concentrated or disbursed. That is, are the impacts of a policy limited to a small number of people or groups or to a much larger sector of the population? To give a nonhealth example of the issue of distribution, consider the price of milk. If the price of milk goes up, say, five cents a gallon, this represents a relatively small increase that many people will pay (those who drink milk). But that nickel a gallon increase represents a significant sum to those involved in the production and distribution of milk.

This concept leads to a fourfold typology. When costs and benefits are widely distributed (diffused), we have what Wilson calls majoritarian politics. Interest groups generally do not arise because no single interest group would gain much of the benefits or pay much of the costs. Social Security is one example of this, as is passage of antitrust legislation.

The opposite situation is when costs and benefits are concentrated. This produces interest-group politics. A subsidy or benefit is given to one group at the expense of another. Labor legislation is a good example of this, as was the passage of the Interstate Commerce Act in 1887.

The third category is client politics, when benefits are concentrated and costs are diffused. Our milk example fits this category. There is considerable inducement for interest groups to form and lobby government. Medicare politics for a long time fit this category. As Feder (1977) pointed out, much of the early concern and interest-group activity focused on how hospitals would be paid.

The final example is entrepreneurial politics, where costs are concentrated and benefits are diffused. The new social regulation fits this category. Some skilled policy advocates and third parties mobilized by advocates are able to overcome what would seem to be the natural inclination of the American political system to limit such policies. Yet the 1960s and 1970s saw much in the way of such new programs. Wilson's major point is that the politics differs depending on the distribution (and magnitude) of costs and benefits.

This insight is not new. Schattschneider (1960) argued that the essence of politics is conflict and that as the scope of a conflict increases, more people become involved and the nature of that conflict changes. Groups seek to confine conflict.

Lowi (1964) expanded on this perception. He argued that politics affected public policy but that public policy also affected politics. Again, as the nature of the policy changed, so would the politics. In his initial classification, Lowi distinguished among distributive, regulatory, and redistributive policies. Distributive policies were concerned with doling out government benefits and were confined to the interests directly involved. Medicare, again, in the early years concentrated on how hospitals would be paid, and so hospital groups were the most concerned about the policies.

Regulatory politics involved restrictions on behavior and thus affected a wider group. If we stay with the Medicare example, consider the institution of the Medicare hospital prospective payment system (diagnostic related groups) in the early 1980s, which limited how much Medicare would pay hospitals for a particular hospital episode. Hospitals would receive a fixed reimbursement for, say, a heart bypass operation. If the patient stayed in the hospital too long, the hospital would lose money. But hospitals do not determine how long patients stay, doctors do, and most doctors do not work for hospitals. So hospitals put pressure on doctors not to keep patients in hospitals for too long. This meant that hospital and doctor groups were interested in the payment system. Medicare patients would also be interested because their care would be affected. Managed care programs have a similar affect.

Lowi's third category, redistributive policy, has the largest scope of conflict (to use Schattschneider's term). More people are affected, conflicts cannot be confined, and so forth. President Clinton's Health Security Act fits this category. Everybody would be covered, and businesses that formerly did not pay for health insurance for their employees would be required to participate (employer mandate). People who did not currently pay into a health insurance pool (for example, self-insured people or working people who received coverage from their spouse's job) would be required to contribute. We should expect, therefore, that a wide variety of interest groups would be involved in the debates during 1993–94. As we see later, that is exactly what happened. The 1995–96 debates (especially over Medicare and Medicaid) did not involve nearly as many interest groups because they focused more on specific government programs and did not directly affect everyone.

What Interest Groups Do

Interest groups engage in a wide variety of activities (we include organizations that are not interest groups per se, such as corporations; they, too, seek to influence public policy). Berry (1997) notes five kinds of activities. Interest groups represent their members before government. They give people a channel in which to participate in politics. They educate people about issues through a variety of campaigns and publications. They bring issues to the attention of the political system, a process known as agenda building. Finally, they engage in monitoring government programs to let their constituents know what is going on and to be able to respond to changes in government policy.

Heinz et al. (1993) offer a slightly different list of activities. Interest groups (and their representatives) testify before congressional committees and regulatory agencies, they work with other interest groups, they engage in election-related activities such as campaign finance through political action committees (PACs), they maintain formal and informal contacts with government officials, they mobilize constituents, they intervene in court proceedings, and so forth.

Critique of Interest Groups

The basic assumption of *pluralism* is that the interaction of interest groups produces public policy. This view suggests that governmental decision makers play a mediating and balancing role among the various groups. A major counter to this pluralistic claim is that decision makers have policy and political goals of their own that they seek to achieve. Consider for a moment those opposed to the Clinton Health Security Act, particularly Republicans. Even in the absence of interest-group opposition, the more conservative Republicans, such as Newt Gingrich, Dick Armey, and Phil Gramm, and the seventy-three Republican freshmen elected in 1994, would have been ideologically opposed to this significant extension of government authority. The Contract with America, after all, was a document that sought on the policy level to shrink government. No interest-group campaign would be necessary to persuade them to oppose the plan. To that we can add the political dimension. We saw in chapter 4 that Gingrich opposed any kind of health care reform because he thought its success would cement a Democratic majority into the twenty-first century and its failure might lead to Republican control of Congress. Finally, in 1995–96 Republican congressional leaders were seeking to influence (and in some cases coerce) interest groups, rather than the reverse. There is precedent for this type of behavior within the Democratic Party in the early 1980s.

But there is another sense in which interest groups are criticized, one that goes back to the Madisonian critique of factions. The mischief of faction, as Madison saw it, was that each group would be focused on its own narrow interests, rather than what was good for the nation as a whole. At the same time, the requirements of political freedom mandated that groups be allowed to follow their special concerns (Berry 1997). That is why interest groups are often derogatorily referred to as *special* interest groups. What happens, it might be asked, if interest groups become so numerous and so protective of their programs that it becomes hard to make difficult decisions. The result could be the gridlock and deadlock discussed in the previous chapter.

Several observers have addressed this issue. One such observer is Theodore Lowi. In *The End of Liberalism,* Lowi (1979) argues that interest-group liberalism has several flaws. First, the idea that there is a self-correcting process to group activity is fundamental to group theory (Truman 1951). Such a view suggests that overlapping membership (people belong to more than one group and therefore face conflicting pressures that balance out) and the presence of competing groups will balance out, and that the interaction of groups produces policy that is ultimately in the public interest in the same way that free competition produces the most efficient use of resources and satisfies the wants and demands of consumers. Lowi disagrees with this view. The larger public interest is almost never served (Lowi 1979). Another argument that Lowi makes is that many groups are integrally involved in the policy-making process, including program implementation. Finally, Lowi asserts that interest-group liberalism is conservative in that it resists reforms that affect programs supported by the groups.

Later in the book, Lowi describes the triumph of interest-group liberalism as the Second Republic and the state of permanent receivership. The Second Republic, with its roots in the policies of the 1930s (New Deal) and the 1960s (Great Society), is characterized by a massive expansion of the federal government, as opposed to what Lowi calls the First Republic, where the federal government did little and most of the governing was by the states. The idea behind permanent receivership is that the government, through regulatory and fiscal policies, provides stability by protecting sectors of the economy from failure. Examples here include the bailouts of Lockheed, Chrysler, and savings and loan institutions. The result was that interest-group liberalism corrupted democratic government.

A similar critique, with a somewhat different emphasis, comes from economist Mancur Olson and journalist Jonathan Rauch. Olson (1982) argues that all economically advanced democratic countries will go through the same process. Countries that have experienced stability will develop an elaborate structure of interest groups. Those interest groups, concerned largely with their own wants and needs, reduce the economic efficiency and growth of the society as a whole.

This idea was developed and carried forward (in a more accessible or readable way) by Rauch (1994, 1996). Rauch originated the concept of *demosclerosis,* which he defined as "government's progressive loss of the ability to adapt" (1994, 123). The comparison Rauch uses is with arteriosclerosis, or hardening of the arteries. Rauch argues that both demosclerosis and arteriosclerosis can be arrested but only by long-term changes in behavior (in the case of arteriosclerosis, diet and exercise). The question that follows from this definition is not why nothing ever gets accomplished but "why is it that what Washington does is less and less effective at solving problems?" (Rauch 1994, 124).

Rauch then notes that because of the deliberate design of the American political system, change is supposed to be difficult. The problem is that change occurs but generally in only one direction: adding programs rather than eliminating them. The result, Rauch observes, is that *"we are stuck with everything the government ever tries"* (1994, 135; emphasis in the original). Demoslcerosis means that we cannot use trial and error with public programs, keeping things that work and abandoning those that do not. As new programs are added, the policy space becomes more crowded and things that need to be done become even more difficult to do. Thus, an activist government, again stemming from the New Deal and the Great Society, results in paralyzing an activist government. It also, as we argue in chapter 7, produces its own reaction in public opinion and among those who oppose an activist government.

Another implication that Rauch points out is that the federal budget deficit increases. He rightly notes that the budget deficit increased from the 1950s (when the average budget deficit as a percentage of GDP was .4 percent) through the 1960s (.75percent), the 1970s (3 percent), and the 1980s (4.1 percent). Rauch (1994, 153) writes:

> Budget deficits help hungry lobbies accumulate, by letting them draw resources from the future when money gets scarce in the present. Returning the favor, hungry lobbies help budget deficits accumulate, by adding to the fiscal demands on politicians and so creating pressure to write IOUs. In that way, deficits and demosclerosis go hand in hand—and in another way, too; demosclerosis makes getting rid of a deficit, once one exists, practically impossible. Balancing the budget would be easy if the government had the flexibility to shut down programs and mover resources around—but, of course, that flexibility is exactly what government does not have.

One should add, perhaps as an endnote, that following the logic of Rauch (and Olson) suggests that little change can occur. Stone (1997, 220), utilizing insights from the field of cognitive psychology, argues in a similar vein that "every political goal can be portrayed both as a good to be obtained and a bad to be avoided. . . . People respond different to bads and goods. They are far more likely to organize around a threatened or actual loss than around a potential gain."

But two examples show that this analysis is overstated. First, the federal budget deficit has decreased significantly. It peaked in 1992 at $290 billion (about 4.8 percent of GDP, the highest proportion was 6.3 percent in fiscal year 1983); by FY 1996, the deficit was $107 billion, about 1.7 percent of GDP. A second example was the welfare-reform bill passed in 1996, which ended Aid to Families with Dependent Children and the sixty-year federal guarantee of federal assistance for the needy.

Our discussion so far seems perfectly cast for a conservative revolution: government, especially at the federal level, should be cut back considerably. But in a more recent work, Rauch (1996) argues that conservatives waiting for government to get smaller have a long wait. "Taxpayers will not allow the government to do much more than it does now. But government's client groups will not allow it to do much less" (Rauch 1996, 1891). If reform comes, it will be incremental in nature. Only some crisis or shock, Rauch writes, will produce the more systemic changes needed.

Following the argument of Lowi and Schattschneider, some scholars have found that the nature of the interest-group network surrounding health care policy has changed. As it moves from distributive to redistributive, we should expect such change. Peterson (1993) argues that the "representation community" in health care has changed from iron triangles, typical of distributive policy (Lowi 1964; Ripley and Franklin 1982) to *issue networks* (Heclo 1978; Kingdon 1995).

Peterson (1993, 400) writes that "the iron triangle was an autonomous policy community, built on close relations between powerful private interests and an oligarchically organized Congress, which organized medicine and its allies could and did thoroughly dominate." (See also Starr 1982.)

Several factors led to this change in the structure of interest groups in health care. These included a decline in insurance coverage because of cost increases by employers and increasing risk rating by insurers (Patel and Rushefsky 1995). A second and related factor Peterson mentions is the increasing cost of the system at a time (early 1990s) when the economy was either gripped by recession or a slow recovery from that recession. Of these and two other factors (allocation of resources and administrative burden) that Peterson discusses, cost has the largest impact because it affects the other three.

Another element in the transformation from iron triangles to issue networks was changes in public views (to be discussed more thoroughly in chapter 7). Because of the factors mentioned earlier (decline in insurance coverage and costs), the public was ready for reform, though perhaps not the specific alterations President Clinton had in mind.

A further aspect of these changes was challenges to the domination of the traditional interest groups in health care. While there were challengers to traditional health care interest groups in the 1960s (with the establishment of Medicare and Medicaid) and in the late 1970s when reform attained the policy agenda, the breakup came in the 1990s. Peterson (1993) notes that the provider community began splitting over health care reform.

For example, the traditional dominance of the American Medical Association weakened as other physician groups (such as the American Academy of Family Physicians) became strong supporters of comprehensive change. Similarly, there was a split between for-profit and nonprofit hospitals over reform. The insurance industry also saw splits as small insurance companies opposed reforms, particularly those based on managed competition, and larger companies supported managed competition. As we see later, the largest of the health insurance companies became active advocates of managed care (though not necessarily of the Clinton plan).

Another set of challengers was the business community, which paid for much of health insurance. Large businesses sought reform, while smallers ones did not. Unions and consumer groups also sought to forward the reform agenda.

The evolution to issue networks was also advanced by changes within Congress. Reforms of the 1970s, with more autonomy for committees and especially subcommittees, made Congress more open and provided additional access points for interest groups. Thus the representational and structural changes occurring in Congress together helped transform the tight iron triangle into the looser issue network. Peterson (1993) concludes optimistically that these changes increase the likelihood of reform.

This line of analysis is supported by Baumgartner and Talbert (1995, 439). They write that the "health care interest-group structure is one of the most diverse, conflictual, and well endowed of any in Washington."

One last theoretical perspective on interest groups should be considered. This is the theory offered by Thomas Ferguson (1995, 1996). Ferguson argues that business interests or elites play the major role in elections and political party behavior. They invest in a party because what government does affects their businesses. In Wilson's terms, business groups face concentrated benefits and costs. Ferguson writes (1995, 22) that "blocs of major investors define the core of political parties and are responsible for most of the signals the party sends to the electorate." Realignment occurs when industrial structures change and the business community becomes polarized. Voters do not have the resources (information or time) to pay much attention to the political system and elections or try to influence it. The only caveat to this occurs when groups with a mass appeal, such as labor unions, are drawn into the fray. Ferguson's theory points us toward the constellation of interests in the three elections that constitute our time period, 1992, 1994, and 1996. It also directs us to examining campaign financing during the two reform periods. In the first (1993–94), characterized by attempts at comprehensive change, we should expect a whole constellation of interests engaged in the policy battle. In the second (1995–96), we should expect the constellation of interest groups, or stakeholders, to use Skocpol's (1996) term, those with occupational or financial interests in an issue, to be much smaller because the nature of the reform (Medicare, Medicaid, and private insurance) was considerably less.

Interest Groups and Comprehensive Health Care Reform Proposals, 1993–94

Design of Reform

As Skocpol (1996) makes abundantly clear (and as discussed in chapter 3), the design of the Clinton administration's Health Security Act was affected by external circumstances. One was the ever-present federal budget deficits. Any program that would increase the deficit would be virtually impossible to enact. A second external circumstance was the growing antigovernment feeling among the public (see chapter 7) and particularly within the Republican Party. Any significant extension of federal government power would likely be opposed. Likewise, any massive increases in taxes, necessary to fund a national health insurance program based on a single-payer plan, would be virtual political suicide.

So the administration chose a strategy that minimized these problems and sought a middle ground between a completely free-market system and total government takeover of health care. This strategy was managed competition with a backup limit or ceiling on insurance premium increases.

But the very design of the program (and to a large extent, the idea of national health insurance itself) contributed to its demise. In Skocpol's (1995) phrase, the plan boomeranged on the administration. Why was this the case?

To avoid a large tax, the plan had to require individuals and groups to undertake certain actions. All employers would have to offer and pay a portion of health insurance for their employees (the employer mandate). Everyone would have to belong to a large organization that would administer health insurance (health care alliances). People were encouraged to join organizations such as health maintenance organizations, which would increase the efficient use of health care resources (managed competition). Limits might be placed on increases in health insurance premiums (insurance caps). Each of these important features would activate particular interest groups. Because it was comprehensive health care insurance reform, no person or group would be unaffected by change.

The task force that created the plan met with interest groups that were willing to meet with them. The Clinton administration attempted to forestall some objections by including provisions that it hoped would entice certain groups to support it. For example, large businesses were concerned about two aspects of health insurance for their employees: the continued increases in health care costs that they faced, and financing early retirees. The Health Security Act promised to restrain costs and to cover the health insurance costs for those early retirees (until they were eligible for Medicare).

Small businesses were an important concern of the Clinton administration. For the first time, many of them would be required to cover their employees, even part-time employees, up to 80 percent of health insurance costs. To mollify them, the Health Security Act called for a sliding scale of subsidies for small businesses. The smaller the business, the larger the subsidy. None of these efforts paid off.

Supporters

The Clinton administration expected that certain groups would naturally support comprehensive health care reform. In general, those would be liberal groups such as unions and senior citizens groups such as the American Association of Retired Persons (AARP). The unions included the AFL-CIO, the American Federation of State, County, and Municipal Employees (AFSCME), and the United Auto Workers (UAW). The administration also hoped that larger businesses and trade associations would support reform. Again, the task force made concessions or created provisions designed to cement the support of these groups. AARP was concerned about Medicare. A prescription drug benefit, absent from Medicare, was put into the program. Medicare itself would remain, though it would sustain cuts (Medicaid would be abolished) and Medicare recipients would not be forced into managed care organizations. AFSCME wanted their members excluded from the mandatory alliances, similar to employees in large businesses (over 5,000 employees).

But there was never a time that the supposedly supportive groups fully endorsed the Clinton plan. Nor were they well organized. Instead, these groups were interested in their particular concern or problem with the proposed legislation. They would then get some concessions but withheld support, hoping to do better when Congress addressed the issues.

In effect, the Clinton administration was never able to obtain closure from any group that presumably supported health care reform. How does closure work? A good example of closure in action was the operations of the House Ways and Means Committee during the debate eventually resulting in the tax reform legislation in 1986. Dan Rostenkowski (D-Ill.), chairman of the committee, asked his members what they needed in the legislation to satisfy their interests. He then would make the change but insisted that if the change were made, the representative would have to support the entire bill (Birnbaum and Murray 1987). This was closure. In the case of the Health Security Act, groups would get the change they wanted but not commit to the entire bill.

Another problem with the lobbying effort on the part of the supporters was that it began late. Those opposed to reform, as we see below, started plotting strategy a year before reform was on the agenda. Further, they coordinated their efforts. There was little coordination among the supportive groups.

The media campaign in favor of health care reform was run largely by the Democratic National Committee (DNC), not an interest group in our terms. In any event, the proreform media campaign was poorly funded.

There was an attempt to bring some of the supportive groups together, particularly through the Health Care Reform Project, run with the help of AARP and the National Health Care Campaign, and eventually by the DNC. It was unable, however, to raise the money necessary to mount an effective media campaign. One reason was that a number of the unions were unhappy with the Clinton administration's push for ratification of the North American Free Trade Agreement (NAFTA), so they did not make the needed contributions.

Perhaps the most interesting supportive group, and perhaps typical of the problems supporters had, was AARP, a potent interest group. It has a large membership base. It is clearly a stakeholder group because many of the things government does affects its membership, particularly programs such as Medicaid, Medicare, and Social Security. Its leadership is politically active, and the elderly in general vote at a relatively high rate. It has a reputation as a powerful interest group. Yet its role in the 1993–94 health care debate was very circumscribed, to the detrimental of the proreform forces.

A major reason for this was the experience with the Medicare Cata-strophic Coverage Act. The legislation was enacted in 1988. The frame-work for the bill was set by the Reagan administration and was designed to cover "catastrophic" or unusually large health care expenses. AARP sup-ported the legislation and worked within the Reagan administration frame-work, as did other elderly groups and unions. The legislation removed some of the limits on the use of home health care, hospital and skilled nursing care services, and added a prescription drug benefit (Moon 1996). The legislation also contained a unique financing provision. Rather than raise revenue from either the Medicare Hospital Trust Fund tax or from general revenues, the legislation called for additional payments by beneficiaries, especially the more affluent ones.

Both the benefits and the financing portions were the law's downfall. Most Medicare beneficiaries purchase supplemental medical insurance (called "Medigap" policies) that covered much of what the new law pro-vided. Further, they were being asked, especially the wealthier beneficiar-ies, to pay for services they were already getting. The combination of benefits and financing created a redistributive situation, the wealthier Medi-care recipients helping to fund benefits for poorer recipients.

Some interest groups opposed the law. The drug companies were afraid of federal intervention in the industry. Some insurance companies opposed the bill. The Committee to Preserve Social Security and Medicare also opposed the law and, along with the pharmaceutical industry, lobbied for its repeal. The outcry among seniors and the groups opposed was so great that the law was repealed in 1989.

How does this story affect AARP? A critical supporter of the legislation, AARP was seen as being out of touch with the membership and was se-verely criticized, especially by the Committee to Preserve Social Security and Medicare (Skocpol 1996). Because of its experience with the Medicare Catastrophic Coverage Act, which should be seen as a catastrophe for the group, it was reluctant to be out in front of its membership on health reform.

In February 1994 the Clinton administration asked AARP to endorse the Health Security Act. Rather than do so directly, AARP called it "the strong-est and most realistic blueprint"; this was seen as a lukewarm endorsement (Skocpol 1996).

Some groups that did support the plan, such as the Kaiser Foundation and the League of Women Voters, engaged in educational campaigns, rather than more forceful direct lobbying (though that is the major purpose of those two groups). Other groups that placed ads in papers or on televi-sion would come out in favor of the principles contained in the Clinton plan but did not directly endorse that plan.

Finally, some groups whose endorsement might be critical to health reform's success, such as the American Medical Association and the U.S. Chamber of Commerce, were influenced by the opposition.

One group whose support would likely have been critical to the success of health reform, big business, came out in favor of the Cooper-Breaux "Clinton Lite" bill discussed in chapter 4.

To summarize, interest-group activity in support of health care reform suffered from several problems: an unwillingness to buy into the entire concept in exchange for key provisions, underfinancing, poor organization, a late start, lukewarm support from supportive groups (such as unions), and the undermining of some group support (such as big business) by opponents. Those opposed to reform faced none of these problems.

A final factor was the issue of salience or intensity. Those who were opposed to reform felt that issue more deeply than those in favor of it. No group seemed in favor of the entire package. Wilson's theory of regulation suggests that, given this perspective, those opposed would work harder than those in favor.

The Opposition

The Clinton administration, especially the president and the first lady, saw two groups as responsible for some of the problems of the health care system. One was the drug industry, which they felt kept the price of medications higher than they should be. That industry, and its trade association, the Pharmaceutical Manufacturing Association, would oppose the plan based on those attacks. The other "enemy" group was the insurance industry, especially with the high costs of insurance and its unwillingness to cover certain groups of people (e.g., high risk or with preexisting conditions). There were even reports of people whose family health insurance was canceled because a member of the family was found to have a genetic defect that might lead to a costly disease (Cowley 1996).

To many of the opposition groups, the Clinton plan was seen as threatening. Small business was unalterably opposed to the employee mandate. So its representatives bitterly fought not only the Clinton plan but any plan that contained such a mandate. The National Restaurant Association and particularly the National Federation of Independent Businesses (NFIB) were among the leaders of the opposition. The NFIB was so opposed to reform, and the increased government involvement that it meant, that it refused to meet with members of the Clinton health care task force.

The insurance industry was somewhat mixed in its response to health care reform. The five largest insurance companies, Aetna, Cigna, Metropolitan Life, Prudential, and Travelers, were in favor of managed competition. They believed that they would be able to form some of the provider plans that would work with the health care alliances. The smaller insurance companies did not think they would be able to compete in this new competitive environment and opposed reforms based on that concept. The "big five" then quit the trade association, the Health Insurance Association of America (HIAA), to form their own group, the Alliance for Managed Competition. The Alliance called for reform. HIAA did not.

HIAA's concern was threefold. First were the changes that would be forthcoming if managed competition took root. A second concern was that the Clinton plan called for a backup strategy in the event that managed competition did not control costs. The administration eventually agreed upon a plan to limit increases in health insurance premiums. This was seen as a form of government price control. It would directly affect the insurance industry; the plan itself again meant an increase in government involvement in the health care system. A third issue was that the Clinton plan, as well as most of the proposals made in 1993–94, required the insurance industry to move from experience rating or risk rating to community rating. That is, insurance companies would no longer be able to charge individuals or groups more if there were preexisting conditions or the group was likely to have unusually high costs.

HIAA was originally supportive of the portions of health care reforms that would benefit its members financially. The trade association favored coverage of the entire population (universal coverage) and an employer mandate. In 1992 it hired William Gradison, a former Republican congressman, to head the organization. Gradison met with Ira Magaziner, the co-head of the Clinton task force, to negotiate HIAA's concerns. None of the three issues of concern to HIAA were settled to the group's satisfaction and eventually negotiations broke off during the summer of 1993. Even during the period of negotiations, HIAA ran the infamous "Harry and Louise" ads (see later and chapter 6). At times HIAA would suspend the ads during negotiations, but they eventually resumed. HIAA and NFIB were among the fiercest opponents of health care reform during 1993–94.

Other groups also opposed reform, overwhelming the supporters in terms of numbers, financial resources, organization, and tactics. One thing opponents did effectively was to form coalitions among themselves. Perhaps the most effective of these coalitions was the unofficial one branded the *No Name Coalition*. It consisted of a wide variety of groups including NFIB, HIAA, and the National Restaurant Association, as well as property rights groups, the National Taxpayers Union, and the Christian Coalition (Johnson and Broder 1996). The No Name Coalition would meet and plot strategy.

One other important part of the opposition groups was that many of them, especially NFIB, worked closely with the Republican Party. Some of these groups saw the debate over health care as an opportunity to work toward a Republican congressional victory in the 1994 elections and to stem what they saw as the tide of big government embodied in the Health Security Act (Johnson and Broder 1996; Skocpol 1996).

Strategy and Tactics

In controversial public policy issues such as health care reform, traditional lobbying techniques by interest groups include testifying in hearings, contacting members of Congress and their staff, and mobilizing their membership to contact their representatives. The strategy and tactics of opponents of reform included these but also included newer and more sophisticated techniques.

Media Campaign

Perhaps the most celebrated set of tactics was television advertising. This was embodied by the HIAA's "Harry and Louise" and "Louise and Libby" ads shown in selected markets. NFIB, while opposed to health reform, refused to join in sponsoring the ads because HIAA favored an employee mandate.

"Harry and Louise" featured a couple discussing the Clinton plan in their kitchen. The burden of the ads was that reform was indeed necessary in the health care system but that there were specific problems that needed to be changed. Depending on the ad, the problem was the alliances (government-run health care) or the insurance premium caps (what would happen if the ceilings were reached). They concluded that they should contact their congressional representatives and ask for changes in the proposals. "Louise and Libby" showed small business partners who had similar concerns.

As we discuss in more detail in the next two chapters, the ads themselves had little impact on public opinion; however, they had a major impact on the Clinton administration. Administration spokespersons denounced the ads as manipulative and inaccurate, and those denunciations were covered especially on television evening news programs. That gave much more publicity to the ads than the ads themselves were able to garner.

Supporters of reform responded by producing ads that parodied "Harry and Louise," which also gave more publicity to the HIAA campaign. The Democratic National Campaign, working hand in hand with the Clinton administration, ran an ad showing the couple getting injured, losing their insurance and their jobs. Supporters of a single-payer plan ran a similar parody.

But supporters did not have the funds to respond adequately. One estimate was that about $50 million was spent on print and electronic ads, about $14–15 million by HIAA alone (Skocpol 1996). This was one indication that health reform was not being treated as just another public policy debate but had the elements of political campaign.

Mobilizing Support

Both HIAA and NFIB worked to mobilize their membership to contact their representatives and lobby against health reform. Their membership responded by sending letters, faxes, and e-mail and inundated Congress.

HIAA set up a group, the Coalition of Health Insurance Choices, to work against the health care alliances. This effort was designed to mobilize business people who had good contacts with their Washington representatives. These included lawyers, accountants, and insurance agents (Skocpol 1996). HIAA particularly targeted states in the Midwest and southern portions of the country. Its total grassroots effort resulted in some 450,000 contacts with Congress (Johnson and Broder 1996).

Provider groups likewise mobilized their membership. The American Medical Association (AMA) had used the grassroots and lobbying technique in previous battles over national health insurance (Starr 1982). The AMA was concerned about any program that would restrict doctors' incomes. Hospital groups, such as the American Hospital Association (AHA) and the Federation of American Health Systems, which represented community and for-profit hospitals respectively, also activated their membership. The federation founded a group called the Health Leadership Council (HLC) made up of "chief executives of 50 of the largest health care companies—drug manufacturers, hospital chains, medical suppliers, managed care and insurance companies" (Skocpol 1996, 140). The chief executive officers would then work to influence local public opinion through newspaper columns and the like. The goal of HLC was to minimize government involvement (Skocpol 1996).

Related to grassroots mobilization was an attempt to create and influence public opinion, a practice sometimes known as *astroturf lobbying* (Fritsch 1995; Johnson and Broder 1996; Victor 1995). Astroturf lobbying is an attempt to manufacture public opinion by giving just one side of the issue and then having the respondent call or fax a comment to his or her Washington representative. The large insurance companies, through the Alliance for Managed Competition, employed this tactic (Johnson and Broder 1996).

NFIB, even more vociferously against health reform than the AMA, employed a variety of tactics in its attempt to defeat the Clinton plan. It held public forums in various states, it generated over 2 million mailings to its memberships, and it held seminars in states targeting key representatives. It also provided interviewees for talk-radio programs (Johnson and Broder 1996).

NFIB, the No Name Coalition, and Citizens for a Sound Economy demonstrated their ability to mobilize opponents. During the summer of 1994, the Clinton administration planned a bus caravan to various cities to rally support for health care reform. Instead, the opponents met the caravan at each of its stops. Using newspaper ads and talk-radio programs, they recruited people against what they called "government-run health care." Citizens for a Sound Economy coordinated with "Newt Gingrich's Capitol Hill office and with Republican senators" (Johnson and Broder 1996). House Republicans, through their "Theme Team," attacked the Clinton caravan in the media, employing language virtually identical to that used by Citizens for a Sound Economy. The protests and media campaign were better organized, planned, and executed than anything the Clinton administration could muster (Johnson and Broder 1996).

As important as all these activities were, NFIB, and to a lesser extent HIAA, attempted to influence other interest groups that might be inclined to support health care reform. This is a process known as *cross-lobbying* (Lance W. Bennett 1996; Johnson and Broder 1996; Skocpol 1996). NFIB lobbied the AMA to drop its support of employer mandates. HIAA and NFIB lobbied the Business Roundtable to reverse its support of the Health Security Act. Drug companies urged AARP not to endorse the Clinton plan (Bennett 1996).

In July 1994 a coalition of groups (AMA, AARP, and AFL-CIO) were getting ready to run a series of ads in favor of comprehensive reform when NFIB and its allies went into action. As Skocpol (1996) tells the story, officials of state NFIB organizations contacted state medical association officials warning them " 'that if employers were compelled to pay for health insurance, they would pressure the government to limit medical fees'" (Skocpol 1996, 162).

In a similar vein, NFIB worked to undercut the Chamber of Commerce's support for health care reform. The Chamber was losing membership and was threatened with greater losses if they supported reform (Skocpol 1996)

The Chamber was also subject to *reverse lobbying*. We usually understanding lobbying as interest groups pressuring a government body such as a legislature to make or not make a decision. In the case of reverse lobbying, elected officials press an interest group to make or not make a stand. It was mentioned earlier that some interest groups opposed to reform worked closely with House Republicans. In the case of the Chamber, House Republicans told them that they must automatically oppose anything that the Clinton administration favored. In the earlier episode, when the AMA was about to join with other groups to sponsor proreform ads, House minority whip Newt Gingrich (R-Ga.) and other conservative House Republicans fired a letter to the AMA complaining about its decision and how it was not following the wishes of the AMA's membership. The combination of cross- and reverse lobbying was devastating. The Clinton administration was hop- ing that business, especially big business, would support the Health Secu- rity Act. But in February 1994 the major big business organizations, such as the Business Roundtable and the National Association of Manufacturers, came out in favor of the Cooper-Breaux bill.

Campaign Financing

Opponents of health care reform employed yet another important interest- group technique, campaign financing. Public elections have become in- creasingly expensive, and senators and representatives are engaged in what Hedrick Smith calls the "constant campaign" (Smith 1988; Bennett 1996). Money, it has been said, is the "mother's milk" of politics. Political adver- tising, especially on television, is very costly. Members of Congress and presidential hopefuls have to raise enormous sums of money. The need for campaign funds creates a wonderful opportunity for interest groups to try to influence the political system.

A report by the Center for Public Integrity (1994) estimated that some $25 million was contributed by interest groups (broadly defined, including companies) in 1993–94, most of it through *political action committee* (PAC) contributions to congressional races. A small portion of that $25 million was given as soft-money contributions to political parties. Johnson and Broder (1996) suggest that this estimate understates the amount of money spent on the health care reform campaign. We have already used the figure of $50 million for advertising. An untold sum was spent on grass- roots activities.

A breakdown of campaign contributions during 1991–94 shows the util- ity of Ferguson's investment theory of party competition. The Center for Public Integrity Report lists eleven categories of industry groups that had some health-related interests (which, given the scope of the Clinton Health Security Act and other proposals, included virtually everyone). It can be assumed that two of the eleven groups, unions and public interest groups, supported health care reform. Unions were especially generous in campaign contributions, almost $30 million over this period, with public interest groups contributing almost $4 million.

The other nine categories of groups (health care providers, administrators and trade associations, insurance, alcohol, tobacco, pharmaceutical, non-health care–related businesses, nonhealth care–related trade associations, hospital associations, and other health care–related businesses) were largely against reform (or at least did little to support it). These groups contributed over $64 million, about 66 percent of the total funds contributed by these groups.

The major question is what does all this money (which probably under-states the amount spent) get the various interests? A report by the Center for Responsive Politics (1997, 1) discussed this issue:

> Campaign contributions can't explain everything that politicians do. Even when money seems to play a role in a policy debate, it is seldom the only factor affecting lawmakers' decisions. Geography, ideology, temperament, party, age, education, personal friendships or rivalries—all can and do affect how a politician will vote. Even following the money trail can be compli-cated, since policy debates often pit one monied interest against another.
>
> That said, in case after case, if lawmakers' votes are examined beside a list of their campaign contributions, a stronger-than-coincidence relationship quickly emerges.

What the study found was that there was a strong correlation between the votes a senator or representative made and the amount of campaign contribu-tions from an interest group. The standard reason offered for making a cam-paign contribution, whether a direct contribution to a candidate or a soft-money contribution, is that it buys access for an interest group. That is, if an issue arises that an interest group or organization wishes to talk to a senator or representative about, that legislator is more likely to listen to a contributor (or potential contributor) than to a noncontributor. This desire for access is a major reason why some interest groups will make contributions to both parties, even if one party or candidate is not especially sympathetic to the interest's concerns. Money buys a foot in the door. A related reason for making contributions is to help elect legislators who will be sympathetic to the interest's concerns.

Not all see contributions in such a mild, public-spirited view. Philip Stern (1992), for one, saw special-interest money as magnifying the influ-ence of the groups, undermining democracy, and little more than legalized bribery (see also Fritsch 1996). While the bribery may be legal, the amounts contributed, especially by business interests, certainly lend support to the investment theory of elections (see also Bennett 1996).

There are several other ways beyond PAC contributions that money enters the scene. So-called soft money, contributions to party activities that are subject to little or no regulation, may be as large as PAC contributions. Interest groups also pay for trips, speeches, and seminars by legislators (see Center for Public Integrity 1994; Bennett 1996). Many of the interest groups that worked to stop health care reform, especially those working closely with the Republicans, also worked for the Republican congressional electoral victory in 1994 (Balz and Brownstein 1996). Those supporting reform were clearly outgunned during the 1994 elections, both in terms of financing, campaigning, and getting out the vote.

Interest Groups and Health Care in the 104th Congress

As we have seen in previous chapters, discussions over health care issues during 1995–96 went in two different directions. Much of the time was spent on Medicare and Medicaid, focusing on attempts to reduce spending on the two programs. As we have seen, this was unsuccessful. The other effort centered on health insurance reform, an expansion of government regulatory authority. This was modestly successful, affected very much by the approaching 1996 elections.

We would expect that the role of interest groups would be much different in this period than in the previous one. For one thing, during the Medicare-Medicaid controversy the positions of interest groups would change. Many of the groups potentially affected by comprehensive health care reform would be only marginally impacted by changes in the two large public-sector programs. Thus we do not see groups such as the National Federation of Independent Businesses heavily involved in the effort. Those groups that favored reform, largely liberal groups such as unions and advocacy groups (e.g., AARP), now opposed what they saw as cutbacks to Medicare and Medicaid. Our theoretical discussion above, particularly concerning demosclerosis, suggests that those groups would be in a defensive posture and better able to achieve their goals. This was partially the case.

Interest Groups and the Medicare/Medicaid Debate

We begin this section by looking at how Republicans, especially in the House, dealt with interest groups. As House Republicans worked closely with interest groups to achieve their electoral goals in 1994 (see above), so they also moved to influence interest groups once they attained power.

Republicans had a major gripe with business groups, which they resolved to fix. Business groups were expected to be sympathetic to Republicans because of a shared belief in a limited role for government (unless it benefited them). And while business groups contributed more to the Republican Party than to the Democrats, they also made substantial contributions to the latter. This was understandable for several reasons.

The Democrats controlled Congress for much of the time since the early 1950s; in the House, there was a forty-year record of continual control. Because Democrats were in control and could affect business profit margins and freedom to operate, the business sector wanted to be able to lobby them. Campaign contributions grease the wheels and get lobbyists a sympathetic ear from legislators. Additionally, the Democrats, especially in the House, told interest groups that they needed to make those contributions if they wanted to get access (Balz and Brownstein 1996). Republicans fumed that interest groups that should naturally be on their side were helping their opponents. They vowed to remedy this.

In 1994, Gingrich and others convinced PACs and individuals to put more money into Republican challengers. Those people and groups gave about four times as much to Republican challengers or candidates for open seats than to Democrats (Balz and Brownstein 1994). Once in office, Republicans sought to cement their majority by convincing interest groups and PACs to contribute to Republicans but not to Democrats (Stone 1995). House Republicans made not especially subtle statements to this effect.

> Bill Paxton, chairman of the National Republican Congressional Committee, issued a report on the four hundred largest PACs, showing how much each had given to Democrats and to Republicans in 1993–94 and identifying them under one of three headings: "friendly," "unfriendly," and "neutral." (Balz and Brownstein 1996, 334)

Other House Republicans would refuse to meet with lobbyists identified with Democrats and warned that campaign contributions and properly credentialed lobbyists (i.e., Republicans) were necessary to get a sympathetic ear (Balz and Brownstein 1996). Background checks were conducted on lobbyists (Berke 1995). This effort was similar to the reverse lobbying that House Republicans employed in 1994. It also belies the image of interest groups trying to force money onto politicians. Instead, politicians were hitting up interest groups (see Common Cause 1995).

Health care industry groups increased their donations to Republicans in the early part of 1995. As a 1995 Common Cause report pointed out, insurance companies and physician political action committees more than doubled soft-money contributions with over three-quarters going to the three Republican Party committees (national, Senate, and House).

Those who did make the required changes were given more than a sympathetic ear. In some cases they were allowed not just to testify at hearings or sit in during markup sessions but to write the legislation. In one instance, Senate Judiciary Committee staffers had a bill on regulatory reform explained to them by industry representatives (Engelberg 1995). Weisskopf and Maraniss (1995, 13) described the interaction as follows:

> Republicans have championed their legislative agenda as an answer to popular dissatisfaction with Congress and the federal government. But the agenda also represents a triumph of business interests, who after years of playing a primarily defensive role in Democratic-controlled Congresses now find themselves a full partner of the Republican leadership in shaping congressional priorities.

At times, the two reporters continued, the line between the lobbyist and legislator roles was clouded (Weisskopf and Maraniss 1995).

The Republican takeover led interest groups to form coalitions to affect legislation and elections campaigns. The two groups on the Republican/conservative side were *the Coalition* and the *Wednesday Group* (Edsall 1996). The Coalition, essentially a successor to the No-Name Coalition opposing health care reform in 1994, consisted of a number of trade associations including the NFIB, the National Restaurant Association, NAM, the U.S. Chamber of Commerce, and the National Association of Wholesaler-Distributors. The Wednesday Group consisted of staffers from groups such as "conservative think tanks, anti-gun control and anti-tax groups, organizations supporting home schooling, term limits proponents" (Edsall 1996, 12–13). Citizens for a Sound Economy, which worked with Republicans in 1993–94 against health care reform, supported the Republican Medicare/Medicaid positions with advertising and mailing campaigns (Serafini 1995e).

On the liberal/Democratic side were the AFL-CIO and other labor organizations, consumer groups, abortion rights groups, and environment groups. There was also a counterpart to the Wednesday Group, the Progressive Alliance, which includes environmental, peace, feminist, and gay groups (Edsall 1996). Both sets of groups ran campaign ads, phone banks, grassroots campaigns, direct-mail campaigns, community meetings, rallies and, occasionally, picketing (Serafini 1995e).

If one sector of the population was concerned about Medicare (and to a certain extent Medicaid), it was the elderly. The elderly as a group benefit from these and other federal programs (such as Social Security) and are protective of their interests. The elderly vote at a higher rate than the overall population and have shown that they will punish those who threaten their programs. When the Reagan administration came into office in 1981 it sought cuts in Social Security to counterbalance proposed tax cuts. Elderly groups mobilized against the cuts and punished Republicans during the

1982 congressional elections. Thus it is not surprising to find that the elderly support Medicare more than any other age group (Rosenbaum 1995). This means that both Republicans and Democrats will attempt to appeal to the elderly and their interest groups.

The Democrats pointed out the large size of the proposed cuts in Medicare (and Medicaid) and constantly mentioned this in campaign events. Republicans sought to neutralize the issue by first noting, as discussed in chapter 4, that they were not reducing Medicare spending but slowing its growth and, second, by appealing to the elderly on other social issues (Rosenbaum 1995).

There were other ways that Republicans sought to defuse the impact on the elderly and their interest groups (especially AARP). One way was to support other elderly interest groups and argue that those groups were more representative of the views of the elderly than AARP (Serafini 1995b).

Apart from AARP, two other interest groups represented the elderly. A group even more liberal than AARP was the National Council of Senior Citizens, which coordinated with the Democrats and unions. The National Committee to Preserve Social Security and Medicare was a third group that opposed Medicare and Social Security cutbacks (Serafini 1995b).

Conservatives started three groups that they hoped would displace or counterbalance the more established elderly interest groups. These were the Seniors Coalition, the 60/Plus Association, and the United Seniors Association. These three groups, though not having nearly the membership of the previous three, were heavily supported by Republicans (Serafini 1995b). By August 1995, the Seniors Coalition had spent about $350,000 to send some 6 million mailings to support Republicans (Serafini 1995c). Some have argued that their visibility in Congress in 1995 and 1996 was limited and that the organizations were largely fund-raising operations ("Seniors' Lobbying Groups Surfacing" July 1995; Serafini 1995e).

A second way that Republicans sought to limit opposition to Medicare cuts was to threaten AARP. A tax-exempt organization, AARP engages in political advocacy and gains much of its revenue from selling services (such as Medigap policies) and products. In 1995 Republicans threatened to investigate whether AARP should maintain this tax-exempt status (Serafini 1995b). Gingrich was also willing to make some concessions to the seniors' organization. In one case, Gingrich had a provision softened in the Medicare changes that would have forced Medicare beneficiaries into health maintenance organizations (Rosenstiel 1995). The result of the combination of threats and concessions was that AARP did not work hard against the Republican budget proposals; they were essentially neutralized. This was in line with other attempts to "defund" liberal or left-wing organizations

(Serafini 1995b). A similar attempt was made to restrict lobbying by groups that received federal funding (Cohen 1995).

Republicans were also very aggressive in dealing with groups that opposed them. In May 1995, Speaker Gingrich held a series of meetings with representatives of the American Hospital Association focusing on Medicare reforms. But when the AHA began its series of attack ads, Republicans reacted very harshly to the attacks. John Boehner (R-Ohio) wrote a letter to the AHA which stated in part that:

> As long as the American Hospital Association chooses to continue this dialogue by mimicking the Democrat line and running a paid fear campaign in the media, I feel it is my responsibility as chairman of the House Republican Conference to keep Conference members assessed of your public actions in opposition to our agenda. (Serafini 1995b)

Similar threats led AARP to limit its attacks on the GOP plans. The Republican House strategy was to work with those who supported them, neutralize potential opponents, and refuse to have negotiations with groups that attacked them (Serafini 1995b).

As we saw in chapter 3, Medicare and Medicaid reductions were embedded in the larger issue of eliminating the federal budget deficit. Medicare and Medicaid were prime targets for reductions. By October 1995, interest activity reached a peak.

Groups were involved in policy debates for the "elderly, for disabled people, for doctors, hospitals, drug companies and all sorts of health care providers" (Pear 1995m). Drug companies, represented by the Pharmaceutical Research and Manufacturers of America, had many concerns. They were worried about having to give Medicare and Medicaid discounts on their products, an issue that also arose in regard to the Health Security Act in 1993. There were numerous tax issues and proposals that would make generic drugs more competitive with brand-name products (Pear 1995m).

Some parts of the proposed reductions pitted interest groups against each other. Providers (doctors and hospitals) lobbied for exemptions from antitrust laws and state insurance regulations so that they could form groups that would compete with health maintenance organizations and insurance companies. The latter groups naturally opposed the changes and were supported by state insurance commissioners (Pear 1995m).

AARP opposed increases on premiums for Medicare beneficiaries. Groups such as the United Cerebral Palsy Association opposed transforming Medicaid into a block-grant program. They wanted a "national standard of eligibility" so that states would not eliminate coverage for certain groups, such as those suffering from AIDS (Pear 1995m). The American Federation of State, County, and Municipal Employees was lobbying both Congress, to defeat proposed changes in Medicare, and the White House to vigorously defend the programs (Pear 1995m). The AFL-CIO spent $1 million in ads in early 1995 to protest proposed cuts in Medicare (Serafini 1995e). In 1996, the giant labor association committed $35 million to the 1996 elections for restoring Democratic control of Congress. Their ads castigated Republicans for voting to cut Medicare (as well as Medicaid, education, and environmental programs).

Other industries within the health care sector were also fighting to defend their interests. Groups such as the National Association of Medical Equipment Services were concerned that the Senate version of the Medicare changes would not increase payments for medical equipment and would cut payments for some services (Pear 1995m). The Corporate Health Care Coalition, representing twenty-five large businesses, opposed a provision in the Republican bill that would raise the Medicare eligibility age from sixty-five to sixty-seven. This would extend the time that businesses would have to cover the health care costs of their retirees (Pear 1995i).

The American Medical Association was originally neutral about Medicare changes and indeed favored portions that reformed antitrust and malpractice law. But when the Republican bills changed the Medicare physician fee schedule, which called for cutbacks in physician reimbursements, they began lobbying against at least that portion of the bill (Pear 1995i). When the AMA lobbying convinced Republicans not to cut their fees and to allow doctors to organize their own plans, they dropped their opposition to Medicare reductions and endorsed the House Republican plan (Pear 1995k; 1995m). AMA's changed position was denounced by President Clinton for putting their interests before those of their patients (Hasson 1995). The *New York Times* described the changed stance as a bribe, which both the AMA and the Republicans denied ("Bribe for Doctors" 1995; Pear 1995l).

But other providers worked hard against the changes. These included the American College of Physicians (internists), the American Academy of Pediatrics, the National Association of Children's Hospitals, and the American Nurses Association. These groups mobilized their constituents, and the Children's Hospital Association began running newspaper ads attacking the Medicaid changes. Some of these and other groups were working with the Clinton administration, using Vice-President Al Gore's Senate office as a headquarters (Pear 1995m).

By December 1995, Republicans made modifications that would help gain the support of elements of the health care industry. In particular, insurers and providers, especially HMOs, won changes that would increase reimbursements for managed care plans. The industry lobby, led by the Group Health Association of America (GHAA), won other important reforms (Gottlieb 1995). For example, the bill approved by the conference committee in December allowed "private plans to receive Medicare money for medical education and care of the uninsured, even when they do not send members to teaching hospitals or to institutions that serve uninsured patients" (Gottlieb 1995). As a result of these and other changes, the savings from reductions in Medicare spending was only $26.9 billion over the seven-year period (Gottlieb 1995).

The Republicans were good about including provisions that would help gather support for their proposals. We saw this in regard to the American Medical Association. These provisions were in the details of the legislation and included easing regulation of doctor-owned laboratories, some tax reimbursements for private hospitals, and benefits for makers of medical supply equipment and pharmaceutical companies. For example, one provision in the House version of the bill prohibited punitive damages for injury from a medical device or drug if that product were approved by the Food and Drug Administration. Other provisions provided for Medicare reimbursement for hospital clinical trials of "investigational devices" (Gottlieb and Pear 1995).

Republicans were also clever in not revealing details of the Medicare and Medicaid changes until October 1995. That way, though there might be opposition to the announced cutbacks based on the amount of proposed reductions, the details could not be attacked.

One group that might oppose the Medicare and Medicaid cutbacks was big business. One analysis suggested that if the proposed reductions had passed, large corporations would face cost shifting and would have to pay another $91 billion in health care costs for their employees over the proposed seven-year period. Yet corporate America, especially the National Association of Manufacturers, supported the changes. The Corporate Health Care Coalition also supported the changes, despite the change in retirement eligibility (Segal 1995).

They did so for several reasons. First is ideology: they prefer a smaller, less intrusive government to a larger, more active one. Second, they saw many of the changes opening up Medicare to private markets and moving away from fee for service. Third, they could pass some of their additional costs on to their employees. Finally, with changes in the health care sector toward managed care, large businesses felt they would be in a position to negotiate hospital fees, rather than just accept them (Segal 1995).

Another part of the health care sector would have been adversely affected by the proposed changes: teaching hospitals. Medicare pays hospitals

$150,000 a year for each doctor trained and pays premiums to hospitals that serve a large number of poor and uninsured patients, often the same hospitals. The proposed cuts amounted to $8.6 billion for teaching hospitals and $7.1 billion for treating the poor (Fein 1995).

The hospital industry as a whole was concerned about cuts in Medicare and Medicaid. In July 1995 they called for a commission to devise a plan to revamp Medicare. Earlier they had opposed the cuts, eventually adopted in the budget resolution in June 1995, and put ads in newspapers attacking the proposals (Serafini 1995e; Toner 1995).

One last aspect related to interest groups needs to be told. In chapters 3 and 4, we discussed a policy proposal known as medical savings accounts (MSAs). We saw that MSAs were mentioned in some proposals in 1994, that they were included in some of the Republican plans for Medicare in 1995, and that they showed up again in 1996 in regards to insurance reform (the Kennedy-Kassebaum bill). The major interest lobbying for MSAs was Golden Rule Insurance Company. Golden Rule gave almost $1 million in campaign contributions to Republicans in 1993–94 and worked closely with Gingrich and other key Republicans. Golden Rule also contributed to political action campaigns, such as Gingrich's GOPAC, and funded groups such as the National Center for Policy Analysis and the Council For Affordable Health Insurance (Common Cause 1995; Dreyfus and Stone 1996). The company's efforts paid off when the Kennedy-Kassebaum bill included money for a trial run of medical savings accounts.

Conclusion

From the early days of the American Republic, the issue of interest groups in the political system has been a concern. Madison, as we have seen, sought ways to curb the "mischiefs" of faction. Some political scientists going back to early years of the twentieth century have seen in the clash of interest groups the very stuff of politics. Others have seen certain groups, primarily business, as having a dominating presence over public policy. Based on the theoretical discussion of interest groups in the first section of this chapter and the examination of interest groups in the two health care periods, what can we conclude about interest groups and the outcome of policy making in the health care area and, more generally, about interest groups in the political system?

Interest Groups and Health Policy Outcomes

Both periods under study were marked by intense interest-group activity. As Wilson's (1980) discussion of the importance of concentrated costs and benefits suggests, those most affected by changes in health policy were the most active participants. As Rauch's (1994, 1996) and Olson's analyses suggest, successful interest groups were those in a defensive mode. That is, they were against change that would adversely affect them, though there were a few exceptions to this. While there were interest groups in favor of change, on the whole they were not as animated or activated about the changes as those opposed to them. This is most clearly seen in the 1993–94 health care reform period.

The effort by the Clinton administration to pass a national health insurance program affected virtually every major sector of the economy. Key interest groups, especially business interests, did not sign on to the entire package, despite attempts made to address some of their concerns. Those in favor of reform were slow to act, never achieved coordination or the level of resources dedicated to defeat of health reform. Groups opposed to reform, such as the National Federation of Independent Businesses, worked long and hard to defeat even modest changes. Further, their efforts were coordinated with Republicans, especially in the House. Health care reform was seen through the larger lens of control of Congress. Passion, commitment, and resources were on the side of opposition. Further, those opposed to reform "used the strategy of portraying concentrated costs to rally support from a variety of interests who might otherwise have benefited from the plan" (Stone 1997, 226).

In 1995–96, the positions were somewhat reversed. It was the Republicans who wanted change in Medicare and Medicaid. Groups that supported health care reform in the previous period—consumer, union, and elderly groups—now opposed changes they thought would hurt them. Even then, the coordination and resources that marked the opposition in 1993–94 was missing. Those opposed to spending reductions were sporadic in their efforts, with the exception of some of the unions, particularly the AFL-CIO, with its commitment to target House Republicans in the 1996 elections.

One explanation for the difference in interest-group behavior was the strategies adopted or not adopted by the Democrats and Republicans. The Clinton administration sought to buy off interest-group opposition by making what it thought was significant concessions. But, as discussed above, the administration could never get those groups to commit to the entire plan. Nor did the administration or congressional Democrats work particularly closely with interest groups.

The Republicans, by contrast, were more masterful in their dealings with interest groups, both those working with them and those against them. In 1993–94, there was clear coordination between House Republicans and allied interest groups. In addition, Republicans engaged in reverse lobbying, trying to convince some interest groups not to support the Clinton plan. In 1995–96, Republicans used both rewards and threats. They worked with industry groups that did not attack them (e.g., the AMA) and refused to work with groups that did attack them (e.g., the American Hospital Association). Groups that by nature would oppose changes in Medicare and Medicaid, such as the AARP, were threatened with loss of tax-exempt status. House Republicans also engaged in reverse lobbying in this period with regard to campaign contributions and the partisan makeup of interest-group lobbyists. Ultimately, the Republican effort failed (at least in this period) because the Medicare/Medicaid reductions were vetoed and became embroiled in the budget battle with the Clinton administration, a battle that hurt the Republicans politically.

The ultimate question is what effect interest groups had on the two efforts, which ultimately resulted in failure to enact legislation? In 1993–94, the impact was likely greater on Democrats than on Republicans. Many Republicans opposed reform in principle and did not need to be lobbied. But the inability of congressional Democratic leadership to carve out a majority in either house in favor of reform must be attributed at least partially to the intense campaign waged against reform. As we see in chapters 6 and 7, though the impact of the "Harry and Louise" campaign on public opinion was limited, the combination of that campaign and other efforts, such as those on talk radio, contributed to a decline in public support for reform.

In 1995–96, not nearly as heated over health care as the previous period, it is more difficult to attribute some portion of success or failure to interest groups. First, the changes did pass Congress but were vetoed by President Clinton, a veto that could not be overridden. Second, the ideological composition of the parties led members of Congress to the positions they took, regardless of interest-group efforts. The battle for public opinion, influenced by interest groups, ultimately led Congress to pass health insurance reform. But in that case the inclusion of the medical savings account provision was helped by the efforts of one company, Golden Rule Insurance.

Much the same can be said about campaign financing. Its impact is difficult to pinpoint, though we can say that recipients of campaign financing tend to vote the way major contributors would like and that candidates with more money have an electoral advantage over those with less money.

But we can conclude one thing about interest groups and health care reform: although there was much heat, as the saying goes, there was little light. Interest groups engaged in considerable manipulation of ideas and did not help forward a deliberative debate over the need for changing health care policies.

Interest Groups in the Political System

We return to the ideas in the beginning section. Interest groups play an important role in the policy-making process. They seek to influence government, efforts that have constitutional protection. But their role is controversial. The theories of Wilson (1980), Rauch (1995, 1996), and Olson (1982) strongly suggest that interest groups will mobilize to protect their programs or benefits, to prevent change that will affect them adversely. The political burden is on those advocating change. Change can occur, and Ferguson's (1995) investment theory suggests one way in which economic interests will promote change. But the overall effect is what Rauch called demosclerosis. This conservative nature of the interest-group system exacerbates the bias against change that is inherent in the structural features of the American political system.

But, as we have also seen, change is not impossible. The insurance reforms passed in the twilight of the 104th Congress, the only tangible result of four years of debate, shows that small changes, even innovative ones such as medical savings accounts, can be made. Democrats were against MSAs and Republicans were less than enthusiastic about new federal insurance regulations, yet both were enacted.

The health care case studies also demonstrate some new, as well as old, interest-group strategies. The older strategies of campaign contributions, testifying, mobilizing support, and so forth were certainly present. But the use of the media, whether through campaignlike advertisements or talk shows, is relatively recent. The tactics of cross- and reverse lobbying are also new. The closeness with which some interest groups worked with elected and party officials is, likewise, an important development. The stakes were high in the health care policy debates and the interest-group activity was equally animated. Whether that activity ultimately served the larger public interests is questionable. The "mischief of faction" reared its head, ugly or otherwise, in this important policy arena.

6 THE ROLE OF THE MASS MEDIA IN THE POLICY PROCESS

The mass media have become a central part of life in general and politics in particular in the United States. In fact, the relationship between communications and politics is so crucial that we must consider communications a key feature in our study of politics. For most individuals in our society, political realities are mediated through mass communications (Nimo and Combs 1993). Our discussion of mass media mainly focuses on newspapers and television and, to a lesser extent, radio.

Today, there are about 1,700 daily newspapers in the United States with a total circulation of about 60 million. Some of the major national newspapers include the *New York Times,* the *Washington Post,* and the *Wall Street Journal.* Most other newspapers are either regional or local in nature and circulation. There are also over 7,000 weekly papers with a combined circulation of about 39 million. Additionally, there are many weekly magazines, some dealing primarily with news while others cater to the highly specialized and segmented markets. Some of the major national news weeklies include *Time, Newsweek,* and *U.S. News & World Report.* There are over 10,000 radio stations. There are about 5,000 commercial AM radio stations, 4,000 commercial and 1,300 education FM stations. There are approximately twenty-three national radio networks. In 1990, there were 1,449 television stations, mostly commercial, while others are educational. About 85 percent of commercial television stations are affiliated with a major national network. The major national networks include the American Broadcasting Company (ABC), Columbia Broadcasting System (CBS), National Broadcasting Company (NBC), Cable News Network (CNN), the Fox Broadcasting Network (FBN), and the Financial News Network (FNN) (Jamieson and Campbell 1992; Bennett 1988).

As can be seen from the above, Americans today live in an information age dominated by enormous communication empires. This, in turn, has raised some concerns about the influence and impact of the mass media on

American politics and the policy process. In fact, in the past ten years or so the mass media have come under increasing attack and criticism for the way in which they cover politics and news. This chapter examines the role of the mass media in the policy process. First, we briefly discuss the development of the mass media in the United States. Second, we examine the theoretical literature that attempts to explain the role of the media in public agenda setting. Third, we utilize the theoretical ideas and concepts of media and public agenda setting to analyze the role of the mass media during the 1993–94 and 1995–96 health care reform periods. We conclude with a discussion of the roles played by the mass media in the policy process.

The Development of the Mass Media in the United States

This section discusses the changes undergone by print and broadcast media (especially newspapers, radio, and television) from their origins to the present day.

The press has played many different roles throughout U.S. history. The present tendency of reporters to "go after politicians" and rake them over the coals, often referred to as "attack journalism," has deep roots in American history (Kerbel 1995). In the beginning of the American Republic the print media were rarely objective. The simple reason for this was that most newspapers were funded by political parties and were sympathetic to a particular partisan or ideological view. Newspapers constantly attacked politicians of the opposition party. Readers knew that when they bought a particular newspaper, they were buying a particular political viewpoint. This alliance between newspapers and political parties was natural because of the economic limitations faced by newspapers—limited technology, high printing costs, and small markets, since there were very few large urban areas (Bennett 1988; Kerbel 1995).

As the nation grew and the population began to move to the cities, a mass audience for news was created. By the 1830s, technological changes made mass production of newspapers not only possible but much less expensive. The establishment of the Associated Press in 1848 was the first step toward creating standardized news. It made possible pooling reporters and selling the same news story to hundreds and thousands of subscribing newspapers. This also created a need for marketing and promotion. Further technological changes, such as the development of the telegraph in 1844 and linotype in the 1880s, gave rise to large-scale news gathering and news marketing organizations (Kerbel 1988). It also produced a natural marriage between newspapers and advertisers. Newspapers became affordable and gained economic independence from political parties. They became profit-making, independent businesses. The partisan press had given way to the "penny press."

The penny press became a forerunner of the modern press dependent on mass circulation and commercial advertising for profit. Daily newspapers soon discovered that readers were attracted by sensational and scandalous political news. This helped increase their readership and thus circulation. The seamy side of politics became the entertainment of the times. The press became more intrusive, giving rise to "yellow journalism." This type of journalism emphasized pictures, comics, and colors. Front-page "editorial crusades" became common. At the turn of the century, yellow journalism was followed by what President Theodore Roosevelt referred to as "muck-rakers," named after a special rake designed to collect manure (Sabato 1991).

The fact that the penny press was markedly less partisan also gave rise to the notion of objective journalism. Successive generations of reporters began to consider their work as a skilled occupation requiring formal education and training, higher status, and better wages. Led by respectable journalists such as Walter Lippmann, journalism came to be viewed as a "profession" by the end of World War I (Bennett 1988).

During World War I, the U.S. military was interested in using electronic communication. Because telegraph wires were vulnerable to destruction, the military saw radio signals as more secure and reliable. Thus, during World War I, the military was given the monopoly over radio. The commercial system of broadcasting began to develop after the war. The General Electric Company (GE) worked to set up a U.S.-owned and controlled communication industry. GE helped create the Radio Corporation of America (RCA) in 1919 to assure control of radio by U.S. corporations. Initially, radio technology was used by RCA to broadcast messages. The popularity of home radio for entertainment and information became obvious and soon led to over-the-air broadcasts of music, sports, news, and talk shows for home receivers. In 1921, RCA merged with Westinghouse and United Fruit to establish a virtual monopoly on radio signals.

The rapid growth of radio also created chaos due to the proliferation of overlapping broadcast signals. This in turn led to demands for government regulation. In 1927 the Federal Radio Commission was established to regulate broadcasting (Kellner 1990). By 1930, more than 600 radio stations were broadcasting to more than 12 million homes with radios, about 40 percent of American families (Czitrom 1982). The Communication Act of 1934 declared that the airwaves were public utilities to be used in the public's interest. Radio helped advance a homogenized set of values in the United States, producing a mainstream culture in a diverse nation (Kellner 1990). Radio also played a major role in mobilizing the country in support of U.S. involvement in World War II.

By the 1930s, radio was developing a national audience, newspaper chains were forming, and national magazines such as *Time* and *Life* were changing America. The United States was beginning to develop a national media network. But the development of a national media network did not truly come to fruition until the advent of television in the early 1950s. Even though television was invented in the 1930s, by 1939 television still remained a mystery to most Americans. The introduction of television to American households was delayed because of World War II. Network television emerged in the late 1940s, and many top radio stars and programs migrated to television. Television used the same format employed by radio: soap operas, situation comedies, crime dramas, quiz shows, and the like. The stampede for television began in 1951 when coaxial cable was laid from coast to coast, making it possible for Americans throughout the country to see the same programs at the same time. Despite this, only 10 percent of the population had a TV set in 1951. By 1963, when the networks started their half-hour nightly news broadcast, 95 out of every 100 American households had a television set. Soon, television replaced newspapers as the nation's most widely used medium of information. Today, a television set is on for about seven hours a day in the typical American household (P. Taylor, 1990).

Since the early 1960s, television has become the main source of information for many Americans. Furthermore, the public rates television higher than print media or radio in terms of credibility and fairness (Lichter, Rothman, and Lichter 1986).

Larry Sabato (1991) argues that press reporting (including television) since the early 1940s has gone through three stages. From 1941 to 1966, journalists engaged in what is called *lapdog journalism,* that is, reporting that served and reinforced the political establishment. Mainstream reporters rarely challenged the existing power structure, accepted at face value what those in positions of power told them, and even protected politicians by not revealing anything about politicians' private lives even when their private vices affected their public performance. *Watchdog journalism* dominated from about 1966 to 1974. During this period reporters closely scrutinized the behavior and spoken words of the politicians by engaging in independent investigations (investigative journalism). The Vietnam War and Watergate encouraged this type of journalism. Finally, Sabato argues that the style of journalism prevalent from about 1974 to the present can be described as *junkyard dog journalism.* It consists of political reporting that is often harsh, aggressive, and intrusive. It is a style of journalism where feeding frenzies thrive. Every aspect of politicians' private lives becomes fair play where the operating motto is "anything goes."

The revolution in communication technology and its by-product—the information age—is reshaping American democracy in ways unimagined only thirty years ago. The dawn of the "electronic republic" (Grossman 1995), made up of television, radio, computers, information highway, electronic mail, fax machines, and cable and digital satellite systems with literally hundreds of channels, electronic town hall meetings, and so on, holds out a promise of direct democracy by bridging the information gap and bringing closer than ever before those who govern and those who are governed. Yet in that same electronic republic airwaves are filled with hot air and the constant chatter of talk shows (Kurtz 1996); news broadcasts take on the appearance of a media show (Diamond 1991); news is embedded in a culture of lying (Weaver 1994); toll-free 800 numbers encourage dial-in democracy (Bolce, Maio, and Muzzio 1996); political advertising, with its thirty-second spots (Diamond and Bates 1992) and sound bites is used as simply another marketing gimmick to sell candidates, parties, ideology and policies; newspapers increasingly take on the appearance of scandal sheets and tabloids; and citizens have become mere spectators consuming thousands of images paraded before them (Ewen 1988). All these things raise a serious threat to the traditional form of democratic government envisioned by the Founding Fathers.

It is not too surprising, then, that in recent years the role of the mass media in American politics and the policy process has come under increased scrutiny and criticism. Who decides what is news and what is not? How is news and its analysis presented to the viewers? What factors influence the mass media of communication as they go about their business? To what extent does what is reported and how it is reported influence public perception of what is important and what is not?

Theories of Media and Public Agenda Setting

The literature on agenda setting has grown dramatically over the past twenty-five years or so. This research has focused on three types of agenda setting. The first is policy agenda setting. Such studies try to explain how issues get on the policy agenda of the government. The media agenda-setting literature examines how the mass media processes news, that is, definition, selection, and emphasis of the news and what factors influence and shape the mass media's agenda. Finally, the research on public agenda setting analyzes the relationship between issues as portrayed by the mass media and issue priorities of the general public. Does the way in which the media present issues influence the public agenda, that is, what the public perceives as important issues that deserve government attention? (McCombs and Shaw 1993; Rogers, Dearing, and Bergman 1993; Kosicki 1993)

Media Agenda Setting

Of literally hundreds of possible news events that happen on any given day, how do the mass media decide what is newsworthy? How and why do they select some stories to report and not others? Which stories should be given more emphasis and which ones less? Do they simply report the events as they happened, or do they also interpret these events in their reporting? Are there factors that interject biases in reporters' reporting of the news? What factors influence news gathering?

Kathleen Jamieson and Karlyn Campbell (1992) argue that news gathering is affected by a variety of external and internal constraints imposed on the mass media. This, in turn, affects what is covered and reported by the news media. The significance of these external and internal constraints may vary from one medium to the other. They argue that these external constraints include access, cost, time, and space. Whether reporters are assigned to specific beats or general assignments, some newsworthy events always fall between the cracks of assigned beats. Furthermore, without access to confidential sources, many news stories cannot be written. It also costs money to gather news and report it to the public. How much resources a particular newspaper, radio or television station have and how much resources it is willing to commit to news gathering and reporting, compared to resources for other programs, directly influences the gathering of news and what is covered. This is all the more true in the coverage of foreign news, which requires foreign correspondents, satellite up-link and down-link facilities, and so forth. Finally, different communications media have different time and space constraints. For example, a network evening news broadcast has a very limited amount of time to report news. News editors must select certain stories to report and others to ignore. There are no objective standards for making such selections; instead, such choices are made on a subjective basis. Similarly, newspapers and magazines are influenced in their selection of news stories to report by available space (Jamieson and Campbell 1992; Graber 1988). According to Jamieson and Campbell, internal constraints include available footage (especially television), strong preference for visual events, a tendency to cover newsworthy people and personalities, a desire not to offend anyone, and a desire not to become part of the news.

Four models of the newsmaking process have been identified in the literature. Each model represents a judgment about what the major forces associated with newsmaking are or ought to be. The *mirror model* argues that news should be a reflection of reality and that reporters should simply report news as accurately and objectively as possible without interjecting their personal and subjective opinions or interpretations in reporting the news. The *professional model* views newsmaking as an activity of very skilled professionals who put together an interesting collection of stories based on their importance. The *organizational model* posits the notion that news selection emerges from pressures found in organizational processes and goals. These include interpersonal relations, professional norms, a profit orientation, legal requirements, and cost-benefit considerations. Finally, the *political model* suggests that news is a product of the ideological biases of individual reporters and journalists and pressures of the political environment in which news organizations operate (Graber 1989).

According to Bennett (1988), four types of information biases are present in news. One such bias is what is called *personalized news*. This results from a tendency on the part of reporters to give preference to individual actors and human-interest angles and to downplay institutional and political considerations that help explain the social context of the news events. The second source of bias results from a tendency on the part of reporters to report those aspects of the story that are easy to dramatize, or *dramatized news*. News drama emphasizes crisis over continuity, conflict over consensus, dissent over agreement, personality conflicts, clashes over honest disagreement over policies, image over substance, present over past or future, and the impact of scandals on personal political careers rather than on institutions. For example, news media tend to view elections as a horserace and politics as a game with winners and losers. Election coverage tends to focus on which candidate is leading and which candidate is trailing, personality conflicts within campaign staffs, character flaws and scandals, rather than on substantive issues facing the country, issue positions of the candidates, and the consequences of choices confronting the voters (Diamond 1991; Patterson 1990; Schram 1990; Cook 1990). The third source of bias is *fragmented news*. Stories are presented in an isolated fashion, ignoring history and context, making it difficult for a reader/viewer to assemble the big picture. Finally, there is a tendency to present *normalized news*. This involves the inclination of the reporters to seek out reassuring, authoritative sources—officials who offer normalized interpretations of the news event.

Another source of possible bias in the reporting of news can arise from the background and composition of the communications industry. The news media are largely populated by white males in their thirties and forties. African Americans, Latinos, Asians, and women are highly underrepresented in the mass media. Only one in twenty is nonwhite and only one in five is female. As of 1990, all minority groups taken together made up only 7.8 percent of newsroom employees. Many African American journalists work for African American newspapers or radio stations. Furthermore, a majority of journalists working for major newspapers and networks are well paid and highly educated with over 90 percent possessing college degrees. In general, they are a rather homogeneous group. It is often said that the way we are brought up and live shapes our view of the world. Is it a coincidence that the poor generally receive coverage only during the Thanksgiving and Christmas holidays? Similarly, African Americans and other minorities are overrepresented in the media when the news stories deal with negative news. Most of the general media emphasize established white middle-class values and neglect concerns of minorities and poor people. They also stress urban affairs more than rural affairs (Parenti 1993; Lichter, Rothman, and Lichter 1990; Graber 1989).

Mass media in America are privately owned businesses interested in making a profit. Profit is influenced by the size of the readership or listeners or viewers. The larger the audience, the more can be charged for commercial advertisements. Thus the basic criteria used to select specific stories to report have much to do with attracting an audience. The most important criterion is to select stories that will have broad audience appeal; another criterion is to use stories that would have a strong impact on readers, listeners, and viewers. A third criterion is stories that contain violence, conflict, or scandal. Additional criteria include familiarity with the story and proximity of the event to home, along with timeliness and novelty (Graber 1989; Jamieson and Campbell 1992). Similarly, talk shows by personalities such as Phil Donahue, Oprah Winfrey, Rush Limbaugh, Larry King, and Don Imus, and discussion groups such as the McLaughlin Group, Washington Week in Review, Journalists' Roundtable, and Cross-Fire on radio and television are contrived and staged "dramas" for mass appeal to increase their audience (Nimo and Combs 1990).

The explosion of talk shows is part of the information revolution. We have come to live in a talkathon culture that overloads our circuits with constant chatter, much of it trivial and little of it important. Such a talk culture is further vulgarized by the popularity of tabloid television. Mainstream newspapers and television seem increasingly willing to follow tabloid newspapers and tabloid-style television shows in order to attract more viewers (Kurtz 1996). Today, the difference in styles of television and newspaper reporting is very small. In general, newspaper stories are longer and provide more detail than television stories. But they have also come to rely on the interpretive style of reporting. For example, campaign reporting is not only straight reporting of what the candidates say, but it also involves investigative reporting and analyses of the campaign (Patterson 1994).

Public Agenda Setting

> The power of the press in America is a primordial one. It sets the agenda of public discussion; and this sweeping political power is unrestrained by any law. It determines what people will talk about and think about—an authority that in other nations is reserved for tyrants, priests, parties and mandarins. (White 1972, 327)

In 1922, Walter Lippman argued that the mass media are the main connection between events in the real world and the images of these events we carry in our minds. He further stated that journalists point a flashlight, rather than a mirror, at the world. Thus the audience, instead of getting the entire political picture, receives only selective glimpses. Since the audience cannot experience the world directly, the media shape opinions and reconstruct reality by providing images or pictures in our minds (Lippman 1922).

Lippman's assertions stimulated significant research in the media's role in influencing and setting public agenda. The public agenda has to do with what the general public considers important issues facing the country at any given time and the priorities it places on these issues. Do the mass media simply reflect the public's thinking about the importance of the issues or do the media influence and shape what the public considers important and the priorities they assign to issues? Is there a positive relationship between what various communication media emphasize and what the general public comes to regard as important?

Public agenda-setting research shares certain common attributes or characteristics: (1) it deals with the importance or salience of public issues; (2) it focuses on media content and audience perception; (3) it deals with a range of issues, ranked in some fashion on an agenda; (4) it focuses on the effect media content and trends have on public agenda setting, rather than the general effect of watching television or reading newspapers or news magazines. Finally, it has followed the legacy of public opinion polling by conceptualizing public issues as broad concepts such as the economy and trust in government (Kosicki 1993).

Research conducted from the 1940s to the early 1960s tended to conclude that the effect of the media on public agenda setting was minimal (Klapper 1960; Barelson, Lazarsfeld, and McPhee 1954; Lazarsfeld, Berelson, and Gaudet 1948). Since the 1970s, research has demonstrated the fairly powerful, if not unlimited, agenda-shaping influence of the mass media (Weaver 1994; Fan, Brosius, and Mathias 1994; Page and Shapiro 1992; Protess and McCombs 1991; Iyengar and Kinder 1987; Gitlin 1980; Shaw and McCombs 1977).

In today's society, people increasingly depend on the mass media for their version of reality. This is the central concept of the *dependency theory* of mass communications. This theory argues that as society grows more complex, opportunities for firsthand social and political experiences decrease. Under this condition, people grow increasingly dependent on the mass media for their understanding of what is real and what is unreal. The more dependent people become on the media for information, the more likely they will change their opinions as a result of that information. Furthermore, the more mass-mediated information satisfies people's needs, the more dependent they become on it. This in turn increases the media's influence. In addition, the more developed a society's media, the more people rely on the media during crises, conflicts, and periods of change (Nimo and Combs 1990).

It has been suggested that the mass media play a gatekeeper role in the American political system. The relatively few people who select news (e.g., editors, news directors, reporters, wire services) are often called gatekeepers because they tightly control access to the publicity arena (Graber 1989). The mass media to a great extent regulate the content of public information and communication in the United States. They exercise a great deal of discretion over whose dreams, hopes, and aspirations are admitted through the gate and into the public consciousness. By regulating the flow of information, the mass media hold considerable power in the American political system (Bennett 1988).

As Denis McQuail (1990) argues, the mass media can influence the public agenda in a variety of ways. The media can attract and direct the public's attention to problems, solutions, or people and events. The media can confer status and legitimacy. The media can be used as a channel for persuasion and mobilization. The media can give publicity and thus recognition to certain individuals or groups. Finally, the media can offer gratification and psychic rewards to the audience.

The mass media can influence the salience (importance) of events in the public mind. The media influence the public agenda when news stories center attention on a problem and make it seem important. They do this by the frequency and amount of time and space they devote to a story, the size of the headlines, and so on. This influence begins when news people decide to publish a particular story. They select what to publish and what not to publish. They also decide how much attention to give to that particular story. The media can manipulate the story so as to influence how people perceive the importance of the issues and evaluate these issues and policies (Graber 1989). By making certain issues or candidates more salient, the media can significantly influence the construction of perceived reality by the audience (Weaver 1994). The way in which an issue is framed also influences how the public thinks about that issue (McCombs and Shaw 1993; Shaw and Martin 1992). Even if the mass media do not mold every opinion, they do mold opinion visibility, that is, they can establish a perceptual framework within which public opinion takes shape (Parenti 1993).

Research also suggests that the news media's power to influence the agenda depends on the concreteness or abstractness of the issues. Influence is greater with concrete as opposed to abstract issues or problems (Yagade and Dozier 1990). Similarly, research also suggests that the president can interfere with the relationship between the news media and the public by presenting an agenda of issues that differ from the press's agenda. Nevertheless, the president is likely to win attention only when his popularity is very high (Wanta 1991).

Bernard Cohen (1963) argues that the mass media may not tell us what to think, but they are very successful in telling us what to think about. More recent research findings on the relationship between mass media and public agenda setting suggest that the mass media not only tell us what to think about, but also how to think about it and, thus, what to think (McCombs and Shaw 1993).

Advertising and the Mass Media

In 1989, $222.9 billion was spent on advertising and promotion in the mass media. Of the total spent, 36 percent was spent on advertising in newspapers, 21.6 percent on network television, 18.7 percent on cable television, 16.7 percent on magazines, and 1.5 percent on radio. The mass media permeate our environment and inundate us with advertisements trying to promote or sell some product or service. Advertisers pay for the time and space to allow them to bring a particular message to an intended audience (Jamieson and Campbell 1992).

Jamieson and Campbell (1992) have identified various types of advertisements (ads) typically found in the mass media. *Product ads* try to market a product or a product line (e.g., Nike's ad for its line of shoes). *Service ads* try to persuade the audience that a particular service is provided with a personal touch and is desirable (e.g., an ad depicting a friendly bank teller or a Kodak representative). *Goodwill ads* are what are often called image advertising. Such ads do not directly try to make a sales pitch for a particular product or a service. Instead, they are designed to create a positive image of the company in the minds of the public (e.g., a gas company ad expressing its concern for a clean environment). In *advocacy ads,* a company or organization takes a public stand on a public policy issue and uses the ad to promote a particular viewpoint or policy alternative (e.g., an ad by the National Rifle Association advocating opposition to a gun-control law). *Infomercials* are generally fifteen- to thirty-minute ads designed to look like a program but are instead selling a product. In the 1992 and 1996 presidential elections, Ross Perot used many infomercials to sell his message and his candidacy to the American voters. *Political ads* argue that the voters should elect candidate A rather than candidate B or urge voters to vote a specific way on an issue. Political ads are generally short-lived and more intense than an ad for a product or product line (Jamieson and Campbell 1992).

Advertising can influence both public agenda setting and mass media agenda setting. Several studies have examined the role of advertising in influencing the perception (how the public views certain issues) and beliefs (what the public thinks are important issues and how they rank them) of the general public, that is, the public agenda (Ghorpade 1986; Sutherland and Galloway 1981). Advertising by political candidates and organizations generally has a dual purpose. One is to influence the public's agenda, that is, the public's perceptions and opinions about candidates, issues, and the like; the other is to influence the mass media's agenda, that is, the agenda of issues advanced by the various news media.

As we have discussed before, the mass media rely on various sources for information. One such source is the political consultant. Political consultants are skilled in manufacturing pseudo events to obtain beneficial news coverage and photo opportunities for candidates. They are also experts at producing highly charged, emotion-evoking advertisements. Political campaigns, in order to generate positive coverage, try to control news coverage by controlling media access, helping set the media's agenda, and increase the credibility of the advertisement's message by trying to blur the line between commercial and news (Jamieson and Campbell 1992). The mass media often become an easy prey for such tactics because of their need for a story and, in case of television, the visuals (Roberts and McCombs 1994). A study of the 1990 Texas gubernatorial campaign revealed that television political advertisements affected the news agenda of both television and newspapers. They reflected the same issue priorities as that of the candidates (Roberts and McCombs 1994).

The Mass Media and Coverage of Health Care News

In the past fifteen to twenty years, there has been an explosion in health care reporting in newspapers and television. A series of major medical stories, such as artificial heart experiments and the herpes epidemic, followed by the AIDS epidemic, made the medical beat a necessity for newspapers and network television (Aumente 1995). Health care has become as hot a topic for coverage as the environment or crime. The proliferation of health databases and health-related journals, news channels on cable television, and audience-specific, specialty magazines; the growth of the elderly population; and increased public concern for healthy lifestyles have made health news almost a daily event. This has led major news media to establish regular forums or columns such as "health watch," "business and health," "your health," and "news from medicine." There is no dearth of health care coverage (Case 1994a). Health and the medical beat have evolved from a haphazard collection of many unrelated stories covered by reporters often lacking in education and health care expertise to a prime assignment handled by well-educated and seasoned medical journalists. Today's reporters bring background and experience to the job. This is all the more true of the major networks (Aumente 1995).

Despite this flood of health care news, most Americans still do not understand concepts such as managed care or managed competition. According to a study conducted by the Kaiser Family Foundation and Harvard University, no more than a fifth to a third of the public had heard of and understood the meaning of these terms. Half the respondents in the study said that the media did only a "fair" or "poor" job of explaining what the different health care proposals mean to them and their families. Only 10 percent said the media had done an excellent job, while only a third called it "good." Respondents in general gave the media high marks for reporting on the "politics" of reform (Cohn 1993).

According to David Satcher, director of the Centers for Disease Control and Prevention in Atlanta, the media give too much attention to isolated occurrences and health matters with tabloid appeal such as "flesh-eating bacteria" distracting the public from real health issues that need attention (Case 1994b). There is a tendency on the part of the media to glorify new medical miracles without discussion of the cost, impact, or side effects or to report too many medical tear-jerker stories without any attempt to put those stories in a broader context that would help the audience to understand systemic problems better (Case 1994b). Furthermore, in order to get the story on the front page or on the evening news, there is a tendency to overstate, to make the story compelling and dramatic (Case 1994b). Given the fact that mass media are often motivated by profit, the health care information that the public is more likely to receive is that which is interesting and entertaining, not necessarily informative and educational.

The revolution in health care coverage and health care news in the mass media also raises the question about the role and the influence, if any, of the mass media on setting the public agenda and health policy development.

Some studies suggest that the mass media play an influential role in setting the public agenda on health care. For example, one study found support for the hypothesis that the public's issue priority was influenced by both media and social interaction (Zhu et al. 1993). Another study that examined the influence of television news coverage with respect to three issues—inflation, Iran, and the Soviet Union—found an agenda-setting effect for all three issues examined, though the forms of the effect varied among the three issues (Watt, Mazza, and Snyder 1993). Still another study found that provocative, anecdotal media stories about problems surrounding shortened hospital stays, that is, "drive-by deliveries" for new mothers and other cost-related problems, had the effect of arousing concern on the part of consumers and legislators, leading to legislative initiatives designed to curb such practices (Bilchik 1996). In contrast to these studies, a study that examined the influence of four newspapers on four different issues found that in three of the four situations studied, newspaper coverage did not lead to changes in health policy. But their potential to have an impact on change became greater when reprints of the news items were widely distributed and follow-up studies were published. Furthermore, national recognition of newspaper coverage and an increase in lawmakers' exposure to the news are also likely to increase newspaper coverage's impact on policy changes (Walsh-Childers 1994).

Mass Media and Health Care Reform: 1993–94

This section discusses the role played by the mass media during the 1993–94 health care reform period. We examine the relationship between the mass media agenda and the public agenda. How did the media cover the health care reform debate? What factors influenced their coverage? Did the mass media influence public opinion and, thus, the public agenda? What role, if any, did political advertisements play in the health care reform debate?

It is important to remember that identifying precise causal linkages is difficult because the relationship between the mass media agenda and the public agenda is rarely linear or unidirectional. More often, the relationship tends to be complex and multidimensional. The relationship between the media agenda and the public agenda is a two-way, mutually dependent relationship whereby each influences the other (Roger and Dearing 1988).

Media Agenda and the Public Agenda

Media coverage of health care reform was practically nonexistent throughout the 1980s. During this period, a total of about forty stories were published on health care reform or national health insurance in three major news-papers—the *Christian Science Monitor,* the *New York Times,* and the *Wall Street Journal* (Hacker 1996). This is in sharp contrast to coverage of health care reform starting with 1991 when the number of articles increased to thirty-five. In 1992 alone, ninety-three articles on health care reform and national health insurance were published in these three newspapers (Hacker 1996). This might suggest that the press was reacting to various political factors.

One such factor was Harris Wofford's dramatic victory for the U.S. Senate in Pennsylvania in 1991, based largely on the issue of national health insurance. Almost all explanations for the outcome of the 1991 U.S. Senate election in Pennsylvania pointed to Wofford's support for national health insurance as a key to his victory (Hacker 1996). The second factor was the presidential primaries, in which all Democratic contenders declared their support for some type of health care reform. Third was the congres-sional agenda, which displayed considerable activity in the area of health care. For example, the number of congressional hearings focusing on health care costs or the uninsured increased significantly in 1991 and 1992 com-pared to previous years. Similarly, the number of bills introduced in Con-gress related to national health care or national health insurance also increased dramatically from 1987–88 to 1991–92 (Hacker 1996).

It is no coincidence that the percentage of Americans who believed that the American health care system needed to be completely rebuilt increased from 23 percent in October 1989 to 42 percent in November 1991, while the percentage of Americans who believed that the American health care system needed only few minor changes decreased from 21 percent to 6 percent during the same time (Thomas 1992). This would suggest that the public's recognition of health care as a national problem was related to the proliferation of media coverage. Even without a clear causal linkage, it is important to note that political events, media coverage, and public aware-ness of health care reform as a national issue seem to have converged at about the same time. When asked by the Gallup poll to name the most important problem facing the country in 1990, only 1 percent of Americans cited health care. This number increased to 6 percent in 1991, 12 percent in 1992, and 28 percent in 1993 (Hacker 1996). By January 1994, the number had climbed to 31 percent (see Table 6.1).

Table 6.1 presents data on the number of speeches dealing with health care given by President Clinton, the number of health care–related stories on television, the number of articles in the *New York Times,* President Clinton's overall job approval ratings, approval ratings for his handling of health care policy, and the level of support for his health care reform plan during 1993–94. A number of interesting observations can be derived from the data.

Table 6.1

Number of Health Care Speeches[a] by President Clinton, Number of Television and *New York Times* Stories on Health Care, Health Care as Most Important Issue, President Clinton's Job Approval Ratings and His Handling of Health Care Policy, and Support for Clinton's Health Care Plan, 1993–94

	Speeches[a]	(n)Television[b] stories (n)	*New York[c] Times* stories (n)	Health care[d] as most important issue (%)	Job[d] approval ratings (%)	Handling[d] of health care policy (%)	Support[d] for Clinton's plan (%)
1994							
December	1	0	4		40	37	
November	5	0	4		43		
October	6	4	10		48		
September	2	9	33		44	36	
August	16	66	84		39	35	
July	18	49	80	29	42	34	40
June	21	50	48	21	44	38	43
May	18	23	36		51	41	46
April	15	16	19		48	41	43
March	16	19	37		51	40	44
February	16	27	47		53	39	46
January	5	12	30	31	58	46	57
Total	139	275	432				
1993							
December	6	7	35		54		52
November	7	17	47		48	51	45
October	20	28	68		48		59
September	24	89	100	28	56	55	
August	11	10	28		44	44	
July	7	10	12		41		

(continued)

Table 6.1 *(continued)*

June	9	12	18		46	51
May	6	39	37		44	
April	6	34	27		55	
March	6	35	52		52	
February	6	15	22		59	
January	3	13	8	18	58	
Total	114	309	454			

Sources: Public Papers of the Presidents of the United States—William J. Clinton—1993, vols. 1 and 2 (Washington, D.C.: Government Printing Office, 1994); *Public Papers of the Presidents of the United States—William J. Clinton—1994* vols. 1 and 2 (Washington, D.C.: Government Printing Office, 1995).

[a]Includes speeches, town hall meetings, media interviews, and statements to Congress in which health care reform, the Health Security Plan, or health insurance were discussed.

[b]Compiled from Television News Archives at Vanderbilt University. Http://tvnews.vanderbilt.edu. Includes ABC, CBS, NBC, and CNN.

[c]Compiled from the analysis of the *New York Times Index* for 1993 and 1994. Letters to the editors and op-ed pieces were excluded.

[d]Compiled from *Gallup Poll Monthly* for 1993 and 1994.

The trend of increased coverage of health care topics started in the early 1990s and increased dramatically. In 1993 television reported 309 stories, while the *New York Times* published 454 articles related to health care. What is interesting is that from January 1993 to May 1993 both television and newspapers (the *New York Times*) reported many more stories than the number of health care speeches given by the president. It appears that the media agenda was not influenced by the presidential agenda or speechmaking. It is also interesting to note that President Clinton's job approval rating stayed in the 50-plus percent range from January to April 1993. His job approval ratings dropped to 44 percent in May of 1993. This was the month the Clinton administration had originally promised to deliver its health care reform package. As the Clinton administration continued to work on developing a health care reform plan during June, July, and August, media coverage declined significantly.

The number of health policy speeches by President Clinton increased significantly in September, culminating with his address to a joint session of Congress on September 23 in which he outlined the major features of his health care reform proposal, the Health Security Act. In response to this, television and newspaper coverage increased dramatically with the major television networks doing eight or nine stories and the *New York Times* publishing a hundred articles dealing with health care during the month of September alone. During the same month, President Clinton's job approval ratings reached 56 percent, and approval for his handling of the health care policy climbed to 55 percent. Support for his proposed health care reform reached its highest level of 59 percent. During October and November 1993 and January 1994, the number of health care speeches given by the president declined significantly as the administration became preoccupied with the crisis in Somalia and congressional ratification of NAFTA. Correspondingly, coverage of health care in the media also declined, though it did continue at a higher pace than the rate of presidential speeches.

As Table 6.1 indicates, the second major increase in the number of presidential speeches on health care and the media's coverage of health care reform occurred between May and August 1994. This was the period when Congress was actively considering various competing health care reform plans, including the Health Security Act. We can see a dramatic increase in the number of reports and articles devoted to health care on the major television networks and in the *New York Times*. This finding is consistent with findings of similar studies (Times Mirror Center for the People and the Press 1995).

By August 1994, 29 percent of the American people questioned listed health care as the most important problem facing the country. Unfortu-

Table 6.2

Number of Stories Published in *St. Louis Post-Dispatch* in Which the Phrase "Health Care Reform" Appeared, 1991–94

	1991	1992	1993	1994
December	2	15	31	15
November	2	14	37	34
October	2	15	43	34
September	4	6	72	38
August	3	11	27	67
July	0	12	16	72
June	1	4	38	48
May	3	6	42	38
April	1	3	41	37
March	1	6	26	42
February	1	4	35	34
January	1	12	24	49
Total	22	108	432	508

Source: Compiled from the *St. Louis Post-Dispatch* on CD-ROM.

nately, for the supporters of health care reform, President Clinton's job approval rating dropped to 39 percent, one of the lowest approval ratings he received since assuming office in January 1993. By August 1994, the approval rating for his handling of health care policy had dropped to 35 percent from a high of 55 percent in September 1993. By July 1994, support for his Health Security Act dropped to 40 percent from a high of 59 percent in September 1993 when he presented his plan to the joint session of Congress.

By August 1994, it was clear that the window of opportunity for major reform of the U.S. health care system had passed. Health care reform was declared dead and buried as Congress recessed. Beginning in September 1994, we see a dramatic decline in the number of speeches on health care by the president and the number of health care reports or articles on major television networks and in the *New York Times*. What this suggests is that the mass media perhaps has a limited attention span and once an issue is perceived as dead or not viable, media attention shifts to some other issue.

To examine the pattern of health care news coverage on a regional level, we selected the *St. Louis Post-Dispatch* as our newspaper. We calculated the number of stories reported in the paper from 1991 to 1994 in which the phrase "health care reform" was used. The results are displayed in Table 6.2. We found a pattern similar to the national media attention. Beginning with 1991, the number of stories dealing with health care reform increased dramatically every year until 1994. For example, in 1991, 22 stories dealing with health care reform were reported in the newspaper. In 1992 this number jumped to 108, an increase of 490 percent. In 1993 the number jumped to 432 stories, an increase of 400 percent from the previous year. In 1994 there were 508 health care reform stories reported, an increase of about 18 percent. The largest amount of coverage on health care reform was provided in September 1993 and during June, July, and August 1994.

As mentioned earlier, while it is difficult to establish causal linkages between media agenda, public agenda, and presidential and/or congressional agenda, it does appear that there is a strong relationship between these factors. It is not by sheer coincidence that many of these factors seemed to come together at a certain point in time. The frequency of presidential speeches and the number of health-related stories on major network television and newspapers appear to coincide. For example, the public's perception of health care as the most important issue facing the nation seems to be related to the frequency of presidential speeches and the intensity of the media's news coverage. Nevertheless, our data do not demonstrate whether the presidential agenda shapes the media agenda, or vice versa, or whether the mass media agenda sets the public agenda, or vice versa. We suspect each influences the other, and the relationship is more mutual rather than unidirectional. Our data also indicate a relationship between presidential popularity as measured by overall job approval rating, approval rating for handling health care policy, and support for his plan to reform the U.S. health care system. Lower overall approval ratings seem to be related to lower approval ratings for his handling of the health care policy and lower support for his health care reform plan. Our data suggest a lack of relationship between presidential popularity and frequency of news coverage.

Mass Media and the Health Care Reform Debate: Education or Entertainment?

Overall, how well did the mass media do in informing and educating the general public about the complex and intricate issue of health care reform? As Tables 6.1 and 6.2 demonstrate, the mass media devoted a significant amount of airtime (television) and print space (newspapers) to the issue of health care reform. A study funded by the Robert Wood Johnson Foundation and conducted by the Annenberg Public Policy Center at the University of Pennsylvania tracked the health care debate in newspapers, television, and radio from January 16, 1994, to October 5, 1994. This study reported that segments longer than five minutes accounted for more than half of the total airtime devoted to health care reform on the nine major broadcast news programs monitored in the study. Among newspapers, the *New York Times* ran significantly more front-page stories about health care reform than the other nine newspapers monitored in the study (Jamieson and Cappella 1995).

While television and newspapers devoted considerable amounts of time and space reporting on the health care reform debate, the quality of coverage left a great deal to be desired. Two major areas of criticism of the mass media's coverage of the health care reform debate include the media's tendency to focus on the "drama" (i.e., politics, disagreements, conflicts, personal tragedies) and a lack of objective reporting, that is, biases in the media's reporting on the health care reform debate.

Politics versus Context

As we pointed out in our discussion of media agenda setting, the mass media have a tendency to dramatize a story to make it more interesting and attractive. Such was the case in the coverage of the health care reform debate. Our own analysis of the reporting of the health care debate in the *New York Times* helps illustrate this point.

Based on the description of health care related stories in the *New York Times Index,* we classified these stories into three types—problem, policy, and politics—following Kingdon's (1995) agenda-building framework. Stories that largely focused on the shortcomings, disadvantages, and/or problems of the U.S. health care system were classified as problem stories. Such stories or reporting can help the reader better understand and grasp the problems of the U.S. health care system and the need for reform. Stories that primarily dealt with discussion of proposed solutions, a systematic examination of competing alternatives and their consequences were classified as policy stories. This type of story helps the reader understand the array of possible policy alternatives. Finally, stories that focused mainly on political and legal conflicts and maneuvering, disagreements, personalities, partisan charges and countercharges, winners and losers, personal tragedies and such were classified as political stories. Such stories dramatize the "politics"of health care reform, but do not inform and educate the reader about complex choices and consequences they faced in reforming the U.S. health care system. The results of this classification are displayed for 1993 and 1994 in Table 6.3.

As the data indicate, during both years political stories far outnumbered problem and policy stories. Of the 432 health care–related stories reported by the *New York Times* in 1993, 70 percent were political stories, 23 percent were policy stories, and 7 percent were problem stories. Of the 454 health-related stories reported in 1994, 54 percent were political stories, 35 percent were policy stories, and 11 percent were problem stories. Stories on the "politics" of health care may be interesting, but such reporting does not inform and educate the general public and help them make informed deci-

Table 6.3

Number of Stories Related to Health Care Reported in *New York Times* by Type of Story, 1993–94

	Problem	Policy	Politics	Total
1994				
December	1	1	2	4
November	3	0	1	4
October	1	3	6	10
September	2	7	24	33
August	0	25	54	84
July	2	17	61	80
June	2	13	33	48
May	3	8	25	36
April	4	2	13	19
March	6	7	24	37
February	2	11	34	47
January	3	4	23	30
Total	29	98	305	432
1993				
December	0	12	23	35
November	4	20	23	47
October	7	22	39	68
September	8	30	62	100
August	5	12	11	28
July	2	7	3	12
June	2	9	7	18
May	3	18	16	37
April	2	12	13	27
March	9	9	34	52
February	4	7	11	22
January	2	1	5	8
Total	48	159	247	454

Source: Compiled from analysis of the *New York Times Index* for 1993 and 1994.
Note: Letters to the editor and op-ed pieces were excluded. Stories that discussed the problems of the U.S. health care system were classified as problem stories. Stories that mainly discussed proposed solutions, policy alternatives or options, and analysis of proposed solutions were classified as policy stories. Stories that mainly focused on personalities, conflicts, disagreements, partisanship, legal conflicts, interest groups, and personal tragedies were classified as political stories.

sions. This may be a factor in the perceptions the public holds about the health care system and its problems, discussed in chapter 7.

Other studies that have analyzed the type of coverage on health care reform provided by the mass media came to similar conclusions. One study analyzed local television coverage of President Clinton's Health Security

Act in California during the week of September 19, 1993. This study found that of the 366 television news stories on health care reform, 57 percent of the local news stories focused on interest-group politics. The study concluded that even though health care reform was the focus of a large number of local television stories, the stories lacked in-depth explanations, largely provided superficial coverage, and were framed largely in terms of the risks and costs of reform to specific stakeholders (Dorfman, Schauffler, Wilkerson, and Feinson 1996).

Another study was funded by the Henry J. Kaiser Family Foundation and conducted by the Times Mirror Center for the People and the Press (1995). This study, a content analysis of media coverage of health care issues from July through mid-November of 1994, concluded that the politics of reform dominated the news coverage. The press chose to concentrate on political aspects, that is, political infighting, counterproposals, and lobbying activities that highlight conflict and attract wider audiences, rather than stories that seek to explain the complexities of providing health care coverage to all Americans. Thirty-one percent of all health care stories focused on politics, while only 17 percent dealt with the impact of reform on individuals and families. Sixty-six percent of the stories were filed by Washington, D.C., based reporters (Schear 1994, 36).

Similarly, a study by the Annenberg Policy Center found that the media was more interested in covering strategy and process than issues. For example, 67 percent of the broadcast news and 62 percent of the print stories focused on strategy and process (Jamieson and Cappella 1995).

Still another study found that of the forty-one articles published about health care reform in *USA Today* during a two-month period in 1994, twenty-seven (66 percent) focused on health care "battles" or "challenges" and who was for and who was against the plan. This journalistic preference for conflict over context is explained by the fact that health care is a vast and complex subject, and journalists who are short on time and patience take the easy way out by doing political stories dealing with personalities, conflicts, and horseraces (i.e., who is ahead and who is behind) (Diamond, Katz, and Matthews 1994). According to the Annenberg Public Policy Center Study, reporters failed to cover areas of agreement among competing plans because they were more interested in conflict and strategy than the content or the pros and cons of various reform proposals. They wrote for the already knowledgeable, not the average citizen, and often viable policy options were prematurely judged "dead" by reporters and not given coverage (Jamieson and Cappella 1995). Thus it is not too surprising that despite the intense coverage given to the issue of health care reform in the mass media, many polls found that the general public did not know some of the basic facts about health care reform, and the public was confused and misinformed about the Clinton plan (Jamieson and Cappella 1995; Blendon 1995; Marmor 1995). After examining the press coverage of efforts by the Truman and Nixon administrations to enact health plans and the 1993–94 health reform efforts, Blendon concluded that in the two historical cases and present-day efforts special interests found an inadvertent ally in the media because news organizations were guilty of neglecting the informational needs of the American public (Glaberson 1993).

Objective or Biased Reporting?

Another criticism that has been raised about the mass media's coverage of health care reform is the lack of objectivity in reporting. While most of the reporting was neutral, examples abound of biased reporting by certain segments of the media at various points in time. The criticism of press bias in coverage of health care reform came from both the left and the right of the political spectrum. For example, Fred Barnes, senior editor of the *New Republic,* in an article published in *Forbes Media Critic,* accused the press corps of accepting and perpetuating many myths about health care, including the notion that the nation's health care system was in "crisis" (Kosterlitz 1994a). On the other hand, the press has been accused of bias in favor of conservative reform plans such as the media's portrayal of conservative Representative Jim Cooper's health care bill as a popular and workable compromise (Kosterlitz 1994a). In fact, the senior editor of *Consumer Reports,* Trudy Lieberman (1994), faults reporters for their failure to point out that Representative Cooper received significant campaign contributions from the health care industry.

The media's coverage was also faulted in the PBS special "The Great Health Care Debate." In the special, the host of the show, Bill Moyers, reported that while recovering from heart surgery he spent the summer listening to a lot of radio and found that almost every talk-radio host was against the Clinton reform plan. According to Thomas Patterson, contemporary Washington journalists aspire to being "anti" instinctively, which leads them to magnify the bad and underplay the good (Diamond, Katz, and Matthews 1994). Similarly, Elizabeth McCaughey's five-page article titled "No Exit" (1994) attacking Clinton's health care reform plan in the *New Republic* was well received by conservatives such as George Will and Bob Dole. Others leveled serious and strong charges of biased reporting. According to James Fallows, many of the claims made by McCaughey in her article were simply false. Furthermore, according to Fallows, McCaughey's pose of impartiality was undermined by her campaign as the Republican nominee for lieutenant governor of New York soon after her article was published (Fallows 1995). Her false assertions and misrepresentations essentially went unchallenged (Weinstein 1994; Marmor 1995).

Even the *New York Times* has been the subject of criticism for its role in the health care debate. Critics have charged that the *New York Times* greatly influenced the debate by wholeheartedly endorsing the concept of managed competition, and thus only the reform plans associated with managed competition. The *New York Times* launched a campaign to back managed competition, and the rest of the media followed suit. Between May 1991 and July 1993, some thirty-five editorials in the *New York Times* boosted managed competition. As early as 1991, long before the debate on health care reform had even started, the *New York Times* opened with a series of editorials that softened the way for managed competition. Originally labeled managed care, it later was referred to as managed competition. The editorials in the *New York Times* referred to managed competition in glowing terms, constantly referring to it as the best answer and often criticized Canada's single-payer system (Lieberman 1993). The *New York Times'* star health policy reporter, Robert Pear, who racked up more than forty front-page health care stories in 1993, was also a recipient of many criticisms for misrepresentation, biased and false reporting. According to one health policy reporter, "he has been really wrong a lot" (Starobin 1993). According to Jack Nelson, the Washington Bureau chief of the *Los Angeles Times,* a story by Pear on September 30, 1993, which claimed that the American Medical Association was urging patients to lobby against Clinton's health care reform plan, was totally wrong. According to one White House aide, Pear was constantly exaggerating and overcreating conflict and misleading the public. Since it was reported in the *New York Times,* however, there was a tendency on the part of editors of other newspapers to follow suit (Starobin 1993). Similar charges of bias or lack of objectivity have also been leveled against major television networks (Orient 1994).

Political Advertising and the Health Care Reform

As we mentioned earlier in the chapter, advertising can influence both the public and mass media agenda settings. Political advertising often has a dual purpose of influencing the perception of the general public about issues and/or candidates (i.e., the public agenda) and influencing the issues advanced by the mass media (i.e., the media agenda). The aim is to generate positive coverage and increase the credibility of an advertisement's message by blurring the line between commercial and news. The mass media often become easy prey to tactics used by advertisers and political consultants because of the media's need for story, drama, and entertainment.

As soon as President Clinton outlined his plan to reform the U.S. health care system, a campaign was started by opponents to derail the plan. Perhaps no other public policy issue in American politics has been subjected to such an intense political advertisement campaign as health care reform. Advocacy ads were run by a wide variety of groups and interests in support or opposition to the various competing reform plans. Do you want your next life-or-death decision to be made by an M.D. or an MBA? Are you willing to put your family's health insurance into the hands of regional alliances staffed by thousand of bureaucrats? Are you willing to accept a federal government-run health care system? Are you ready to limit your choice of doctors? Are you ready to accept the federal government setting a global budget for health care and the rationing that will follow? These were the kinds of questions raised by opponents of health care reform in their political advertisements. Such ads had the immediate potential to appeal to a large number of viewers because they dealt with emotional issues such as illness, injury, life and death, and thus preyed on the vulnerability of the health care consumer, the patient. Just as in political campaign advertising, at work in many of these policy advertisements or policy advocacy ads was the basic imperative of all advertising: whoever defines the candidate or the issue (health care plan) wins. As Kathleen Hall Jamieson stated at the time, "public policy is now being conducted the way we conduct campaigns for elective office—with all the flaws" (Toner 1994a).

Two of the most important groups that launched an intense campaign against President Clinton's Health Security Act were the Health Insurance Association of America (HIAA) and the National Federation of Independent Businesses (NFIB). The HIAA, in coordination with its member organizations, alone spent more than $17 million to wage a campaign against the Clinton plan. Aside from ads, they also spent money on extensive polling, focus groups, and direct mail, among other activities. The bulk of the money, however, about $13.5 million of the $17 million, was spent on TV, print, and radio advertising (Scarlett 1994).

The most interesting of the political advertisements run by the HIAA were the "Harry and Louise" commercials that showed a white, middle-aged, middle-class couple sitting at a dinner table at home reading President Clinton's Health Security Act, lamenting the complexity of the Clinton plan, and wishing that there was a better way to reform the U.S. health care system. Some of the themes addressed by these ads included the notion that consumers will pay more under the Clinton plan; that an army of bureaucrats will intrude on the intimate relationship of doctor and patient; the possibility of the Clinton plan's limiting consumers' choice of doctor; and price control and rationing. Two of the central features of the Clinton plan that came under attack the most were regional alliances and the system of price controls on insurance premiums to be administered through the alliances (Toner 1994b).

To a great extent, HIAA's advocacy ads engaged in classic doublespeak. On the one hand, HIAA publicly maintained the position that it was for health care reform and that it favored universal coverage and employee mandates. On the other hand, they spent millions of dollar attacking the Clinton plan, which provided both universal coverage and employer mandate, arguing that there has to be a better way (Kosterlitz 1994b).

What is interesting about the HIAA ads is that the ads were very carefully targeted. First, they were to a significant extent aimed at the national media and, through the media, policy makers in Washington D.C. Second, they aimed at the targeted public, especially CNN viewers (a large majority of the "Harry and Louise" ads were run on CNN) because CNN viewers are the ones who most frequently contact their elected representatives, discuss issues with their friends, and often succeed in transmitting their opinions to them (Scarlett 1994).

Newspaper ads also played a role in the advertisement campaign. One of the clever ads featured quotes from President Clinton's controversial surgeon general, Joycelyn Elders, on topics such as condoms in schools. The ad ended with the tag line "President Clinton picked this doctor. Now he wants to pick your doctor" (Scarlett 1994).

Another major critic of the Clinton reform plan was the NFIB, which mainly focused on attacking the employer mandate provision. The American Medical Association (AMA) spent more than $2 million on a series of newspaper and magazine ads raising questions about the bureaucratic nature of the proposed new health care system (Scarlett 1994).

In contrast, the Clinton administration and the supporters of the Health Security Act wasted considerable time getting out their political ads. When they did, it was too little and too late; the damage had already been done. Originally, the Clinton administration was scheduled to propose its health care reform plan within the first 100 days. But it was not until September 1993 that the plan was finally presented to the Congress. Even before the plan was formally presented, major features of the plan were leaked to the press. Inaction on the part of the Clinton administration throughout the spring and summer of 1993 turned out to be a big boon for the HIAA. It gave them a lot of time to refine their message and raise money (West, Heith, and Goodwin 1996).

Opponents spent a considerable amount of resources on the ads very early in the debate. For example, during the crucial period of October to December 1993, opposition groups had a field day. The HIAA, in the fall of

1993 alone, spent about $10.5 million for television spots, while the Pharmaceutical Research and Manufacturers of America (PERMA), which represents the drug industry, spent about $7 million on print ads (West, Heith, and Goodwin 1996).

By early 1994, the Democratic National Committee (DNC), recognizing that they were losing the political ads war, decided to abandon its elaborate campaign to gain grassroots support for President Clinton's plan in favor of a media blitz. The DNC spent about $3 to $4 million in a belated attempt to counter the ad war launched by the HIAA. The ads were pitched to senior citizens by talking about how the Clinton plan would strengthen Medicare and provide new coverage for prescription drugs ("Dems Health Care" 1994). Groups that traditionally supported the Democratic Party and national health insurance were not in a position to spend much money in support of the Clinton plan. For example, the AFL-CIO, which was in favor of the Clinton's Health Security Act, had already spent a considerable amount of their resources fighting the administration's support of NAFTA. In January 1994, the Health Care Reform Project, a coalition of labor unions, corporations, League of Women Voters, and other pro-Clinton groups began airing TV ads in favor of the reform, but they had very little impact (Scarlett 1994).

By March 1994, it was clear that the Clinton forces were losing the paid media war (Scarlett 1994). The damage was done. Opponents of the plan had succeeded in defining the issues. Ads directed against the Clinton plan played a crucial role in the public's attaching a negative connotation to some of the key elements of the plan. Groups opposed to the Clinton plan outspent the supporters by a 2.2–to-1 margin (West, Heith, and Goodwin 1996). The largest share of lobbying efforts went to political advertising. An estimated $50 million, more than half of the overall spending on health care reform lobbying, was devoted to advertising (West, Heith, and Goodwin 1996). By March 1994, the public's approval rating for Clinton's handling of the health care policy dropped to 40 percent, from a high of 55 percent in September 1993. Similarly, the public's support for the Clinton plan dropped to 44 percent in March 1994, from a high of 59 percent in September 1993 (see Table 6.1).

The mass media paid considerable attention in their news to the political ads, giving interest groups and their political views additional, free exposure. The "Harry and Louise" commercials received extensive coverage from the news media. Between January 15 and July 12, 1994, 324 seconds of network evening news time was devoted to the HIAA ads, compared to 122 seconds for the DNC spots (Jamieson 1994). Furthermore, almost every major newspaper and television network ran stories about the ads. The *New*

York Times provided front-page coverage on October 21, 1993 (Kolbert 1993).

Furthermore, there was no attempt made by the mass media to check for the accuracy in these political ads and debunk advertising claims. After the 1988 elections, there was a feeling that the mass media had failed the electorate. This led to changes that saw the advent of ad watchers. In the 1992 elections, the mass media engaged in analyses of ads to point out to voters the distortions and unsubstantiated claims made in the ads. This practice was totally absent with regard to political advertisement about health care reforms. The mass media rarely raised questions of truth, fairness, and/or accuracy in its coverage of the health care reform ads. Rather than analyze ads in the context of the actual debate, the mass media showed more interest in discussing these ads as creative marketing efforts. The Annenberg Public Policy Center analyzed TV stories using ad footage between January 25 and July 12, 1994. It found a total of thirty-seven such stories. Of these, thirty stories were descriptive in nature, six others were he said, she said variety, and only one addressed the issue of accuracy (Jamieson and Cappella 1995).

Thus the mass media, while they provided ample coverage of health care reform news and advertisement, failed to inform and educate citizens about the choices confronting them in the health care reform debate and the consequences of competing alternatives.

Mass Media and Health Care Reform: 1995–96

By September 1994, two months before heading into the 1994 congressional elections, President Clinton's Health Security Act was declared dead and buried. No reform proposal had been even voted on the floor of either house of Congress. The window of opportunity for a major overhaul of the U.S. health care system had closed. President Clinton's job approval rating stood at 44 percent, while his approval rating for his handling of the health care policy stood at 36 percent. The Republican Party used the Health Security Act as a campaign issue, portraying the President as an apologist for tax and spend, liberal, big government. Their campaign platform, captured in the Contract with America, did not mention health care reform. The result was a stunning victory where, after forty years of Democratic control, the Republican Party captured a majority in both houses of Congress, putting them in control of the congressional agenda.

During the 1993–94 reform debates, Republicans had argued against comprehensive and fundamental reforms and for slow or incremental reforms designed to address specific ills of the U.S. health care system. Public opinion polls conducted after the 1994 elections showed that the general public preferred an incremental approach to health care reform. By January 1995, only 12 percent of Americans considered health care the most important issue facing the country. By January 1996, this had dropped to 10 percent (see Table 6.4). The pressure to pass major and comprehensive health care reform had passed; however, the need to address some specific problems through the incremental approach remained.

At the urging of the president, and due to some bipartisan efforts, the 104th Congress (1995–96) dealt with and passed small yet important legislation designed to reform the U.S. health care system. This included the Health Insurance Portability and Accountability Act of 1996 designed to enhance insurance portability and limit preexisting condition exclusions. Congress also passed a few protections for managed care enrollees. For example, insurers offering plans in either group or the individual market were prohibited from restricting hospital stays for mothers and newborns to less than forty-eight hours for vaginal deliveries and ninety-six hours following a cesarean section. Finally, group health plans that offer both medical and surgical benefits and mental health benefits could no longer impose a more restrictive lifetime or annual limits on metal health benefits than is imposed on medical or surgical benefits. This helped bring about some parity in coverage of mental health, medical, and surgical benefits ("Health Legislation Enacted by the 104th Congress" 1996). Congress defeated a proposal to turn Medicaid into block grants to the states, and it failed to restructure Medicare to address the problem of the program's long-term viability.

What role did the mass media play in the health care reform debate during 1995–96? The 1995–96 reform period was not characterized by as intense a debate as occurred in 1993–94. This is understandable in view of the fact that most of the reform proposals during 1993–94 were comprehensive in nature, designed fundamentally to overhaul the U.S. health care system. The reform proposals introduced and discussed during 1995–96 were more modest and incremental in nature. Thus, one would expect the mass media to have played a more modest role in the health care reform debate of 1995–96.

Media Agenda and the Public Agenda

Table 6.4 provides us some insight regarding media and public agendas during the 1995–96 reform period. The data in Table 6.4 stand in sharp contrast to the data provided for 1993–94 in Table 6.1. For example, during 1993–94 reform period President Clinton made a total of 239 speeches dealing with health care (114 in 1993 and 139 in 1994). This was the period of presidential initiative in health policy. Clinton proposed a major plan, the Health Security Act of 1993, to reform the U.S. health care system, and was trying to sell his plan to the American public and Congress. This is in stark contrast to the 1995–96 reform period during which time President Clinton made 169 speeches dealing with health care (88 in 1995 and 81 in 1996). This was the period of congressional initiative in health policy. President Clinton largely stayed out of the fray as Congress debated health insurance reform. He jumped into the battle over the issue of Medicare and Medicaid reform. Most of his health care speeches during 1995–96 dealt with Medicare and Medicaid. He portrayed himself as a champion of the elderly and the poor, fighting the draconian spending cuts proposed in these programs by the Republican-controlled Congress as a way to balance the federal budget.

What is even more striking is the pattern of news coverage during the two reform periods. During 1993–94 the major television networks did a total of 584 stories dealing with health care in their evening news broadcasts. During 1995–96 the major television networks did a total of only 93 health-related stories in their evening broadcasts. This represents a drop of 628 percent. Similarly, during 1993–94, the *New York Times* reported 886 health-related stories in contrast to 312 during 1995–96, a drop of about 284 percent. Clearly, comprehensive reform proposals designed to overhaul the U.S. health care system during the 1993–94 reform period provided the mass media with more "drama" for their news coverage than did the incremental reform proposals navigating through the often dull, dry, and lengthy legislative process of 1995–96.

The same pattern holds when we examine regional health reform news coverage in the *St. Louis Post-Dispatch,* as displayed in Table 6.5. During the 1993–94 reform period, the *Post-Dispatch* reported 940 stories in which the phrase "health care reform" was used. During the 1995–96 reform period, the number of such stories had dropped to 175, a drop of 540 percent. This also suggests that the mass media often demonstrate a short attention span. When an issue becomes, or comes to be perceived as, a front-burner issue the media provide intense coverage to the issue, but the media's coverage drops just as rapidly when the issue moves to the back-burner or comes to be perceived as dead.

The data in Table 6.4 again demonstrate a relationship between the presidential agenda, mass media agenda, and the public agenda. The smaller number of speeches by President Clinton on the topic of health care seem to be related to a smaller number of stories related to health care in the mass media. Similarly, fewer speeches by the president and fewer news stories related to health care seem to be related to whether the public perceived

Table 6.4

Number of Health Care Speeches by President Clinton, Number of Television and *New York Times* Stories on Health Care, Health Care as Most Important Issue, President Clinton's Job Approval Ratings, and His Handling of Health Care Policy, 1995–96

	Speeches[a] (ⁿ)	Television[b] stories (ⁿ)	*New York* [c] *Times stories*(ⁿ)	Health care[d] as most important issue (%)	Approval[d] rating (%)	Handling[d] of health care policy (%)	Handling[d] of Medicare (5)
1996							
December	1	2		58	58		
November	4	2	13		54		
October	6	0	9		60		
September	7	4	13		53		
August	13	5	6	8	58	42	44
July	8	6	11		52		
June	8	1	11		53		
May	7	3	10	10	56		
April	6	7	14		52		
March	5	2	9		53		41
February	9	2	15		52		
January	7	2	7	10	52	44	47
Total	81	36	118				
1995							
December	10	7	14		51		
November	4	4	14		53		
October	8	4	52		49		
September	14	18	31		48		
August	8	1	15		46		
July	6	6	16	7	46		

(continued)

Table 6.4 (continued)

June	16	3	13		47
May	7	8	16		51
April	9	2	11		51
March	2	1	1		44
February	2	2	6		42
January	2	1	5	12	47
Total	88	57	194		

Sources: Public Papers of the Presidents of the United States—William J. Clinton—1995, vols. 1 and 2 (Washington, D.C.: Government Printing Office, 1996); *Public Papers of the Presidents of the United States—William J. Clinton—1996*, vols. 1 and 2 (Washington, D.C.: Government Printing Office, 1997).

[a]Includes speeches, town hall meetings, media interviews, and statements to Congress in which health care reform, the Health Security Plan, or health insurance were discussed.

[b]Compiled from Television News Archives at Vanderbilt University. Includes ABC, CBS, NBC, and CNN. Http://tvnews.vanderbilt.edu.

[c]Compiled from the analysis of the *New York Times Index* for 1995 and 1996. Letters to the editors and op-ed pieces were excluded.

[d]Compiled from *Gallup Poll Monthly* for 1995 and 1996.

Table 6.5

Number of Stories Published in *St. Louis Post-Dispatch* in Which the Phrase "Health Care Reform" Appeared, 1995–96

	1995	1996
January	20	8
February	10	7
March	12	12
April	12	7
May	10	6
June	8	1
July	6	3
August	6	6
September	1	3
October	2	9
November	5	16
December	2	3
Total	94	81

Source: Compiled from *St. Louis Post-Dispatch* on CD ROM.

health care as an important issue. During 1993–94, when the number of presidential speeches and mass media health stories was very high, any-where from 28 to 31 percent of the general public viewed health care as the most important issue facing the country (see Table 6.1). As Table 6.4 shows, during 1995–96, when the number of speeches and the number of stories related to health care in the mass media were few, the percentage of the public who viewed health care as the most important issue facing the country ranged from only 7 to 12 percent. While the nature of the causal linkage remains unclear, we believe that all three agendas—presidential, media, and public—tend to influence each other, and that the relationship is bidirectional rather then unidirectional.

Politics versus Context

An examination of health care related stories in the *New York Times* during 1995–96 and the classification of these stories into problem, policy, and politics categories demonstrate the same pattern as the one during the 1993–94 reform period (see Table 6.6).

Of the total of 194 health-related stories reported in the *New York Times* during 1995, 50 percent dealt with the politics of health care reform, 40 percent with policy alternatives and consequences, and about 10 percent with the problems of the U.S. health care system. Similarly, during 1996, of

Table 6.6

Number of Stories Related to Health Care Reported in *New York Times* by Type of Story, 1995-96

	Problem	Policy	Politics	Total
1996				
December				
November	2	2	9	13
October	3	2	4	9
September	0	5	8	13
August	0	3	3	6
July	1	3	7	11
June	1	2	8	11
May	4	1	5	10
April	3	7	4	14
March	1	7	1	9
February	2	4	9	15
January	0	6	1	7
Total	17	42	60	118
1995				
December	1	5	8	14
November	1	6	7	14
October	3	21	28	52
September	1	16	14	31
August	1	2	12	15
July	3	6	7	16
June	2	9	4	13
May	1	6	9	16
April	2	5	4	11
March	0	1	0	1
February	3	2	1	6
January	1	1	3	5
Total	19	78	97	194

Source: Compiled from analysis of the *New York Times Index* for 1995 and 1996.

Note: Letters to the editor and op-ed pieces were excluded. Stories that discussed the problems of the U.S. health care system were classified as problem stories. Stories that mainly discussed proposed solutions, policy alternatives or options, and analysis of proposed solutions were classified as policy stories. Stories that mainly focused on personalities, conflicts, disagreements, partisanship, legal conflicts, interest groups, and personal tragedies were classified as political stories.

the total of 118 health-related stories reported in the *New York Times,* 50 percent dealt with politics of health care reform, 36 percent with policy analysis, and 14 percent with the problems of the U.S. health care system. This again demonstrates that even such a major national newspaper as the *New York Times* has a tendency to report more about the "politics" (i.e., conflicts, personalities, disagreements, partisan squabbling, etc.) than informative discussion of policy alternatives, their consequences, and the problems facing the U.S. health care system.

Mass Media and Political Advertisement

Compared to the 1993–94 reform period, the amount of advertisement as well as the amount of money spent on advertisements regarding health care reform during 1995–96 was minor. The advertisements mainly dealt with the Republicans' proposal to save $270 billion from projected Medicare expenditures over a seven-year period. After the defeat of the Health Security Act in 1994, the Clinton administration realized that one of the mistakes they had made was that they had allowed the opponents of reform to define the terms of the debate through the use of television, lobbying, and grassroots efforts to capitalize on the public's fear of change (Mitchell 1995). Taking a lesson from that experience, the Clinton administration used the same tactics, such as political commercials and speeches by the president and his cabinet members to fight the Republican plan to cut projected expenditures of the Medicare and Medicaid programs. The Democrats allocated about $850,000 to broadcast political commercials targeted in thirteen states. One of the political ads asserted that Republicans were wrong to want to cut Medicare benefits and that preserving those benefits "is moral, good and right by our elderly." Another ad charged that the Republican plan would increase the cost of medical care for the elderly by $600 and $1,700 for home care annually. Democratic television advertisements used pictures of happy elderly people playing with children and of Mr. Clinton in the Oval Office along with the shadowy images of Speaker Newt Gingrich and Senate Majority Leader Bob Dole (Clymer 1995e). Organized labor also went on the offensive, and the AFL-CIO ran damaging ads accusing Newt Gingrich of wanting to eliminate Medicare (Clymer 1995b).

The Republican National Committee and the National Republican Congressional Committee refused to say how much they spent on their commercials. Republicans largely relied on radio advertisements during commuting hours and talk shows. The ads cited the Medicare trustees' report and how their plan would put Medicare on a sound footing. Republican radio spots were specifically targeted at eleven congressional districts, including that of the House Minority Leader, Richard A. Gephardt. The ads stated that politicians like Gephardt were ignoring Medicare's looming bankruptcy, that Medicare's survival was at stake, and urged listeners to call Gephardt and implore him to stop playing politics with Medicare (Clymer 1995e).

During the 1995–96 reform period, Democrats were successful in raising the public's fear about Republican plans for Medicare, just as Republicans were successful during 1993–94 in raising the public's fear about the changes in the U.S. health care system implied in the Health Security Act. The Republican proposal on Medicare and Medicaid ultimately failed. Throughout 1996, President Clinton enjoyed a job approval rating that ranged from 52 to 60 percent (see Table 6.4). President Clinton, portraying himself as a champion of the elderly standing-up against the Republican-controlled Congress, was easily able to win reelection in 1996 against the Republican challenger, Bob Dole.

Conclusion

This chapter has examined the role of the mass media in the policy process with specific reference to the health care reform periods of 1993–94 and 1995–96. The mass media, wittingly or unwittingly, have become major players in the policy process. The result has been more scrutiny and critical analysis of the mass media for the role they play in our political and policy processes.

The scholarly literature suggests that the mass media agenda, that is, what is considered news and how it is presented, is influenced by a variety of factors that include access to news, cost, time, space, preference for visual events, and a tendency to emphasize conflicts over agreement, among others. The bias present in the news includes a tendency on the part of reporters to give preference to individual actors and human-interest angles without providing the context, the tendency to dramatize news by emphasizing crisis over continuity, image over substance, presenting isolated stories without any continuity, and providing normalized news. The literature also suggests that the mass media agenda in turn influences the public agenda, that is, what the public perceives or views as important issues at a given point in time. The mass media play the role of "gatekeeper" by controlling the public's access to news and the type of information it receives.

Our analysis of the role of the mass media in the health care reform debates in 1993–94 and 1995–96 suggests that the media indeed played a significant role in shaping and influencing the nature of the debate. Nevertheless, a great deal of the role played by the mass media was of a negative variety, and the media must be given a low grade for their performance. As our analysis has demonstrated, the mass media's agenda was influenced by access, cost, time, and space. While in general the mass media dedicated extensive coverage to health care stories, the stories were fragmented, normalized, personalized, and dramatized, emphasizing the politics of health care reform, rather than offering an explanation and analysis of the problems of the U.S. health care system, competing alternatives for reforming the system, and the consequences of each of the competing alternatives. As a result, the mass media failed to inform and educate the American public about the choices facing them and the importance of their choices. In fact, surveys have indicated that the extensive coverage of the health care reform debate in the mass media produced confusion rather than clarity among the general public about reform.

There is also evidence to suggest that reporting on the health care debate was not always objective, often reflecting biases of the reporter or the news medium. For example, an overwhelming majority of radio talk-show hosts were against Clinton's Health Security Act. The *New York Times,* long before the debate over health care reform and the various competing plans began, had already endorsed the notion of managed competition as the only viable answer, and as a result gave little coverage to reform plans such as a single-payer plan, despite the fact that over seventy House members co-sponsored this plan. Similarly, the "town hall" meetings on television tended to have unbalanced representation of different viewpoints. Finally, it was clear that the mass media readily became a tool to be used by political advertisers willing to pay big bucks to run advocacy ads favoring or opposing different reform plans. Not only did the mass media not act as watchdogs scrutinizing health reform ads for their accuracy and exposing false claims, but the media provided political advertisers free additional exposure by reporting and discussing these ads as clever marketing gimmicks worthy of treatment as news in their news shows.

Finally, our analysis also suggests that there is a relationship between the media agenda and the public agenda. The mass media agenda seems to influence the public agenda, that is, more health reform coverage seems to be associated with more people perceiving health care as an important issue facing the country. Yet it is quite possible that the public agenda influences the media agenda, that is, as more and more people think of health care as an important issue, the media increase their coverage of health care stories. Furthermore, it also appears that the high frequency of presidential speeches on a given subject may translate into more news coverage on that topic, that is, presidential agenda influencing mass media agenda. We have not attempted to establish and thus do not make any claims to causal relationship, that is, whether one causes the other. The relationship between these factors tends to be bidirectional, with each influencing the other.

7 PUBLIC OPINION AND HEALTH CARE POLICY

> The ethical imperative that government heed the opinion of the public has its origins, thus, in democratic ideology as well as in the practical necessity that governments obtain the support of influential elements in society. (Key 1961, 4)

> Americans are deeply ambivalent toward reforming government involvement in health care: they are simultaneously supportive of significant reform and uneasy about expanding the government's role. (Jacobs 1993, 629)

Democracy is a Greek word meaning rule by the people. It means that government operates on the basis of consent of the governed and the governed have some role in making decisions. The original form of democracy, direct democracy, began with the ancient Greek city-states, such as Athens. Citizens would meet and vote on policy decisions (Hudson 1995). In the United States, New England town meetings and Congregational churches, both dating back to colonial times, embodied direct democracy. Voting mechanisms, such as the initiative and the referendum, developed during the Progressive era in the early years of the twentieth century, are more current forms of direct democracy. One important implication of the idea of democracy is that the majority of the people should be able to have its way.

The United States, however, is not a direct democracy. Despite the existence of the initiative and referendum, the system created by the Founding Fathers in 1787 made clear efforts to limit democracy as they understood it. Their understanding of democracy was the direct form: the people themselves should rule. But the Founders were largely fearful that such a political system would not last long and did not trust the judgment of the common person. They were particularly concerned about what they saw as the irresponsible behavior of the state legislatures as being overly responsive to the wants of the people and not the needs of the political system and the economy (Dye and Zeigler 1987; Hudson 1995). They were also distressed by the weakness of the national government set up by the Articles of

Confederation. So the problem was twofold: limit what they saw as the tyranny of the majority, and at the same time establish a national government that could rule effectively.

The Constitution of 1787 dealt with both problems. First, it gave the national or federal government substantially more, though limited, powers and ability to act than it had under the Articles of Confederation. The Constitution was written in such a fashion that the powers of the federal government could grow, largely through the "necessary and proper" clause of Article I.

At the same time, it created a representative form of government, known variously as indirect democracy, representative democracy, or a republic. The essential idea was to limit direct participation by the population or the masses. This was done through several mechanisms.

The Constitution provided for the indirect election of the president through the electoral college. Voters in presidential elections actually vote for a slate of electors pledged to a candidate, rather than for the candidate himself. The original Constitution gave the power to elect senators to the state legislatures. It was not until 1913 with the passage of the Seventeenth Amendment that direct election of U.S. senators was allowed. The only representatives that the people could originally vote directly for were congressmen for the U.S. House of Representatives.

Thus, as far as the federal government was concerned, the major role for the people was to vote for representatives (sometimes directly, sometimes indirectly). This was also largely true at the state and local levels. Elected officials were to make decisions with the good of the people in mind. That, at least, was the theory.

But an indirect democracy is nevertheless a democracy. The will of the people, the consent of the governed, with due regard for the rights of minorities, was still to have some force. The question that remained was how elected officials were to know that will.

The obvious mechanism is elections. But elections come only on an infrequent though regular basis: every two years for the House of Representatives, every four years for the presidency, and every two years on a rotating basis for the Senate. Members of the federal judiciary are appointed for life (nominated by the president and confirmed by the Senate). Further, as we see, the meaning of elections is not always obvious. Elected officials can claim a mandate to undertake one policy or another, but mandates seldom emerge clearly. This was the case for the presidential elections of 1992 (and the 1991 special senatorial election in Pennsylvania) and for the 1994 congressional elections that produced Republican majorities in the House and Senate.

There are other mechanisms by which the population can let its elected representatives know its desires. Protests and marches may be used. Another is through membership in interest groups, discussed in chapter 5. Constituents can directly contact their representatives through letters, electronic mail, faxes, phone calls, and so forth. But group membership and direct contact seldom represent the public as a whole or give a sense of what a majority of the public wants. To get a feel for what the public as a whole wants requires some other mechanism. That mechanism is the public opinion poll.

Polling

Public opinion polling, undertaken to gain a sense of where the public stands on issues and candidates, has a long history in the United States. Newspapers in the early nineteenth century tracked public support for presidential candidates and in the early twentieth century conducted straw polls among their readers (Light 1997). Modern scientific public opinion polling has its origins in the 1930s, and by the 1960s played an increasingly important role in American political life.

The other major mechanism for understanding public opinion is the focus group. Originally developed for commercial advertising ("Madison Avenue"), a focus group is a small group of people who are brought together to react to and discuss issues and ads. While a public opinion survey provides a broad view of where the public stands on an issue, survey instruments preclude a detailed understanding of the reasons behind those views. Focus groups provide the detailed understanding but sacrifice the breadth. Both public opinion surveys and focus groups played important roles in health policy debates.

One important consistent finding of public opinion surveys is the low level of knowledge about politics and public policy among the general public. Most Americans have little knowledge of the basic facts of American political life and are often misinformed about public policy (see "Details of Constitution Escape Many" 1997; Patterson 1997). This is true in health care as well.

An important question, then, is how to take account of public opinion, given the massive level of ignorance and relatively low levels of political participation (see Times Mirror Center for the People and the Press 1993a). One could argue that public opinion should be ignored because of ignorance, indifference, and inconsistency in policy preferences. Such a conclusion would be unwarranted.

Scholars such as Benjamin Page, Robert Shapiro (Page and Shapiro

1992; Page 1994), and James Stimson (1991; Stimson, MacKuen. and Erikson 1994) have argued that the public, taken as a whole, has clear preferences, often based on deeply held values, and is rational in its opinions. What these scholars have done is to aggregate public opinion over time. They find stability in preferences and change occurring when the public is presented with information. Page and Shapiro (1992, 1) argue that "collective public opinion has properties quite different from those of the opinions of individual citizens, taken one at a time."

Stimson (1991) found that collective public opinion is orderly and meaningful and has structure. He defines *policy mood* as "shared feelings that move over time and circumstance . . . changing *general* dispositions" (Stimson 1991, 18). He found that the policy mood of the American public was becoming more liberal toward the end of the 1980s.

In a later piece, Stimson, MacKuen, and Erikson (1994) define the problem of representativeness and responsiveness of political leaders to the general public by pointing out that the public has preferences at a fairly general level, but that policy makers have to deal with the details of policy proposals and public programs.

Policy Congruence

Given these notions of policy mood and collective public opinion, we can raise the vital question of the relationship or congruence between public policy and public opinion. This is, after all, one of the key ideas of representative democracy, that our elected officials be responsive to the public or the governed.

Several scholars have addressed this issue (Monroe 1979, 1983; Jacobs and Shapiro 1997; Page and Shapiro 1992). Monroe (1979) found an overall consistency of 64 percent between public opinion and public policy. When the public wanted to maintain public policies as they are (maintain the status quo), the consistency rose to over 76 percent. When the public wanted change, consistency fell to about 60 percent. Monroe also found that when an issue was of considerable importance to the public (salience was high), consistency was higher than among policies for which salience was low. Thus Monroe's data suggests much of what we have discussed in previous pages. First, there is a bias against change. This does not mean that change is not impossible, merely that it is difficult. Second, those preferences held most strongly are likely to produce some policy coherence. Wilson's (1980) theory of regulation, focusing on the distribution of costs and benefits, as discussed in chapter 5, supports this finding.

In a later study, Monroe (1983) found that political party platforms were generally consistent with public opinion preferences. Both parties took positions that were frequently harmonious with public opinion, though Monroe points out that the Democratic Party was slightly more likely to take stands in favor of change when public opinion opposed change than was the Republican Party. He also found that Democrats were closer to the public on economic and welfare issues than Republicans.

Page and Shapiro (1992) established that public policy often corresponded with public opinion and that changes in public opinion are followed by changes in policy about two-thirds of the time. Jacobs and Shapiro (1997; see also Morin 1997) found that policy congruence varied over time. During the Great Depression/World War II period, policy congruence was about 64 percent. It declined to about 54 percent during the 1960s and reached a peak of about 75 percent during the 1970s.

They then examined policy congruence in more recent periods: the second Reagan administration, the Bush administration, and the Clinton administration (through 1995). They found that policy congruence declined during this period: 67 percent during the second Reagan administration, 40 percent during the Bush administration, and between 26 and 36 percent during the Clinton administration, depending on what was included. Jacobs and Shapiro do not conclude, however, that elected officials at the national level became unresponsive to public opinion. They noted, as we discussed in chapter 4 on Congress, that the latter months of the 104th Congress (1996) saw legislation that the public wanted, including health care. So while policy congruence may have declined in the 1990s, the desires of the public remain important. We return to this issue later.

One important issue that needs to be addressed is why public opinion or policy mood changes. Page and Shapiro (1992) contend that collective public opinion changes when "circumstances," such as the state of the economy, changes. Durr (1993) likewise notes that economic expectations will move policy sentiment ("policy mood" in Stimson's terms). He argues that as economic expectations increase, the economy is growing and the outlook is good, then public sentiment is more likely to support a liberal agenda. He, like Stimson (1991; Stimson, MacKuen, and Erikson 1994), finds a public increasingly supportive of liberal policy initiatives. Conversely, of course, when economic expectations decline, policy sentiment becomes more conservative. Durr also contends that the more intrusive government becomes, the more domestic policy sentiment declines as well (see also Samuelson 1995a). The view of the public toward government is one we shortly address. We also see that a counter to Durr's argument about economic expectations and policy sentiment, at least in the health care area, is possible.

The remainder of this chapter covers four areas. First, we explore public opinion on health care in the years prior to 1993. This gives us some basis for looking at what the public wanted and how it viewed health care problems in the United States. Second, we look at public opinion during 1993–94 when comprehensive health care reform was on the policy agenda. Next we consider public opinion during the latter period of budget battles, proposed cuts in Medicare and Medicaid, and passage of health insurance reform. We end the chapter with observations about the role of public opinion in policy debates.

Laying the Foundation: Public Opinion Prior to 1993

The United States is the only major Western industrialized country without some version of a national health care system (Skocpol 1995). For strong advocates of a welfare state, health care remains the one major failure (see Marmor, Mashaw, and Harvey 1990). National health insurance had been on the policy agenda several times before 1993, only to fail each time (see Patel and Rushefsky 1995; Starr 1982). Much of the blame for this failure was laid at the feet of interest groups, particularly the American Medical Association (AMA) (see Starr 1982). But where does the public stand on health policy issues? The answer, it turns out, is quite illuminating.

Looking at data that in some cases goes back to the 1930s, it can be seen that there was a high level of support for national health insurance. An early poll by the Gallup organization in 1938 found over 81 percent of the public favored government being responsible for the health care of those who could not afford that care (Yankelovich 1995). During the Truman administration, 50 percent of those surveyed supported national health insurance, until the AMA's blistering attacks (Page and Shapiro 1992). The public supported spending more money on health care, helping, in particular, those without private health insurance. To the public, health care was a right, an entitlement. This public support for a federal role in health care remained strong and consistent into the 1990s (Bowman 1995; Yankelovich 1995).

A second set of findings from the public opinion data and literature is also enlightening. First, the public, by and large, is satisfied with the quality of health care it receives. It is not as certain, however, about the quality of care that other people have. Nor was the American public as satisfied with their health care as people were in other countries (Blendon and Donelan 1991). Related to this was a growing sense of crisis in the health care system and the need for change as we approached 1992. By 1992, a clear majority of those surveyed felt that the health care system should be completely rebuilt (Bowman 1994; Yankelovich 1995). Support for change was present and growing. The question is why.

The answer appears to be economic anxiety. The 1990–91 recession brought growth to a temporary halt and, combined with cutbacks in large corporations ("downsizing"), resulted in a decline in the number of workers covered by private health insurance. In 1980, over 65 percent of the population were totally insured through the private sector; by 1991, that figure dropped to a little over 60 percent (Patel and Rushefsky 1995).

Related to the drop in private health insurance coverage was apprehension about maintaining health insurance in the event that a job switch occurred. This was the issue of portability of insurance coverage that eventually produced legislation in 1996.

That anxiety showed itself in the 1991 special senatorial election in Pennsylvania. Harris Wofford, the victorious Democrat, campaigned on the issue of health security. His most effective television ad stated that if people had the right to a lawyer, they should have the right to health care. Wofford's campaign transformed the health care issue into an economic issue, in this case economic insecurity (Altman 1995). Wofford's unexpected victory convinced Bill Clinton and President George Bush that health care was an important issue to the public (Jacobs and Shapiro 1995).

Consultants for Wofford found concern among members of focus groups about costs and access. Wofford then aired his commercial about a right to lawyer/right to doctor, and his victory signaled the importance of the issue. Consultants for Wofford worked for Clinton in 1992 and helped shape an emphasis on health care. Indeed, those who supported Clinton felt that national health insurance was a particularly important (salient) issue. There was clear and strong support for broadening health insurance to cover the entire population with a government guarantee of coverage and strong strong support for a Canadian type of system (Jacobs 1993). The growing support for doing something about health care reform was part of a larger trend within public opinion, moving toward more liberal policies and favoring a more activist government (Durr 1993; Schlesinger and Lee 1993; Stimson 1991).

The Public's View of the Health Care Problem

As promising as these trends were for advocates of comprehensive reform, there were also considerable warning signs. The contrary major indications were, first, what the public perceived as the cause of health care problems as well as their definition of what those problems were and, second, the public's view of government.

If the public, as measured by surveys and focus groups, was going to influence debates over health care reform in the 1990s, then it became important to understand how the public understood the problems of the health care system. It was equally important that those involved in the debate, policy experts and policy makers, comprehended the public's viewpoints. And, if the experts' and policy makers' understanding of health care problems and needed reforms differed from public understanding, then support for public policy initiatives might be lacking. This turns out to have been very much the case.

One of the most careful and targeted studies of the public's view of health care was conducted in 1991 and 1992 by the Public Agenda Foundation (Johnson and Kernan-Schloss 1992). Its report, with the alarming title of *Faulty Diagnosis: Public Misconceptions about Health Care Reform,* utilized both national surveys and fifteen focus groups in different parts of the country. The authors of the report wrote that the debate over health care reform in the early 1990s was taking place among leaders but at the same time the public was confused:

> But among the public, confusion, misunderstanding, fear, frustration, scapegoating, and wishful thinking characterize a discussion poised to go nowhere. While Americans care deeply about this issue and bring an important perspective and list of concerns, most approach health care from a radically different starting point than do leaders. (Johnson and Kernan-Schloss 1992, 2)

The study found that leaders and the public saw the same health care problems, though the problems were not defined in the same way by the two groups, nor were the causes of those problems seen in the same way. The major problems seen were cost and access to care.

For leaders and experts, the cost problem was that the country was spending too much on health care. For the public, the problem was that their own costs were too high. The Public Agenda report said that the public overestimates what they pay and underestimates what national health care costs are. The public was also not aware of the indirect costs of health care, such as higher taxes and lower wages.

The second health care problem is access to health insurance. For leaders and experts, the problem is seen as employees in companies that do not provide health insurance and people who cannot afford health insurance but make too much to qualify for Medicaid (the working poor and their dependents). By contrast, the public thinks that the elderly and very poor have no coverage, when in fact, as the Public Agenda report pointed out, these are the two groups covered by government programs (Medicare and Medicaid). This is a nice example of what the report labels the misperceptions of the public about health care.

Another question asked leaders and the public why health care costs were rising. Leaders and experts offered a set of explanations: defensive medicine, duplication of services, aging of the population, new technology, and the health impacts of drugs and crime. The public had a much different perspective. Health care costs were rising because of waste, fraud and greed, blaming providers, malpractice lawyers, and pharmaceutical companies seeking high profits. To the public, there is a *"profits* problem, not a *costs* problem" (Johnson and Kernan-Schloss 1992, 4). A related aspect was that leaders saw the need to limit the development and expansion of technology; the public, with its emphasis on greed and waste, refused to think about limiting technology (Johnson and Kernan-Schloss 1992, p. 4; for a discussion of waste and fraud in Medicare, see Serafini 1997a; for a discussion of waste and fraud in health care in general, see Sparrow 1996)

A further question addressed the role of the elderly as a contributor to the cost problem. To experts and leaders, the demographic inevitability of an aging population is a significant problem, leading to a disproportionate amount of spending on the elderly. The public does not see aging as a cause of increased health care costs, nor does it wish to consider the implications of an aging population (though see "Special Issue: Ageism on the Agenda" 1997).

While leaders and experts agreed among themselves on a definition of national health insurance ("universal system paid for by taxes covering a majority of health care costs for every citizen"), they disagreed on whether national health insurance (NHI) was necessary (Johnson and Kernan-Schloss 1992, 5). As other polls have repeatedly shown, the public strongly supports (75 percent in this study) NHI. But only about a third of the public defined such a program the same way that leaders did. Many of those polled thought that national health insurance would be optional or would not be the responsibility of the federal government.

Finally, the public was unfamiliar with a major proposal that was part of the health care reform debates in 1991 and 1992: play or pay.

Johnson and Kernan-Schloss (1992) observe that because the public's view of the problems are related to inefficiency, greed, and profits, they support changes reducing profits in the system but not those that would reduce the quality or the quantity of care they receive from the system. With that kind of mindset, they write, the public is unlikely to support any reform that would result in higher costs or higher taxes or reduce access to the system. Sacrifice, in other words, would find little appeal among the public.

The Public's View of Government

Recall what national health insurance is. It is a program of universal coverage paid for by taxes. There are a variety of different ways of running a national health insurance system, ranging from a system where the national government owns health care facilities and providers are government employees to one that mandates that private employers cover employees and government covers those missed by the private insurance network (White 1995). Whatever the system, expanding access to health care and controlling costs would inevitably require an enhanced role for government. Given this requirement, the view of the public toward government would be critical as a base of support for or opposition to comprehensive health care reform. To say the least, the public does not have much confidence in government, especially the federal government.

Public opinion surveys ask questions relating to trust, efficacy, and governmental responsiveness. Typical trust questions ask whether the respondent thinks government will do the right thing, whether taxes are wasted, whether government is run for the benefit of a few or for the benefit of all the people, and whether those running government are mostly crooks. Efficacy and responsiveness refer to whether people think government pays attention to their views. As Figure 7.1 shows (looking at the 1964 to 1992 period), responses to questions about trust, efficacy, and responsiveness show a dramatically declining faith in government. Political discontent was on the increase (Craig 1993; see also Tolchin 1996).

One major question to ask based on these data is why the decreasing faith in government and increasing political discontent. Samuelson (1995a) offers one explanation. He argues that government leaders in the 1960s made enormous promises that cannot be fulfilled. For example, the rhetoric of the War on Poverty during the Johnson administration implied that government could wipe out poverty. Other social and economic ills would also be eliminated. In addition, Americans have come to expect more from government (and business), what Samuelson calls an "age of entitlements." Samuelson asserts that while things have gotten better, the perception is one of unfulfilled expectations and failed government (see Schwarz 1988). With government's perceived failure, faith in government diminished.

Samuelson's argument, however, lacks empirical support; that is, he provides little data to back up his major assertion. Craig does provide that support. Utilizing the American National Election Study, he finds that political discontent is partially a result of perceived inconsistencies between one's political values and government policies (see Craig 1993). In other words, people see a lack of policy consistency between public demands and government policy. The literature discussed above suggests that such policy coherence varies during different administrations.

But Craig and others suggest that something related to policy consistency is also going on: political leaders are not listening to citizens; representative

Figure 7.1 **Trends in Trust, Responsiveness and Efficacy, 1976–1992**

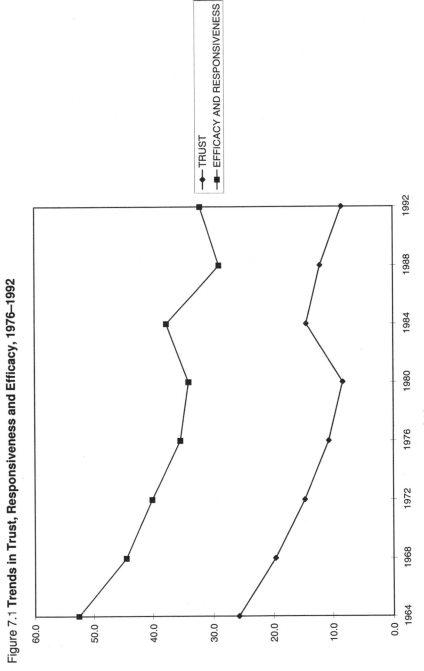

Source: Calculated from Craig (1993), pp. 11 and 13.

government is no longer working. The Kettering Foundation concluded, based on a series of focus groups conducted in 1990 and 1991 (when economic anxiety appeared to reach a peak), that the country was undergoing

> a widespread public reaction against the political system. This reaction is more than the familiar attacks on individual politicians, incumbents, big government, party politics and corruption. It is a reaction against a political system that is perceived as so autonomous that the public is no longer able to control and direct it. People talk as though our political system has been taken over by alien beings. . . .
>
> Americans . . . describe the present political system as impervious to public direction, a system run by a professional political class and controlled by money, not by votes. What is more, people do not believe this system is able to solve the pressing problems they face. (Kettering Foundation 1991, iii–iv; quoted in Craig 1993, 83)

This declining support for political leaders may have led to an increasing reliance on direct democracy mechanisms such as the initiative and referendum at state and local levels, tax limitation amendments to state constitutions, term-limitation ballots, the desire for new leadership (Ross Perot and Colin Powell), and Republican victories in 1994 (at the state and congressional levels).

Tolchin (1996) makes a more assertive claim. Where Samuelson says that Americans are discontent and Craig sees rising levels of cynicism and mistrust, Tolchin sees, simply, angry voters:

> "Anger" has become the political watchword of the 1990s: Leaders from parties worry about the absence of civility, the decline of intelligent dialogue, and the rising decibels of hate in political discourse. Polls reveal that Americans are angrier at government than at any time in recent memory. Disputes that traditionally gravitate toward centrist compromises instead move to opposite extremes, where they divide into intransigent stances. A political form of bipolar disorder has emerged that is a symptom as well as a cause of anger. At peace for the first time in almost a century, Americans question the legitimacy of their own democracy. They are "mad as hell," and political leaders constantly ask why. (Tolchin 1996, 3)

This new atmosphere affected the elections of 1992 (the Clinton victory and the Perot campaign) and 1994 (Republican victories) and led to numerous retirements from Congress.

Tolchin sees this anger based on several legs. Like Samuelson, Tolchin sees an entitlement mentality as part of the problem. The reality of government benefits has not met public expectations. High taxes (or at least the perception of high taxes), a chronic issue in American politics (see Makin and Ornstein 1994), are also a factor. People see their taxes going up (at all levels of American government) but do not see any connection between those taxes and their well-being. George Bush's very public promise in his 1988 acceptance speech at the Republican National Convention that he would not raise taxes lasted a scant two years and was likely a contributing factor to his defeat in 1992.

Tolchin also identifies economic anxiety as a factor in increasing voters' anger. The recession of 1990–91 helped develop this issue and the downsizing of corporations in the 1990s continued to fuel it. Stagnant or declining wages and increased income inequality were also factors (Rushefsky 1996), as was the globalization of trade.

Another factor Tolchin identifies is a cultural divide, a cultural war. This was the values issue that seemed to take prominence in the early 1980s and at least through the 1994 elections (Aaron, Mann, and Taylor 1994; Hunter 1991). This, along with economic insecurity, helped fuel the growth of talk radio, perhaps the nation's most utilized outlet of political discontent and anger.

Summarizing Public Opinion

The above discussion focused on several dimensions of public opinion that laid the foundation for the policy battles of 1993–94 and 1995–96. First, health care is important to the public, which supported greater spending for health care. But people also want to maintain the quality of their care (which they rate quite highly) and were unlikely to approve of policies that would raise their taxes, curtail their choice of doctor, or in some other way decrease the benefits or quality of care they receive. The public identified health care problems as largely due to greed and waste; thus any changes in the health care system could, in a sense, be self-financing. Greater sacrifice would be unnecessary. Nor was the public likely to support a federally run system. Page and Shapiro noted that the public prefers the mixed system we have now with the role of government limited to where "government oversees, regulates, and perhaps subsidizes or acts as a provider of last resort" (Page and Shapiro 1992, 121). They warned, in 1992, not to read too much into public support for reform.

A second, related lesson from the above discussion was the growing distrust of government. That distrust of government in general would translate into repudiation of any complex program that would appear to change the health care system. Republicans would thus have a solid base for their opposition to Clinton's Health Security Act or any other similar proposal.

A third lesson from public opinion polls and focus groups was ignored by congressional Republicans in 1995–96. The public likes entitlement programs, especially Medicare and Medicaid (the former more than the latter perhaps, but Medicaid pays for a substantial portion of nursing home expenses). Perceived attempts to cut those programs to balance the budget or reduce the size of government would thus not find public support.

But a fourth lesson was finally absorbed by both Republicans and Democrats. The public was anxious about the security of its health insurance and the rationing implied by managed care. Faced with the looming 1996 elections, politicians from both parties would eventually be responsive to the public's demands.

Public Opinion and Comprehensive Health Care Reform, 1993–94

Drafting the Health Security Act

The first question we can ask is the extent to which the Clinton Health Security Act was crafted with public opinion in mind. We have seen previously that much of the proposal was developed with the purpose of gaining the support of interest groups. For example, while the plan had an employee mandate, it also called for a sliding scale of subsidies aimed at smaller businesses. It also sought to cover early retirees and lift the burden of paying for health insurance from large employers.

Several elements of the proposal had public opinion in mind, or at least would seem likely to garner public support. One element addressed taxation. Covering the entire population would inevitably require additional spending. The question was how to raise the revenue. The public had clearly shown a dislike for additional taxes; President Bush had been defeated for reelection partly because of taxes, and states were facing various forms of tax revolts. Further, Democrats have been continuously labeled by Republicans as "tax and spend" liberals (see Edsall and Edsall 1991). The big deficit-reduction agreement between President Clinton and the Democratically controlled Congress (the agreement had little Republican support) contained tax increases, though many of them targeted at the upper-income classes. Another large tax increase, even if for expanded health care coverage, would have lost public support. The Clinton task force chose, therefore, to rely on increased taxes on cigarettes, a "sin tax" that was much more popular than income taxes (Skocpol 1996).

A second part of the Clinton plan that was designed to appeal to the public had to do with cost control. Cost control was one of the six major principles of the Health Security Act, and public opinion polls identified health care costs as a major public concern. But as we have seen, for the public, the concern was not the overall level of spending, that national health expenditures were too high; if anything, the public thought we spent too little on health care. Instead, the public was concerned about increased health care costs to themselves. Further, the public did not think that federal regulation would be able to control costs (Johnson and Kernan-Schloss 1992). As Skocpol (1996) pointed out, the Clinton administration sought a path of cost control that would involve less overt federal regulation. The authors of the Health Security Act hoped that managed competition (competition among organized groups of providers, insurers, purchasers, etc.) would be sufficient to control health care costs. As a backup measure, the act called for a cap or limit on increases in insurance premiums. Controlling the cost of health insurance would appeal, presumably, to a public concerned by personal health care expenses.

There was a third element to the Health Security Act that should have appealed to the public. The public likes the ability to choose providers (Blendon and Donelan 1990). The Clinton plan required that subscribers be offered a choice of at least three plans: a managed care, health maintenance organization type plan; a fee-for-service plan that would preserve choice of providers though be more expensive than the managed care plan; and a mixed plan. In other words, the Clinton plan maintained the freedom of provider choice so cherished among the public. ABC News/*Washington Post* polls in September 1993 and February 1994 demonstrated this support. Given a choice between an inexpensive plan that does not allow choice of provider and a more expensive plan those does, the public overwhelmingly selected the more expensive plan (58 percent to 32 percent in September and 62 percent to 26 percent in February) (Bowman 1994). The public's awareness of this was another question.

The Ups and Downs of Public Support

Public opinion in early 1993 was optimistic about the prospects for health care reform during the Clinton administration. A Gallup poll found that 68 percent of those sampled were sure that President Clinton could make health care available and affordable to the entire population. ("Clinton: How Will Handle Specific Problems" 1993). The Gallup poll showed that the confidence in the new president (the poll was taken prior to Clinton's 1993 inauguration) was across the board. Majorities of Democrats, Republicans, and independents expressed that confidence (though only a slim majority of Republicans took that choice). Those who voted for Perot also expressed confidence, though a majority of those voting for George Bush in 1992 were not so confident.

Similarly, when President Clinton appointed his wife to head the health care reform task force, a large majority (59 percent) approved of the appointment. An even larger majority (75 percent) said that the appointment either gave them more confidence that the Clinton administration would be able to reform the health care system or that it did not affect their views ("Hillary Clinton and Health Care Task Force" 1993).

One could detect in the polls public momentum building for health care reform. The Gallup poll regularly asks the public what they think is the most important problem facing the United States. The economy is generally rated the number-one problem. But among noneconomic problems, health care made a dramatic increase, even faster than that perennial favorite, crime. In November 1991, 6 percent of the public polled listed crime and health care as the most important problem. By March 1992, 5 percent picked crime and 12 percent picked health care. In January 1993, 18 percent selected health care and 9 percent picked crime. By September 1993, the month that Clinton made his health care reform address to Congress, 28 percent picked health care and 16 percent picked crime. The 28 percent figure for health care was also higher than for any specific economic problem (Newport 1993).

The President's September 1993 speech was a major success, at least as far as the public was concerned. Fifty-nine percent of those polled favored the president's plan, and 56 percent approved of how he was handling his job as president (see Figures 7.2 and 7.3). This was a 10 percent increase over the previous poll taken about two weeks earlier and the highest approval level for the president since February. The health care speech seemed to spill over into other areas, as the president's approval of handling the economy and foreign affairs also increased. A majority of the public wanted health care reform; 52 percent said that the health care system was unsound and needed major changes, and another 21 percent said the system was unsound and should be rebuilt (Newport and Moore 1993). The public was more interested in the Clinton plan than in other news stories in September and thought that universal coverage was the most important aspect of the Clinton plan (Times Mirror Center, October 1993). These results would seem to be very encouraging for the administration.

Lurking within the same Gallup poll, however, were intimations that while the public wanted change, they were not completely sold on the Clinton approach. Eighty percent of the respondents felt that the Clinton plan did not have enough financing to cover everybody (and provide new benefits), and 51 percent thought they would pay more for their health care as a result of the Clinton plan. When the Gallup pollsters asked respondents whether Congress should accept the Clinton plan as proposed or make major changes first, only 23 percent said pass as is, while 54 percent said

Figure 7.2 **Percentage Approving Clinton Presidency**

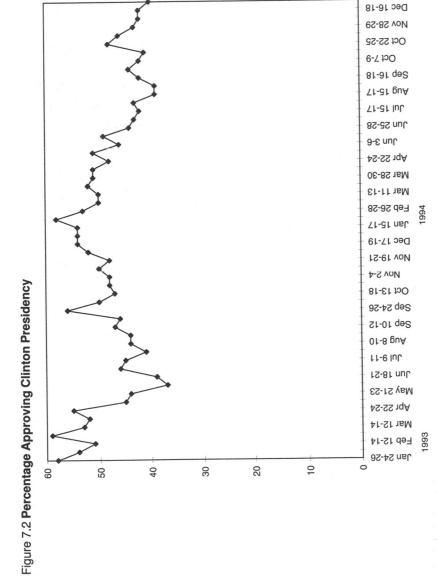

Source: Gallup Polls.

228

Figure 7.3 **Percentage Approving Health Security Act**

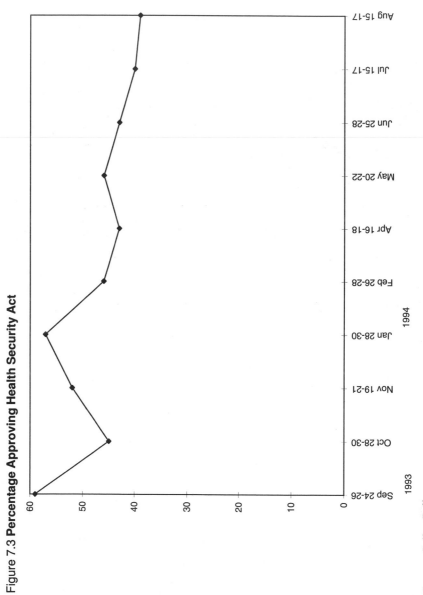

Source: Gallup Polls.

make major changes first. In February and September 1993, Gallup asked the public whether the Clinton plan would solve the problems of the health care system. In February, 61 percent said it would; by September, right after Clinton's speech, only 50 percent thought so. What was going on?

One possibility is that, as we have seen, the assault on the Clinton plan began before the Clinton speech. It is possible that attacks such as the "Harry and Louise" ads sponsored by the Health Insurance Association of America had an impact. We return to this issue below.

Another possibility is raised by Bowman (1995). She notes that Clinton's support increased after his September 1993 speech. But she interprets this to mean support for the speech (acknowledging concern) rather than for the specific plan.

By October 1993, one could see weaknesses in public support for the Clinton variety of health care reform. The Gallup poll showed that 57 percent of the public thought the United States as a whole would benefit from the Clinton plan, but only 28 percent thought they would benefit personally. About 40 percent thought the plan was directed at the poor. More alarming for the Clinton administration, support for the plan dropped from 59 percent in September to 45 percent in October. The public now thought it unlikely (by a two-to-one margin) that Clinton would be able to solve the country's health care problems. Clinton's job approval rating also declined, from 56 percent just after the September speech to 47 percent by mid-October (Newport and Saad 1993). People also had concerns about costs to them and about the preservation of choice (Times Mirror Center 1993b).

A majority of those polled in October 1993 still supported guaranteeing health care to the entire population, even if it meant higher taxes. But much of the public saw the plan through the lens of individual self-interest. People thought that, if the Clinton plan passed, their own costs would increase, they would lose some choice of provider, and the quality of their health care would decrease (Newport and Saad 1993).

The year 1994 would not provide more encouragement for the Clinton health care reform effort. By January 1994, the percentage of the public polled that felt confident Clinton would be able to make health care available and affordable to the population was still high (60 percent) but had declined by 8 percentage points since January 1993 (*Gallup Poll Monthly,* January 1994).

Fifty-one percent of the public polled thought that the Clinton speech in September 1993 was more symbolic than serious. The public still wanted reform. A majority thought the health care system faced a crisis. And a large majority (79 percent) was so strongly in favor of guaranteeing coverage that they favored Clinton vetoing a bill that did not guarantee coverage. Still, 55 percent favored Congress passing the bill after making major changes (*Gallup Poll Monthly,* February 1994).

By April 1994, only 43 percent favored the Clinton plan, a decline of sixteen percentage points since September 1993 (Moore 1994a; Blendon, Brodie, and Benson 1995). Some more specific questions asked in autumn 1993 and spring 1994 added detail to the deterioration of support for the Clinton plan. An increasing number of Americans (48 percent in April compared to 42 percent in October) thought the Clinton plan would result in fewer choices of provider. There was an 8 percent increase in the percentage of the public who thought the quality of care would decline as a result of the plan (39 percent compared to 31 percent). A small majority of the public thought health care costs would increase. And whereas in October 1993, 53 percent of the public thought the Clinton plan involved too much government, 63 percent thought so in April 1994 (Moore 1994a; Blendon, Brodie, and Benson 1995).

By June 1994, support for the Clinton plan had dropped to 40 percent. And a majority of the public thought that Congress should consider health care reform over a period of several years and make gradual changes, rather than pass comprehensive reform in 1994 (*Gallup Poll Monthly,* June 1994).

The Gallup polls in June and July 1994 asked some very specific questions about health care reform (*Gallup Poll Monthly,* July 1994). Those who supported the Clinton plan were asked what they liked most about it. The overwhelming choice was guarantee of universal coverage; no other response amassed more than 8 percent of the respondents (*Gallup Poll Monthly,* July 1994).

Those who opposed the plan were asked what they most disliked about it. The responses were more evenly distributed. Twenty-eight percent referred to financial considerations: it cost too much, taxes would increase, hurt small business, disliked employer mandate, would cost jobs and hurt the economy. Eighteen percent picked a variety of choices that could be labeled antigovernment: too much bureaucracy and government involvement. Another 28 percent had problems other than financial or bureaucratic. These included restrictions on choice and that it simply would not work (*Gallup Poll Monthly,* July 1994).

The same poll saw fewer people perceiving the health care system as in crisis and more seeing just problems. Sixty percent of those polled felt they needed more information about the Clinton plan. A very interesting question asked respondents which of a list of groups had a positive or negative effect on the health care reform effort. Sixty-two percent said that the Clinton administration had a positive effect, and 52 percent said that congressional Democrats also had a positive effect. Majorities of respondents thought the following groups had a negative effect on the reform effort: the media, doctors and hospitals, congressional Republicans, insurance companies, and lobbyists and lawyers (*Gallup Poll Monthly,* July 1994).

The public was clear about what it wanted. It wanted guaranteed coverage and cost control. And it thought that cost control was more important than guaranteeing coverage. Americans wanted employers to pick up much of the cost of health care, and there was concern about covering catastrophic illnesses, nursing home care, and prescription drugs (Moore 1994b).

By August 1994, as health care reform was dying in Congress (see chapter 4), the public also turned its back on reform. While the desire for reform remained, the public was clearly moving away from the Clinton plan. Only 39 percent supported the plan. The public did not like any of the congressional Democratic plans and were more concerned (54 percent) that Congress might pass something that would hurt coverage. There was also concern that Congress would pass a bill that would result in too much government involvement in health care (53 percent). Ominously, 53 percent of those polled trusted Congress to reform the health care system; only 26 percent trusted President Clinton to do so. This represented a significant drop in trust for Clinton from October 1993, when 38 percent trusted him, compared to 42 percent who trusted Congress (Saad 1994).

The public was also becoming increasingly supportive of the Republican Party and health care policy. In December 1993, 53 percent of respondents thought the Democrats would do a better job in dealing with health care policy, compared to 32 percent for the Republicans. Forty-eight percent opposed the Democratic alternatives, and more people (45 percent) thought Congress was moving in the wrong direction on health care than thought it was moving in the right direction (41 percent). More people (48 percent) were concerned that Congress might pass something than would be worried if no reform was passed (32 percent) (*Gallup Poll Monthly,* January 1994).

By September 1994, 52 percent of respondents thought Congress was headed in the wrong direction. A month earlier, only 32 percent thought so. Sixty-one percent said that in the coming elections, opposing health care reform would either make voters more likely to vote for candidates (22 percent) or would not make any difference (39 percent). Forty-three percent felt that Congress should make only minor changes, and another 27 percent said to leave the health care system alone (*Gallup Poll Monthly,* September 1994). By October 1994, a majority of respondents, 53 percent, were relieved that Congress had taken no action.

Explaining Public Opinion and Comprehensive Reform

The lack of public support for the Clinton Health Security Act or any of the congressional Democratic alternatives was certainly one factor that led to the defeat of comprehensive health care reform in 1994. The question is why public support was lacking.

One possible explanation can be dismissed: the ad campaigns run by opponents of reform, particularly the Health Insurance Association of America (HIAA). The "Harry and Louise" ads that made such a big splash in the media (news) and caused great consternation in the White House seem to have had little effect on the public.

The "Harry and Louise" ads were developed based on findings of a number of focus groups and several public opinion surveys (West, Heith, and Goodwin 1996). The focus groups were used to help develop the message the ads were meant to emphasize and the set or environment in which "Harry and Louise" would discuss health care reform. West, Heith, and Goodwin (1996) examined three public opinion surveys that asked about health care reform and about the ads. According to a *New York Times*/CBS News survey, about 19 percent of respondents saw the ads, a relatively high number compared to ads from previous political campaigns, but still relatively low. Those who saw the ads did not think they were especially accurate. Only a little more than a third of those seeing the ads were able to identify the ads' sponsor (HIAA). Jamieson's focus-group studies (Jamieson 1994a, 1994b; West, Heith, and Goodwin 1996) likewise found little familiarity with the ads, and some confusion. Further, the focus groups were confused about who "Harry and Louise" were; focus-group members thought they were real people rather than actors. The only apparently significant impact of the ads was that they increased knowledge about health care issues (West, Heith, and Goodwin 1996).

Another possible explanation has considerably more backing: public ignorance. As mentioned at the beginning of this chapter, the public is often ignorant of the details of public policy proposals and issues. It may have a general sense of where it wants to go, but no road map; a number of studies document this statement.

West, Heith, and Goodwin (1996) argue that the polls showed that few people knew much about health care reform or details of plans. They point out, for example, that few among the people knew what health care alliances, an important component of the president's plan, were. The 1992 Public Agenda survey (Johnson and Kernan-Schloss 1992) found that the public had an unrealistic view of the problems of the health care system, one that would make it unlikely that it would accept sacrifice. Yankelovich

(1995) asserts that in effect there was no debate as far as the public was concerned. Our analysis of the media role (chapter 6) supports this statement. We found that the print media, using the *New York Times* and *St. Louis Post-Dispatch* as our examples, tended to focus more on political aspects and less on discussion of problems or policy alternatives. Because much of the public relies on television as its source of news, this trend was exacerbated. The very nature of television news, with its severe time constraints on stories and its emphasis on the dramatic and conflictual, leads it to concentrate on political aspects. Thus the public ignorance over health care issues becomes more understandable. Yankelovich further claims that had there been the kind of public deliberation needed in this kind of public policy debate, the public would have rejected the Clinton plan because it called for changes the public was not prepared to make (we return to this point in the conclusion).

Blendon, Brodie, and Benson (1995) found that a key conflict within the public among three key beliefs helped sink the health care reform, especially the Clinton plan. The three beliefs are support for reform, judging reform on how it personally affected individuals, and growing cynicism about government (discussed above). They further argue, as does Skocpol (1996), that the choices the Clinton team made about reform led to its demise. Skocpol argues that those choices (limited taxes and limited reforms) led the president to choose features that the public would either oppose or not understand (such as health care alliances and managed competition). Blendon, Brodie, and Benson (1996) also point to political or strategic factors that hurt reform. These included foreign policy crises and passage of the North American Free Trade Agreement (NAFTA); the use of a task force that was working behind closed doors and perceived as not engaged in public, open discussion; and the complexity of the plan. Fallows (1995) asserts, however, that none of these elements was important in explaining the failure of the Clinton plan.

One of the more interesting aspects was how the public identified health care reform with President Clinton. Given the importance and publicity candidate and then President Clinton gave to the issue, this was not unreasonable. The problem was that as Clinton became more unpopular, so did *his* health care plan. A *Wall Street Journal*/NBC News poll conducted in March 1994 found that there was considerable public support for elements of the Clinton plan at the same time that public support for that plan was eroding (Stout 1994). The poll found that 76 percent of those surveyed liked (a "great deal" or "some" appeal) a description of the Clinton plan, almost thirty points higher than four proposals circulating in Congress at that time. The kicker was that the plan was not identified as the Clinton plan. Jamieson and Cappella (1994) write that the public was not well informed about the Clinton plan.

We close this section by noting that regardless of confusion or ignorance about health care reform, the public was unlikely to support a massive change of the health care system. As discussed previously, the public saw greed and waste as the prime factors in soaring health care costs and was concerned about those who lacked insurance, the insecurity of those who had insurance, and personal health care costs. To the extent that the Clinton plan, or any other proposal, addressed those issues, it would receive public support. Anything beyond that was unlikely to gain the support needed to counteract the intense interest-group and partisan campaign against reform.

Public Opinion and Health Care: 1995–96

As we have seen, there was support for health care reform in 1993–94. That effort resulted in failure and contributed to the 1994 electoral victories for the Republicans. They now had the policy initiative and would set the agenda. The question is how the public would respond to proposed changes.

The Republican agenda, at least in the House, was contained in their Contract with America (Gingrich et al. 1994), essentially a campaign platform. The Contract, discussed in earlier chapters, called for, among other things, a balanced budget via a balanced budget amendment to the Constitution. Health care programs, such as Medicare and Medicaid, were not mentioned.

An important question is how much support was there for the Contract and the Republican agenda. The Contract was highly publicized and discussed in the media, and a version of it was placed in one of the most heavily read magazines, *TV Guide*. With all that exposure, we might expect public knowledge and perhaps support for the proposed changes. Perhaps Republicans could expect public support for achieving their stated goals.

Unfortunately for the Republicans, the 1994 elections and public opinion provided little evidence for a mandate for those changes. Republicans employed focus groups, not to develop the ideas contained in the Contract, but to come up with catchy slogans that the public would respond to. At first, Republican pollster Frank Lutz claimed that the Contract was the result of polls and focus groups. Later surveys found that some specific elements of the Contract were actually opposed by a majority of the public, and Lutz refined his claim that the provisions of the Contract were test-marketed with focus groups (Morin 1996; Balz and Brownstein 1996; Stone 1995).

Caraley (1996) argues persuasively that there was little if no mandate for the Republicans. The Contract was released in its early form before the election, containing less than a thousand words; the more elaborate book version came out after the November 1994 elections. Neither version said anything about Medicare or Medicaid. Caraley also cites polling data showing that more than 70 percent of respondents had not heard of the Contract. At best, many Republicans were running on a plank to limit or shrink the federal government, general ideas that would occur should the provisions of the Contract be approved. Caraley concludes:

> The results of the 1994 congressional elections could not have been read as a mandate to enact "Contract with America" specifics, since such specifics hadn't been developed by election day and all Republican candidates for the House had not even signed on to the abbreviated document. The results of the 1994 elections were much more a vote of no confidence in the Clinton administration's first two years and no confidence in the Democratic party more generally, because the Democrats had won unified control of the White House and both Houses of Congress for the first time since 1976 but could not deliver an end to gridlock and statement. (Caraley 1996, 240–41; see also Balz and Brownstein 1996; Tolchin 1996)

From a public opinion perspective, Congress and the president saw improved public opinion ratings early in 1995. Clinton's approval rating exceeded 50 percent for the first time since the death of the health reform effort (see Figure 7.4). The approval level for Congress, jumped from 21 percent in October 1994 to 42 percent in February 1995 (Morin 1995).

But ominously, *Washington Post*/ABC News polls held warnings for the Republicans. In December 1994, one month after the November elections, 60 percent of respondents said they had more trust in Congress than in the president to take care of the country's problems. In January 1995, 54 percent selected that choice. In the February poll, that number was down to 46 percent. Clinton's numbers were rising. A further finding was that a majority of respondents thought the Republicans were working against, rather than with, Clinton, while a huge majority thought Clinton was trying to work with the Republicans. Finally, Speaker of the House and architect of the 1994 Republican congressional victories Newt Gingrich (R-Ga.) saw his disapproval ratings soar to almost 50 percent (Morin 1995).

The Republican Congress, especially in the House, sought to enact its agenda. The provisions of the Contract were voted on within the first 100 days of the 104th Congress. But the balanced budget amendment failed to get the two-thirds votes needed in the Senate, and Congress had to provide its own budget to end the deficit. As we have seen, they picked the year 2002 and the major provisions of the budget resolution passed in June 1995 (see chapter 4) called for the balanced budget, $245 billion in tax cuts, $270 billion of spending reductions in Medicare, and $180 billion of cuts in Medicaid spending, among others.

Figure 7.4 **Percentage Approving Clinton Handling of Presidency**

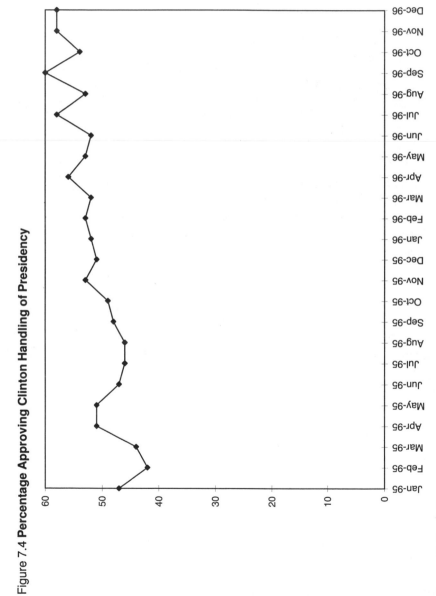

Source: Gallop Polls.

But Republican efforts to cut the Medicare and Medicaid programs (see chapter 4) did not resonate well with the public (Times Mirror Center 1995a). An early 1995 poll conducted for the American Hospital Association by a Republican and a Democratic pollster found that the public strongly supported a balanced federal budget. When asked if they would favor the balanced budget if it meant cuts in Medicare, the public, again by strong majorities, said no. A follow-up question told respondents that under the Republican proposals spending on Medicare would still increase by 50 percent over present (1995) spending levels. Respondents were then asked, given this information, what they would tell their member of Congress. Thirty-six percent chose not to cut Medicare and search for cuts elsewhere in the budget; 25 percent said to allow Medicare spending to keep up with inflation and the growth in the Medicare population; 16 percent favored restraining Medicare growth to the 50 percent increase; and 13 percent said cut Medicare spending (Kolbert 1995).

A May 1995 Gallup poll found that the public still approved efforts to balance the budget and cut spending and even thought that Medicare needed major revision. The public saw financial problems with the Medicare Part A trust fund, but did not want cuts in that program. Fifty-nine percent of those surveyed thought that Medicare was a "special program that shouldn't be cut even if it increases the deficit" (Newport, Moore, and Saad 1995). The public also had more confidence in President Clinton in dealing with Medicare than in congressional Republican leaders (Newport, Moore, and Saad 1995). Clinton's approval rating remained over 50 percent.

By July 1995, the focus on Medicare was assisting Clinton's reelection efforts. The public was asked whether Medicare should be cut to reduce the budget deficit or whether it was more important to prevent significant Medicare cuts. By a 70 to 25 percent margin, the public chose preventing Medicare cuts (though this was actually a closer margin than in an earlier February 1995 poll, 78 percent to 19 percent). The Medicare issue was seen as helping Clinton and hurting the Republican presidential front-runner, Senator Bob Dole (R-Kans.) (Moore 1995a).

The focus on Medicare was clearly having an impact on the public. A study by the Times Mirror Center for the People and the Press found that more people were closely following efforts to reduce Medicare spending (27 percent) than any other story (welfare reform was a close second, 26) (Hernandez 1995; see also Times Mirror Center 1995b). The focus on the budget and Medicare would help Clinton (and to a lesser extent congressional Democrats).

This focus on Medicare was combined with the budget battle between Congress and the president that led to Clinton's vetoing budget bills and eventual shutdowns of the federal government. The public, by and large, supported Clinton. His approval rating climbed to 53 percent, his highest level since January 1994. The November 1995 Gallup poll did show somewhat of a generation gap. The Republican line that the balanced budget was important to reduce later debt payments seemed to resonant with those under thirty, as half that group wanted the president to agree with the Republican budget bills. On the other hand, 59 percent of those between thirty and fifty wanted Clinton to veto the bills, and 64 percent of those over fifty supported the veto (Moore 1995b).

The public was clearly unhappy about the budget standoff and the closing of the federal government. By November 1995, the public had clearly shifted over to the Democrats in the dispute between the two parties, saying that they preferred retaining Medicare to cutting spending to balance the budget, also preferring the Democrats' approach to balancing the budget. But the public saw both Republicans and Democrats using the budget battle as political posturing for the 1996 elections (Saad 1995).

A January 1996 poll produced an interesting result, paralleling the findings of the *Wall Street Journal*/NBC News poll discussed earlier. When presented with budget plans along with the sponsors (Clinton plan and congressional Republican plan), respondents tended to support the plan that fit with their party identification. Forty-three percent preferred the president's proposal to balance the budget (which included smaller cuts in Medicare spending), and 41 percent supported the Republican proposal. This pretty closely mirrored the partisan breakdown (party identification) within the country. When the two proposals were described without mentioning sponsoring, however, the public supported the Clinton plan over the Republican plan, 65 percent to 26 percent (Moore and Saad 1996).

The early 1996 polls indicated the problem that policy issues were raising for Bob Dole. A Gallup poll found that the best predictor of voting choice was a candidate's position on Medicare, followed by the budget deficit and the economy (Moore 1996). As we have seen, the public supported the Clinton positions on the related issues of Medicare cuts and balancing the federal budget; the continued growth of the economy also helped Clinton.

The Democrats and their allies (primarily labor unions such as the AFL-CIO) took advantage of these survey results. The Clinton/Gore team kept repeating their mantra that they wanted to preserve Medicare, Medicaid, education, and the environment. The AFL-CIO and the Democratic Party ran ads against Republican representatives accusing the Republicans of seeking to cut Medicare and the other programs.

Explaining Public Opinion and Entitlement Cutbacks

A major explanation for the failure of the Republican effort to reduce spending (or reduce the rate of increase in spending) in Medicare and Medicaid can be attributed to public opinion. From our discussion in chapter 5, we learned that groups (and presumably the public) strongly support programs already in existence. Defense of public policy, as we said then, is stronger than offense (trying to cut or eliminate programs).

We also saw in this chapter that the public likes Medicare (and to a lesser extent Medicaid, which it tends to identify with welfare). Further, we saw that the public's perception is that the elderly, those covered by Medicare, in fact do not have much coverage. So if the elderly have little health care coverage, cutting back Medicare spending (however it was labeled) would reduce coverage for a group seen as deserving. A further finding is that the public saw the problem of health care spending as mostly greed and waste and therefore sacrifice would not be necessary.

A more recent study reinforces this view of the public and its perceptions (or misperceptions) about Medicare and the budget. The poll, conducted in March 1997, found that the public was largely against cuts in Medicare (and Social Security) and thought that the federal budget could be balanced without touching those two programs. Further, the public agreed with forecasts that both programs would go broke (Medicare considerably sooner than Social Security) but tended to favor solutions that would crack down on abuse and waste. The public seemed unaware that entitlement spending (including these two large programs) constituted over 60 percent of the federal budget. The most interesting finding of this survey was that the public was asked which program constituted the largest area of government spending. Sixty-four percent of respondents selected foreign aid ("Poll Shows Most Against Cuts in Medicare, Social Security" 1997). In reality, less than $20 billion was spent on foreign aid in fiscal year 1997 (about 1.2 percent of the federal budget); by comparison, the federal government spent $210.1 billion for Medicare (about 12.9 percent of the federal budget) and $105.6 billion for Medicaid (about 6.5 percent of the federal budget) for the same fiscal year (see Office of Management and Budget 1996). Add to this that the public largely blamed the Republicans for the two government shutdowns. Given these perceptions, the Republicans had a virtually impossible task of convincing the public that the proposed cutbacks were necessary.

Conclusion

Our trek through public opinion and health care policy leads us to several conclusions. First, the public sees some problems with the health care system and supports increased spending on health care and security of insurance at the same time it supports cracking down on waste and abuse. The public likes the health care it is receiving and does not like change that would hurt the quality or cost of that care. Its understanding of the financial status of the health care system and insurance coverage of the population is flawed, though consistent over time.

This finding explains the failures in our two periods of health care policy making. The attempt at comprehensive health care reform during the first two years of the Clinton administration, 1993–94, was unlikely to gather public support. The public had little understanding of the Clinton plan (for example, perceiving that it would reduce choice of provider) and even less understanding of congressional alternatives. Its perceptions were that the Clinton plan or any comprehensive plan would cost them more and reduce the quality of their care. The Clinton plan in particular was seen as changing a system that the public, by and large, liked. In 1995 and 1996, the Republicans were attempting to reduce spending on Medicare and Medicaid, programs that the public strongly supported. Both sets of proposals, comprehensive reform and program cutbacks, were moving against public sentiment. That sentiment could be seen in pre-1993 public opinion polls. In both cases, moving against public sentiment hurt advocates of change at the polls. It helped fuel the Republican congressional victories in 1994 and helped Clinton win reelection in 1996. It also likely contributed to the decreased Republican majority in the House as a result of the 1996 elections.

A second important conclusion is that the public is ignorant of the details of public policy. This is not a new finding (Page and Shapiro 1992; Stimson 1991), but it does seem to affect public support for policy changes. If people do not see a problem in a given public policy area, it is unlikely to support change that might be perceived as adversely affecting them. This was the case in both periods. The Clinton plan, relatively complex, could be pictured as increasing government bureaucracy and limiting choice. The Republican proposals faced misperceptions about the size of Medicare and Medicaid.

One way to handle this problem is to present the public with information. One interesting suggestion is to make use of deliberative polls, where a group of people are surveyed, then presented with information, discuss that information, and then are polled again. The assumption is that under these conditions, deliberative democracy will lead to more knowledgeable choices (Fishkin 1992). Yankelovich (1995) states that no such deliberative debate occurred in 1993–94, nor would it have made a difference in public support for the Clinton plan. But a small effort at deliberation was made in the health care field in 1993. The Public Agenda Foundation (Immerwahr and Johnson 1994) conducted a series of deliberative sessions in thirteen cities, with nearly 600 participants. Their findings suggest that information and deliberation can cause some change.

Recall the 1997 poll discussed earlier where the public thought that more was spent on foreign aid than on Medicare. In the Public Agenda pretest, the numbers were 72 percent (humanitarian aid) to 18 percent (health care for the elderly). The posttest showed a dramatic reversal, with 44 percent of participants selecting humanitarian aid and 44 percent selecting health care for the elderly. The public was also somewhat more likely to look at structural changes as necessary in the health care system (such as managed care and managed competition) in the posttest. Rationing remained unacceptable and regulating insurance premiums became a bit less acceptable as ways to cut costs. The public viewed employer mandates less favorably after deliberation but showed somewhat increased support for additional income taxes to support expansion of coverage. The view toward government in reforming health care remained negative. Finally, the public does not like bureaucratic health care, as the Clinton administration plan was painted. This might apply to managed care as well (Immerwahr and Johnson 1994). In short, deliberation did produce some change, but probably not enough to support either comprehensive change or entitlement cutbacks.

A third conclusion is one that comes from an intriguing study by Jacobs and Shapiro (1996). They examined the congruence between public policy and public opinion. They found that congruence had decreased, dropping to 36 percent during the Clinton administration. Their conclusion was that our elected officials were not pandering to the public, as some have argued (see King 1997).

But Jacobs and Shapiro went further than looking at the simple congruence of opinion and policy. They interviewed 114 people in Washington, 23 of whom worked in the Clinton administration and 91 of whom were senior congressional staffers. The results of the interviews with the two groups were the same. Both groups said that policy decisions were not driven by public opinion. In the case of the Clinton Health Security Act, the president's pollster, Stanley Greenberg, was not part of the policy formulation or adoption process. Instead, both groups said they looked to public opinion polls and focus groups for ways to sell the policy or frame the issue. So public opinion's role was fairly limited in policy formulation or in voting decisions. Jacobs and Shapiro (1997, p. 8) conclude:

> The pandering politician is a myth; it neither enjoys empirical support nor conforms with the current incentive local and national structure in American politics. The current polarization of Washington policy makers in a divided

national government encourages contending political leaders to focus on directing public opinion to build support for their own ideological or policy goals.

The danger is that the charge of pandering politicians may lead to the erroneous conclusion that the public is to blame ultimately for the ills that afflict America's politics. More leeway, it may be implied, ought to be given to the few who have superior training and knowledge. The evidence suggests, however, that the current state of American politics cannot be blamed on excessive responsiveness to public opinion and insufficient discretion and latitude for political leaders.

Our final conclusion contradicts, to a certain extent, the conclusions of Jacobs and Shapiro (1997) and supports King's (1997) analysis. We argue that the policy results in the health care area conformed fairly closely to the public's desires. The public was against the Clinton plan, as it understood it, and the Clinton plan and other reform proposals failed. The public was against cutbacks in Medicare and Medicaid, and the Republican Congress failed in that attempt (acknowledging that it passed the legislation but could not override the president's veto).

But more important is what did pass in the waning days of the 104th Congress: the Kennedy-Kassebaum bill that provided protection for insurance coverage for people changing jobs (the portability issue) and the legislation mandating coverage of two-day hospital stays for normal maternal deliveries and four-day hospital stays in the event of a cesarean section. A glance at the 1993 and earlier polls shows the public concerned about the quality of care and maintenance of coverage. In other words, facing a looming election in 1996, Congress passed legislation that was popular with the public, if not within the Republican Party. The president signed the legislation. Whether this is pandering will be not addressed here, but it is responsiveness to the public's desires. But we do note that public opinion may set the boundaries for policy changes. The public at large is not capable of, nor is it receiving sufficient information, to address the details of public policy. But it knows what it wants. This is the ultimate lesson of Stimson (1991) and Page and Shapiro (1992). Public opinion sets the boundaries within which policy change may occur.

We leave this exploration of public opinion and health care on one final note. A Louis Harris poll in late 1996 asked the public whether the country would have been better or worse off if the Clinton plan had passed. By a 54–37 percent margin, respondents said better off (Opinion Outlook 1996).

8 POLITICS, POWER, AND POLICY MAKING

The United States remains the only major industrialized nation in the world without a national health insurance system. The failed attempt to adopt comprehensive health care reform and establish a system of affordable health care for all Americans during the 1993–94 reform period stands as yet another tombstone on the long and torturous road to health care reform in the United States in the twentieth century. Previous attempts at comprehensive reform of the U.S. health care system during the Progressive era, the New Deal, and the Fair Deal met a similar fate. The epitaph on the tombstone of the last comprehensive reform effort might as well read "Here lies yet another effort to establish a national health insurance system—1993–94."

The same road to health care reform in the United States in the twentieth century is also marked with several milestones, small as they may be, each representing piecemeal and incremental reforms of the system. The names on these milestones read Medicaid, Medicare, health maintenance organizations (HMOs), certificate of need (CON), Prospective Payment System (PPS) or the Diagnostic Related Groups (DRGs), and the Medicare Catastrophic Coverage Act of 1988. The 1995–96 reform established a few new milestones, notably the Health Insurance Portability and Accountability Act of 1996.

In this book, we have used the efforts to reform the U.S. health care system from 1993 to 1996 to help illustrate and illuminate the role of power and politics in the agenda-setting and policy-making processes. In so doing, we have utilized theories and concepts to help students understand our case studies; indeed, help explain the real world. Agenda setting and policy making in the U.S. political system involve a wide variety of political actors, inside and outside government, made up of individuals, groups, and institutions. These political actors bring their own set of unique attributes to bear on the policy-making process.

At any time, the political system is faced with many issues that demand the attention of policy makers. Not all demands become issues, and not all issues move from the systemic agenda (broad consensus among citizens about issues or problems facing the country at a given point in time) to the institutional agenda (i.e., policy agenda of the government). Not all issues get elevated to the policy agenda of the government because of institutional "gatekeepers." These gatekeepers include powerful actors—individuals, interest groups, mass media, power elites, public opinion, and others—who may help or hinder an issue from getting on the policy agenda.

For an issue to get on the policy agenda of the government, it generally requires an internal or external triggering device, or systemic indicators combined with a focusing event, accompaniment, and feedback that suggest the existence of a problem. The coupling of a problem stream (problem recognition) with that of a policy stream (availability of proposed solutions in the policy community) and a political stream (change in administration, personnel, public opinion, partisan realignment in Congress, etc.) opens a window of opportunity for major policy changes or innovations. As we demonstrated in chapter 2, the merging of the three streams did open a window of opportunity for major reform of the U.S. health care system.

Once a problem gets on the policy agenda, there is no guarantee that it will be acted on by the policy makers. A variety of factors led to the closing of the window of opportunity on the issue of health care reform. The opportunity for major policy innovations in American politics does not come around too frequently, and when it does, it exists only for a short time. In the twentieth century, in the field of health care a window of opportunity for major reforms has come only four times: during the Progressive era of the early twentieth century, during the Roosevelt administration and the New Deal, during the Truman administration and the Fair Deal, and during the Clinton administration from 1993–94. Each time the window of opportunity stayed open only briefly.

Among the various political actors, the president is a major political player in policy agenda setting and policy making. He can set the policy agenda by helping focus the attention of the public and the media on the problems that he perceives to be important. But a president's role in policy making is also ambiguous and full of contradictory expectations. On the one hand, the U.S. Constitution gives the president not only a limited set of powers but it also requires him to share many of those powers with Congress. On the other hand, the president is expected to be a legislative leader, that is, he is expected to propose laws and policies to Congress, and Congress is supposed to deliberate and act on presidential proposals. As president, he is expected to be nonpartisan and to act as a leader of all the people; yet, as leader of his party, he is expected to champion and promote its goals. The American political system combines two different roles—head of state and head of government—into one person, the president. In almost all other countries of the world, these two roles are occupied by two different individuals.

The American political system, with its separation of powers and checks and balances, or coequal branches of government sharing powers, creates a built-in jealousy and competition among the various branches of government for preeminence in policy making. During a period of divided government, when one party controls the White House and the other party controls Congress, chances for successful adoption of programs and policies become even more problematic, requiring careful negotiations, bargaining, and compromise. Even when the same party controls the White House and Congress, there is no guarantee that a president will get what he wants from Congress because of a lack of party discipline, ideological cohesiveness, and decentralized party structure. The president has no formal power to discipline the members of his own party in Congress.

Such limitations on presidential powers and contrary expectations of the president have led some to argue that the president's real power is his power to persuade, and his ability to persuade depends on his reputation in the Washington establishment as a skillful negotiator, his popularity with the general public, and the size of his electoral mandate. Presidents who were successful in bringing about major policy innovations, for example Franklin Roosevelt and the New Deal and Lyndon Johnson and the Great Society, succeeded because they came into office with a large electoral victory and enjoyed considerable public support. Some presidents, such as Ronald Reagan, were able to go to the public and rally strong public support behind their programs and policies. Presidents such as Reagan also used presidential rhetoric and communication skills to their advantage. Furthermore, they undertook major policy initiatives during the traditional honeymoon period between the new president and Congress (first hundred days) when Congress is most likely to be receptive to the new president. Others have suggested that the U.S. political culture, with its strong belief in egalitarian ideology, produces antihierarchical and antileadership sentiments, and that the only way for a president to succeed is to hide or mask his strong leadership and operate more behind the scenes.

With respect to health care reform, President Clinton deserves a great deal of credit for placing the issue of health care reform on the national policy agenda. Nevertheless, he and his administration also deserve considerable blame for several miscalculations and missteps, and for the failure of the Health Security Act of 1993. Clinton's administration got off to a very rocky start. After promising to produce his health care reform plan in the first 100 days, he failed to deliver on it and did not produce the reform plan until September 1993, giving opponents of reform the opportunity to mobilize their resources and attack his plan. President Clinton was also not in a position to persuade and bargain with Congress because he had not won an electoral mandate, having been elected with only 43 percent of the popular vote. In addition, he did not enjoy a very high public approval rating. He also failed to persuade the American public about the need for comprehensive reform because he failed to communicate clear, coherent, and consistent policy goals. Many of these missteps are directly related to his personality and leadership style, which is characterized by a highly ambitious policy agenda that lacks focus and discipline. It was only when he suffered public rebuke and humiliation in the form of the loss of Democratic control of the Congress after more than forty years that he showed some discipline and focus and succeeded in defeating Republican attempts to cut Medicare and Medicaid (including transforming Medicaid into a block grant and turning the program over to the states), and successfully pressured Congress into passing health insurance reforms.

Separation of powers and checks and balances result in competition between the president and Congress for preeminence in policy making, and this often leads to inaction (i.e., gridlock), rather than action, on the part of Congress when it comes to major policy proposals. Furthermore, the two separate chambers, with their own set of rules and the committee and subcommittee structure in Congress, produce overlapping and conflicting jurisdictions that lead to diffusion of power and responsibility. It is much easier to kill a bill than to pass a bill in Congress. Opponents have many opportunities to "kill" a bill. The necessity of winning reelection, the logic of election cycles, dependence on various interest groups and political action committees (PACs) for campaign funds for congressional elections, differing terms of office for Senators and House members, and the ideological and partisan distribution in Congress place a premium on political calculations when it comes to matters of major public policy issues. Congress, especially the Senate with its loose structure and relaxed procedures, is also a slow and deliberative body, which operates at its own pace. Under these conditions, major policy innovations are difficult to accomplish, while small incremental changes resulting from bargaining and compromise are more feasible.

The history of health care reform in the United States illustrates this point. Every attempt at major reform of the U.S. health care system in the twentieth century has failed. Some comprehensive reform proposals never even made it to Congress, while others that did died an agonizing death.

President Clinton's Health Security Act was no exception. This was the most ambitious attempt to overhaul the U.S. health care system and to establish a national health insurance system since the 1940s. At least five major alternative plans, ranging from very liberal to very conservative, emerged to compete with President Clinton's Health Security Act of 1993. A multitude of committees claimed jurisdiction over these competing plans. Partisan and ideological considerations, combined with electoral calculation, made it impossible for any plan to muster a majority. Indeed, not a single plan got voted on in either house of Congress. Democrats in Congress were not united. Liberal, conservative, and moderate Democrats could not find a middle ground to form a united front. Among Republican ranks, some moderate Republicans (more in the Senate than in the House) were willing to work with congressional Democrats in Congress and President Clinton. With the passage of time, however, Republicans came to view opposition and defeat of all major comprehensive reform plans, including the defeat of President Clinton's Health Security Act, as their best strategy for congressional elections in 1994. By the summer of 1994, this position had solidified in the Republican Party, and most Republicans came to accept the view that their best strategy was to not compromise and defeat all health care reform proposals. This strategy paid off for Republicans, and they gained control of both houses of Congress after more than forty years of Democratic dominance. The renewed divided control of government did produce some compromises and bargaining between congressional Democrats, Republicans, and the president, resulting in some incremental health care reforms during 1995–96.

Another important player in the policy-making arena is the interest group. An interest group is a collection of individuals with common interests (economic, political, religious, etc.) that try to protect and promote its interests in the political system. The U.S. Constitution guarantees citizens freedom of speech, expression, the right to peaceful assembly and to petition the government. These rights provide the basis for much of the interest-group activity in the United States. Yet, some of the Founding Fathers were acutely aware of the dangers posed by such interest groups. James Madison, in *Federalist* #10, argued that factions (i.e., interest groups), united by common interest and passion, can undermine democracy by promoting their own narrow and selfish interests at the cost of public interest or the common good. They often promote their narrow or parochial interests using the rhetoric of public interest. Madison recognized the dilemma of factions confronting a democratic society. On the one hand, you cannot eliminate faction because to do so would destroy the very democratic principle on which the nation was founded (i.e., freedom). On the other hand, factions can engage in devilment. The answer, according to Madison, was to control the mischief of factions. More than 200 years later, we are still confronted with the issue of mischief played out by factions in our democratic system.

As our examination of the role of interest groups (i.e., factions) during the health care reform debate suggests, they played a very crucial role in shaping public perception and opinion and, thus, the direction of health care reform. Interest groups were very active in their support or opposition to the various health care reform proposals. They also spent a considerable amount of time, money, and energy in attempts to influence the outcome of various alternative reform proposals. During the 1993–94 health care reform period, a number of interest groups worked feverishly to defeat President Clinton's Health Security Act because they concluded that the adoption of such a reform would work against their economic interest. These groups used a variety of tactics—political advocacy ads on television and radio, astroturf lobbying, cross-lobbying, and reverse lobbying, along with campaign contributions—to influence the policy-making process. They succeeded in defeating any health care reform. During 1995–96 interest groups such as the American Association of Retired Persons (AARP) and the AFL-CIO succeeded in defeating Republican attempts to reform both Medicare and Medicaid. What this suggests is that a few powerful and determined interest groups can often successfully defeat policy proposals they perceive as harmful to their interest. We should note that the power of interest groups in the American political system is largely confined to blocking or vetoing proposals they do not like. In this sense, the role they play is largely a negative one. Interest groups are not as successful in bringing about passage of policy proposals they like.

The mass media also have come to play an important role in public agenda setting and policy making. We live in an information age, and the general public relies on both the electronic and the print media for their sources of information. Of the electronic media, television has become perhaps the most important source of news and information for the general public. The mass media's agenda setting (i.e., what is considered newsworthy and how the news is presented) is influenced by factors such as availability of time, space, resources, and the need to attract larger listeners/viewers/readers by presenting news in an entertaining manner. The mass media also help draw the public's attention to the problems by the frequency and manner with which they report (interpret) societal problems. In so doing, the mass media influence the public's perception of what they view as the most important problems facing the country and what they think about these problems. In this sense, the mass media play the role of "gatekeepers" in the American political system. How did the mass media do its job during the health care reform debate?

Our analysis of the role of the mass media during the two health care reform periods indicates that they did play an important role in helping set the public agenda. The mass media, especially newspapers and television, reported on health-related stories in large numbers. This was especially true in 1993 and 1994. The high frequency of reporting on health care stories did to some extent shape the public's perception that health care was an important problem facing the country. While the media deserve a lot of credit for their extensive coverage of the health care reform debate, they failed to educate the public about the complex issues and choices confronting the American citizens. Health care news coverage tended to place too much emphasis on the "politics" of reform—personality conflicts, disagreements, partisan politics, winners/losers—and less emphasis on explaining the problems of the U.S. health care system and various policy alternatives and their consequences. In this sense, the mass media failed to educate and inform the American citizens in ways that would have allowed them to understand better and thus make more informed choices. In fact, the mass media presented many reports without providing the context necessary to understand the debate. They also engaged in some biased reporting and allowed political advertisers to use the media to pursue their objectives without the mass media's acting as the public's watchdog. It is not too surprising that, according to public opinion polls, the general public gave a very low rating to the mass media for their coverage of the health care reform debate.

Finally, public opinion plays a significant role in shaping the policy agenda and policy making in a democratic society. It is important to remember that the Founding Fathers were never interested in establishing a direct democracy at the national level where citizens directly ruled themselves. They viewed direct democracy as mob rule, and thus they established a representative democracy where people would elect representatives who in turn would make informed decisions after careful deliberation. Public opinion and the passions of the time would be filtered through the calm and deliberate body of wise representatives. But modern communication technologies and research methodologies have made public opinion polling very easy, more frequent, and more scientific. A variety of mass media outlets, as well as private polling firms, engage in survey research where they poll the American public on their views about anything and everything from the president's job performance and important issues facing the country to the eating and sexual habits of citizens. What survey research also shows is that when people are asked their opinion on matters about which they know very little, they still freely express their views. In other words, many citizens who are ill informed or uninformed or just plain ignorant respond to polls by expressing an opinion. This raises a question: should elected representatives rely on the views and opinions expressed in polls in guiding public policy direction, even though those views and opinions are not based on well-informed deliberation? Research suggests that, in general, public policy in the United States often corresponds with public opinion (though this varies over time) and changes in public opinion are followed by changes in policy most of the time. While the public is largely ignorant of the details of public policy, public opinion in the aggregate appears to be rational and consistent. From a policy standpoint, public opinion sets boundaries that limit policy alternatives.

Our analysis suggests that public opinion played a major role in the outcome of health care reform. Prior to President Clinton's assuming the office of the presidency in January 1993, support for health care reform was gaining momentum. By the time President Clinton delivered the outline of his Health Security Act in September 1993, a strong majority of Americans expressed support for the health care reform. The general public recognized some of the problems facing the U.S. health care system (cost and access), and expressed support for reducing waste and increased spending to provide health insurance coverage to everyone. Most were also satisfied with their own doctor and the health care they personally receive. Throughout much of late 1993 and the early months of 1994, however, support for health care reform in general and support for Clinton's Health Security Act in particular declined, as did President Clinton's job approval rating. This was because, to a significant extent, the Clinton administration allowed opponents of his reform plan to define the issue. As attacks on President Clinton's reform plan increased, support continued to decline. By late summer 1994, support for health care reform and President Clinton's reform plan had dropped down to the 40 percent range. The general public had little understanding of the Clinton plan or many of the congressional initiatives. What this suggests is that the more uninformed or ill-informed public opinion is, the easier it is to influence it through carefully targeted strategy. The fact that public opinion declined significantly for any major reform plan helps explain the failure of health care reform. It allowed members of Congress to back away from reform. Public opinion polls after the 1994 congressional elections indicated that the general public was in favor of slow, incremental health care reforms and was strongly opposed to significant cuts in Medicare and Medicaid. The 1995–96 reform period reflected prevailing public opinion. Republicans in Congress who were interested in reducing the growth rate in Medicare and Medicaid failed to get this accomplished (the public likes both programs). At the same time, some incremental reforms did pass Congress, especially making health insurance portable and prohibiting insurance companies from denying coverage for preexisting conditions (issues that were highly salient to the public). Thus, during both reform periods, success or failure in health care reform closely reflects the prevailing public opinion.

What can we conclude about policy making in the United States? The failure of health care reform has led some to argue that the American way of politics is rapidly reaching a breaking point and that the American political system failed the people it was designed to serve. The goal of providing affordable health care for all is farther from realization today than it was at the beginning of the decade (Johnson and Broder, 1996). Referring to the goals of providing affordable health care for everyone, competition among insurance companies, and limiting medical inflation, Haynes Johnson and David Broder (1996, 609) concluded that the "failure to achieve any of those possible changes was a failure of The System and every one of its parts: the presidency, the Congress, the political parties, the interest groups, and the press."

Similarly, after examining the failure of the American political system to deal effectively with such issues as the oil shortage, budget deficits, and crime, Anthony King (1997) argues that American officeholders are too often enslaved to public opinion polls, they singlemindedly worry about their electoral future, they are constantly running scared, and they spend too much time running for office and too little time governing the nation. He argues that the American system is too democratic and suggests lengthening terms of office, eliminating off-year elections, and reducing primary challenges as solutions.

Pessimistic accounts of American democracy such as the above argue that it is no longer possible to govern the country effectively; that political parties are too factionalized to be effective; ever increasingly powerful interest groups have made gridlock the prevailing metaphor for American politics (demosclerosis); and the future of America's liberal democracy is at stake.

In sharp contrast to such a pessimistic view, Kelly Patterson argues that talk about crises in American democracy is misguided. After surveying the developments of political parties in America over a forty-year period from Eisenhower to Clinton, she rejects the idea that policy formulation has little to do with the campaign process. And she concludes that modern presidents do not face insurmountable odds in governing (1996).

We believe that the American political system, in general, works the way it was intended to work. But there are a few new twists in American politics that do make the task of governing more difficult today than in the past. Overall, the Founding Fathers created a limited national government by deliberately limiting its power to act. This was accomplished through separation of powers, checks and balances, a federal system of government, a bicameral legislature, and an independent judiciary. This fragmentation of political power among many competing power centers makes fundamental changes and innovations difficult in American politics. Nevertheless, it does not make it impossible to bring about fundamental changes (see Baumgartner and Jones 1993). Welfare reform in 1996 is a case in point. Most of the time the American political system works at a very slow pace, generating incremental changes in policy.

The new twist in American politics that has made the task of governing the nation more difficult is the significant role played by public opinion and the mass media. American politicians have come to rely too much on public opinion polls to make many policy decisions. Public opinion polls, more often than not, reflect opinions of people who are uninformed or ill-informed. American politicians, instead of becoming leaders who lead and shape public opinion, have become too reactionary, responding to every change in public opinion polls. Similarly, the mass media, and television in particular, today play a major role in shaping public and policy agenda. The mass media agenda is influenced by factors that make it difficult for them to play the role of an educator informing, educating, and helping citizens make better choices. Television, which is the medium least equipped to play this role, has become the main source of information for a large majority of Americans. In most American households, the television set is on for six to seven hours a day! News shows, talk shows, town halls, sound bites, infomercials, and visuals are all designed to entertain the viewers—not to engage them in serious public discourse or to encourage reflective thought (Cappolla and Jamieson 1997).

While we do not share the pessimism of some about the failures of the American political system, we do note that the result of the 1993–96 policy deliberations addressed only a small portion of the problems of the health care system. Millions of Americans remain without health insurance. Health care cost increases moderated in the mid-1990s, perhaps in response to the policy debates, but the concerns about costs remain. Medicare and Medicaid still take large bites out of federal (and state in the case of Medicaid) budgets. Even the legislation that passed, such as the Kennedy-Kassebaum bill, has its weaknesses. While it provides more insurance security for those changing jobs and/or with preexisting conditions, it says nothing about the cost of those policies.

1997 saw a somewhat changed politics and policy making, largely as a result of the 1993–96 battles over health care and balancing the budget and the 1996 presidential elections. The first session of the 105th Congress saw agreement between Congress, still Republican controlled, and the reelected President Clinton to balance the budget by 2002 and perhaps even produce a surplus (Clymer 1997). The major provisions of the deal included $90 billion in targeted tax cuts; some $115 billion in program cuts, mostly from Medicare; a $24 billion program to cover uninsured children; and policy changes in Medicare. The Medicare cutbacks come largely from reductions in provider (doctors, hospitals, HMOs) reimbursements. The policy changes involve providing Medicare recipients with a wider range of choices than currently exists. This includes medical savings accounts and privately contracted fee-for-service, a more expensive option that contains few restrictions on provider charges (Serafini 1997).

But even here, the general agreement and the specific Medicare changes do not ultimately conclude the story. Samuelson (1997a, 1997b) argues that the 1997 budget agreement actually postpones a balanced budget by increasing spending (youth insurance) and cutting taxes. Difficult policy choices have been put off until the latter years of the agreement (2000–2002), when the budget cuts would take place. Additionally, the reduction of the deficit to $27 billion in FY 1997 was enabled largely by a growing economy. The occurrence of a recession would call into question all economic assumptions.

Even with Medicare, the most difficult policy decisions were discussed, but ultimately deferred. The two most difficult Medicare policy changes would be to increase premiums paid by more affluent recipients and to raise the retirement eligibility age (Wildavsky 1997). At least the policy discussions have moved in these new directions (Pear 1997). Nevertheless, the integrity of the Medicare Part A trust fund, especially in the long run, remains an issue.

The problems remain, the policy debates will resume, our story will continue.

CHRONOLOGY

1991

January 28	Report that employee health care costs continue to increase.
February 2	President Bush to ask Congress for $23 billion in cuts in Medicare.
February 19	AFL-CIO endorses national health insurance as well as modest reforms in short term.
March 6	Harris poll finds Americans satisfied with health care system (though less satisfied than Canadians) but concerned about costs.
April 1	Federal report of Medicare and Medicaid shows that Medicaid physician reimbursement considerably lower than Medicare or private insurance reimbursement; result is doctors increasingly turning away Medicaid patients.
April 4	Senator John Heinz (R-Pa.) dies in private plane crash; Democrat Harris Wofford appointed to replace Heinz until November 5 election.
April 7	Poll of chief executive officers of country's largest companies show very strong support for significantly changing health care system, with government intervention necessary to carry it out.
April 10	Massachusetts plan for universal health care, adopted in 1988, fails implementation because of opposition of Governor Weld and small businesses and increasing costs.

April 16	Office of Management and Budget Director Richard Darman warns Congress about increasing costs of Medicare and Medicaid.
April 17	Comptroller General Charles Bowsher testifies before House Ways and Means Committee calling for limits on total spending for health care; state budget officers point to Medicaid as contributor to state fiscal problems.
April 22	Office of Technology Assessment report points to many adolescents not receiving needed health care because they lack public or private insurance.
April 30	White House appoints task force to examine why Medicaid costs are soaring.
May 24	Senate Democrats to propose limits on spending and employer mandate "play or pay" proposal, replacing Medicaid.
June 3	General Accounting Office report states that replacing current health care system with government insurance plan would save sufficient dollars to cover the entire population; health insurance companies oppose plan.
June 5	Senate Democrat leaders propose legislation to cover entire population, including 34 million uninsured, and increased government involvement in health care system; congressional Republicans and Bush administration oppose proposal.
June 8	Bush administration proposes standardizing fees for hospital outpatient care as way of controlling Medicare costs.
June 18	National Commission on Children proposes program ("play or pay") to cover all children and pregnant women; Bush administration and congressional Republicans assert program would accelerate increases in health care costs and would lead to poorer-quality health care.
June 23	Secretary of Health and Human Services Louis Sullivan asks American Medical Association to help slow down increases in health care costs or risk imposition of government program.

July 28

Panel appointed by Secretary Sullivan calls for expanding Medicaid to cover physicians' services for poor people not covered by Medicaid; universal access previously enorsed by American Medical Association, American Hospital Association, Blue Cross and Blue Shield Associations, and the Health Insurance Association of America.

July 31

Physician Payment Review Commission reports that new physician fees under Medicare are so low that it might hurt the access of the elderly to health care.

August 2

House Ways and Means Chairman Dan Rostenkowski (D-Ill.) proposes plan that includes price controls, lowers eligibility for Medicare, and new taxes to finance insurance for those currently not covered.

August 12

National Governors Association develops policy statement calling for universal access to health care within ten years and that federal government should assume costs of long-term care.

August 18

National Governors Association conference, with health care as major topic; says health care hurting state budgets, debates topic, and says Medicaid system is broken.

August 20

After sharply partisan debate, National Governors Association approves statement calling for health care reform and universal access.

August 24

Private insurers pushing managed care as means to avoid federal program.

August 26

Federal officials reduce cuts in Medicare physician reimbursements in response to complaints.

September 17

American Medical Association opposes new Medicare physician fee schedule.

September 23

Health insurers to campaign for state laws mandating that small businesses provide health insurance for employees as means to forestall federal program.

September 26

New York Times poll shows that 30 percent of Americans are staying in job because of fear of losing health insurance; 50 percent say health care system should be changed; 29 percent say they lacked health insurance for at least some time in past twelve months.

October 10   Bush administration official defends administration against charges that it is neglecting problems with health care system.

October 24   Rostenkowski and Senate Finance Chairman Lloyd Bentsen (D-Tex.) introduce legislation to guarantee health insurance for employees of small business.

October 26   Union and management representatives concur that health benefits are major stumbling block in reaching collective bargaining agreements.

October 29   Congressional Democratic leaders and governors agree to push for program guaranteeing access to entire population at reasonable cost.

October 30   Republican Richard Thornburgh, campaigning in special Pennsylvania senatorial election, calls for deregulation and competition as means to contain costs; Democratic opponent, Harris Wofford, moving up in polls against Thornburgh, attributed to his call for national health insurance.

November 5   Wofford wins election.

November 8   Democrats and Republicans in Congress propose health care legislation; Republican plan would cover the 34 million uninsured people at cost of $150 billion over five years, but does not say how it will be financed.

November 11   Bush administration increasingly looking at health care reform; Democrats charge three years of negligence.

November 12   National Leadership Coalition for Health Care Reform (large business-labor coalition) proposes "play-or-pay" plan; proposal includes health spending goals and uniform rate setting.

November 15   Medicare physician fee schedule issued with increased payments for family practitioners and reduced payments for specialists.

November 17	Some twenty health care reform bills before Congress.
December 10	Bush administration to propose increasing Medicare premiums for affluent recipients.
December 18	Study released saying that high premiums and failure to cover high-risk people led to increase in number of uninsured in 1990 to 34.7 million.
December 20	Federal panel proposes covering 20 million uninsured people with plan to cost $6.5 billion a year; labor unions and consumer groups attack plan as inadequate.
December 21	Democratic members of the House of Representatives announce that they will hold "town meetings" in their districts to discuss health care issues.
December 29	Commerce Department reports says health care spending for 1991 should increase by about 11 percent, the fifth consecutive year of double-digit increases.

1992

January 4	Bush admission to ask for tax credits to help uninsured as part of budget message.
January 8	White House Chief of Staff Samuel K. Skinner meets with American Medical Association top executives to discuss President Bush's proposed health care plan; Bush plan is based on tax system: credits for purchase of insurance and incentives to join managed care organizations.
January 9	Members of President Bush's cabinet assert that a study shows that Democratic health care plan would increase taxes and unemployment and mandate huge costs for employers.
January 15	Democratic members of the House of Representatives hold town meetings in their home districts publicizing Democratic health care plans and criticizing President Bush.
January 22	Senate Labor and Human Resources Committee approves, along party lines, reform of health insurance system.

January 27	Office of Management and Budget Director Richard Darman ordered by White House staff to revise parts of President Bush's health reform plan to meet objections from congressional Republicans. Study says business health care costs rose by 12.1 percent in 1991, about four times higher than increases in cost of living.
January 28	President Bush delivers State of the Union message proposing using tax system to help people purchase health insurance.
February 4	Paul Starr, in column in *New York Times,* proposes health care reform system based on managed competition.
February 6	President Bush proposes health reform plan largely based on tax incentives; five-year costs of program estimated at $100 billion.
February 9	National Association of Manufacturers President Jerry Jasinowski says Bush plan is inadequate to prevent large increases in health care spending.
March 3	*New York Times*/CBS News poll shows support for increased taxes to support national health insurance if there would be no other health care costs.
April 10	President Bush announces at news conference that he will not send health reform bill to Congress because administration has not yet decided how to finance it and Congress would not pass it in a presidential election year.
June 6	Republicans in House of Representatives offer health insurance reform plan, including provisions for medical savings accounts.
June 25	Democrats in House of Representatives offer health care plan, authored by Pete Stark (D-Calif.) plan to cut costs, insure about half of those without insurance, and regulate health insurance.
August 4	Democratic senators accuse President Bush of neglecting the problems of the uninsured; Bush campaign aides attack proposals of Democratic candidate Bill Clinton.

August 31   Congressional Budget Office report suggests that managed care has not reduced total national health care costs.

September 14   American College of Physicians proposes cap on national health care spending.

September 23   Senate adds provision to tax-increase bill that would increase tax deductibility of insurance, limit increases in insurance premiums, and prohibit certain insurers from denying coverage for preexisting conditions.

September 24   Bill Clinton announces proposal for health care reform based on managed competition within a budget.

October 15   Clinton, in presidential debate, promises to propose health care reform bill within first one hundred days of his administration.

November 3   Bill Clinton wins presidential election with 43 percent of the popular vote in a three-way race.

December 2   Health Insurance Association of America calls for universal coverage, a basic set of insurance benefits, and limits on tax breaks for purchasing insurance.

December 8   American Medical Association rejects limits on health care spending but would consider other possibilities.

April 10   Representatives Jim Cooper (D-Tenn.) and Mike Andrews (D-Tex.) introduce managed competition plan.

1993

January 24   Bill Gradison, President of HIAA, meets with White House officials to see if they could work on Clinton health plan together. Simultaneously, the HIAA begins ad campaign against the Clinton plan.

January 25   President Clinton announces formation of task force to develop health care reform proposal.

February 9   Representative William Clinger (R-Pa.) asks General Accounting Office to see whether task force invokes Federal Advisory Commission Act.

February 11   Business Roundtable policy committee endorses managed competition.

February 16   Executive committee of AFL-CIO says that labor will support consumption tax to pay for reform.

February 17   President Clinton's State of the Union address calls for health care reform.

February 18   Health Insurance Association of America (HIAA) endorses health care reform.

March 8   U.S. Chamber of Commerce endorses managed competition.

March 10   Federal district court judge orders that official task force meetings be open to public.

March   Representative Jim McDermott (D-Wash.) introduces single-payer plan.

Spring   Democratic National Committee (DNC) allocates funds to support health care reform.

April 6   Harris poll finds strong support for Clinton plan.

May 20   National Federation of Independent Businesses (NFIB) issues press release claiming Clinton plan will result in significant job loss.

Summer   Battle over deficit-reduction plan delays release of Clinton proposal.

August   Over twenty health reform bills introduced in Congress.

September   Minority Leader Robert Michel (R-Ill.) introduces bill to reform insurance reform including medical savings account provision; John Chafee (R-R.I.) announces individual mandate bill.

September 22   President Clinton addresses Congress and formally introduces plan; early poll shows strong support for plan.

September 24   American Medical Association (AMA) sends letter to President Clinton stating its support for health care reform but outlining its objections to specific provisions.

September 28–30   Hillary Rodham Clinton testifies before House and Senate committees on health reform proposal.

October 6   Cooper-Grandy bill introduced with bipartisan support.

October 19   Poll conducted by Kaiser Family Foundation finds public confused about health care reform issues.

October 27   Clinton proposal sent to Congress.

November 20   Clinton proposal formally introduced in Congress.

November 22   Senators Daniel Patrick Moynihan (D-N.Y.) and Edward M. Kennedy (D-Mass.) introduce separate health reform bills so that they can be referred to their committees; Chafee introduces bill announced in September, though with fewer cosponsors.

December 2   First of a series of memos from Republican strategist William Kristol suggesting Republicans not support Clinton plan or any amendments to it.

December 7   AMA House of Delegates withdraws support for employer mandates.

December 21   Report shows health care cost increases declining.

1994

January   Polls show declining public support for Clinton plan.

January 25   Clinton State of the Union message; warns will veto plan not containing universal coverage.

February 2   Business Roundtable endorses Cooper proposal; U.S. Chamber of Commerce and National Association of Manufacturers oppose Clinton plan within next two weeks.

February 8   Congressional Budget Office (CBO) report on scoring of Clinton plan; report says will increase deficit in first six years (though will decrease deficit after that) and that employer contributions should be considered taxes.

March   Polls show continued decline in support for Clinton plan though strong support for most elements of the plan.

March 2	Two House Commerce subcommittees considering health care reform fail to produce a bill.
March 8	House Ways and Means Health Subcommittee Chair Pete Stark offers a proposal to move uninsured workers into a Part C of Medicare.
March 15	Representative Fred Grandy (R-Iowa) offers amendment in Ways and Means Health Subcommittee to delete employer mandate; amendment defeated 6–5.
March 23	House Ways and Means Health Subcommittee approves bill 6–5; votes down McDermott, Cooper, Michels, and Clinton plans.
April	Congressional Republicans fail to decide how to deal with health care reform.
April 21	House Education and Labor Subcommittee on Labor-Management Relations begins consideration of health reform; markup takes six weeks.
May	Senate Labor and Human Resources Committee begins consideration of health reform; Chairman Kennedy makes changes to solicit Republican support; only one Republican, James M. Jeffords (R-Vt.), goes along.
May 4	Robert Reichauer testifies before Senate Finance Committee that the Cooper bill would not provide universal coverage nor would it contain sufficient funds to subsidize low-income families.
May 12	House Education and Labor Subcommittee on Labor-Management Relations defeats attempts to limit coverage of abortions in health reform bill.
May 25	House Education and Labor Subcommittee on Labor-Management Relations approves measure 17–10 (straight party-line vote).
May 31	House Ways and Means Chairman Dan Rostenkowski (D-Ill.) indicted; Sam Gibbons (D-Fla.) takes over as committee chair.

June 9	House Education and Labor Subcommittee on Labor-Management Relations approves a modified single-payer bill.

June 9   House Education and Labor Subcommittee on Labor-Management Relations approves a modified single-payer bill.

June 14   House Ways and Means Committee defeats attempt to delete employer mandate; Senator Robert Packwood (R-Ore.) announces opposition to employer mandates.

June 16   *Washington Post* story that House Ways and Means Committee member Fred Grandy complains about orders from Minority Leader Newt Gingrich (R-Ga.) not to support amendments to Ways and Means bill.

June 21   President Clinton reasserts support for universal coverage.

June 23   House Education and Labor Committee reports liberal bill by 26–17 vote after eight days of markups.

June 27   Senate Finance Committee holds public markup.

June 28   House Commerce and Energy Committee Chair John Dingell (D-Mich.) sends letter to House Speaker Tom Foley (D-Wash.) that committee was unable to report a bill.

June 29   Senate Minority Leader Robert Dole (R-Kans.) achieves agreement among forty Republican senators behind proposal calling for subsidies for poorest Americans, incentives for purchasing cooperatives, and banning discrimination on the part of insurance companies against those with poor health.

June 30   House Ways and Means Committee reports bill by 20–18 vote; McDermott threatens to withdraw support for reform unless benefits strengthened; Senate Finance Committee rejects employer mandate; Finance chairman incorporates into his own proposal a bipartisan proposal that had no spending controls or employer mandates.

July 21   Clinton meets with congressional leaders, who agree that changes are needed in health reform bills.

July 22   Bus caravans begin nationwide tour to push for health care reform; Citizens for Sound Economy establishes counterdemonstrations.

July 29	House Majority Leader Richard Gephardt (D-Mo.) introduces bill that included employer mandate, Medicare Part C proposal, and new taxes.
August 2	Senate Majority Leader George Mitchell (D-Me.) introduces bill to cover 95 percent of population by 2005 with triggers for mandated action if target not met.
August 3	Clinton announces support for Mitchell bill.
August 11	House leaders indefinitely postpone debate over health care reform.
August 19	Bipartisan Mainstream Coalition introduces health care reform proposal similar to Senate Finance Committee bill.
August 22–24	Senate debates crime bill.
August 25	Senate recesses until September 12.
August 26	Senate Majority Leader Mitchell states that there was insufficient time to consider comprehensive reform and would work on incremental bill with Mainstream Coalition.
September 13	*New York Times* poll show 57 percent favor incremental change and half of those polled favor a veto of bill that does not cover the entire population.
September 20	House Energy and Commerce Chairman John Dingell (D-Mich.) tells Clinton in letter that committee cannot produce bill; Congressional Republican leaders meet with Clinton and tell him that any action on health care reform in Congress would lead to blocking the General Agreement on Tariffs and Trade (GATT).
September 26	Senate Majority Leader Mitchell pulls the health care reform bills.
September 27	367 House Republican challengers and incumbents sign Contract with America.
November 8	Republican victories in midterm elections; win control of both houses of Congress for the first time in forty years.

1995

January 4	First day of 104th Congress; Republicans assume control of Congress, 230–204 in House and 53–47 in Senate.
January 24	Clinton State of the Union message, theme is the "New Covenant," trying to establish position between liberals and conservatives.
February 6	Clinton unveils budget with no cuts in Medicare or Medicaid.
February 16	Speaker Gingrich announces that only plans with balanced budget by 2002 would be considered on House floor.
May 9 and 10	House and Senate Budget committees offer plans to balance federal budget by 2002.
May 17	House approves FY 1996 budget resolution; President Clinton casts first veto against budget recissions bill.
May 25	Senate approves budget resolution.
June 14	President Clinton on national television says he will propose budget that will be balanced by 2005, would include smaller cuts in Medicare ($98 billion) and insurance reforms.
June 22	House-Senate conferees approve budget resolution to achieve balance by 2002, with $245 billion in tax cuts and $270 billion in reductions in Medicare spending.
June 29	House approves modified budget recission bill.
July 20	Senate approves modified budget recission bill.
July 27	President Clinton signs budget recission bill.
September 28	Congress and White House agree to keep government open through November 13.
October 1	Fiscal year 1996 begins, with most appropriations bills not passed by Congress.
October 19	Medicare bill brought up before House, separate from reconciliation bill, passes House by 231–201.

October 24	Democrats run ad quoting Speaker Gingrich saying that Medicare should be left to "wither on the vine." Senate Majority Leader Bob Dole says in speech to American Conservative Union that he had voted in 1965 against the enactment of Medicare "because we knew it wouldn't work."
October 26	House passes reconciliation bill by vote of 227–203.
October 28	Senate passes reconciliation bill 52–47.
November 8 and 9	House and Senate approve continuing resolution and debt ceiling bill; continuing resolution eliminates drop in Medicare premiums.
November 10	Clinton vetoes continuing resolution.
November 14	Partial shutdown of government begins.
November 15	Speaker Gingrich complains of snub by President Clinton on Air Force One while on trip to attend funeral of slain Israeli Prime Minister Yitzhak Rabin; says budget resolution made tougher because of snub.
November 16	Compromise FY 1996 budget reconciliation bill approved; Medicaid would become block grant and rate of growth would be cut in half; taxes cut by $245 billion, Medicare spending reduced by $270 billion; Republican freshman insist on keeping Medicare provisions in reconciliation bill.
November 19	White House and congressional leaders agree on continuing resolution that reopens government through December 15 and commits to a balanced budget by 2002.
November 28	White House and congressional leaders resume budget talks.
December 5	White House agrees to submit budget that balances by 2002; Clinton vetoes reconciliation bill.
December 7	White House makes budget proposal.
December 15	A second partial shutdown of the federal government begins.

1996

January 3	First session of 104th Congress ends and second session begins.
January 5	House passes continuing resolution.
January 6	47 Democrats sign letter saying they would support $168 billion in Medicare cuts, majority in House now support position; Republicans lower tax cuts to $185 billion and Medicaid cuts to $85 billion.
February 2	Clinton State of the Union supports Kennedy-Kassebaum bill; health insurance industry objects to portions of proposal.
February 3	At National Governors' Association conference, Republican governors propose reform of Medicaid, including turning program into block grant.
February 4	Medicare Hospital Insurance Trustees report that Medicare Part A lost money in 1995 for the first time in over twenty years.
February 5	Bipartisan agreement on Medicaid reform at National Governors' Association meeting, and progress on agreement on welfare reform. American Academy of Actuaries accuse health insurance industry of exaggerating impact of Kennedy-Kassebaum bill.
February 6	Governors endorse Medicaid and welfare reform proposals; Gingrich, Dole, and Clinton applaud proposals. Senate Republicans agree to schedule debate and vote on Kennedy-Kassebaum bill.
February 13	Civil rights groups attack Medicaid and welfare reform proposals, arguing that it will disproportionately hurt blacks and increase poverty among children and families.
February 28	Clinton administration warns that unless action is taken, Medicare trust fund will go bankrupt by 2001.
March 4	House leaders say that they will start considering health insurance reform (Kennedy-Kassebaum) but warn they will add provisions dealing with medical malpractice

reform, medical savings accounts, and tax deductions for self-employed people.

March 8   House leaders offer modified health insurance reform package containing additional provisions.

March 14   House Commerce Subcommittee approves health insurance reform package.

March 19   House Ways and Means Committee approves health insurance reform.

March 20   House Commerce Committee unanimously approves health insurance reform.

March 28   House of Representatives approves health insurance reform; proposal contains provisions opposed by President Clinton.

April 17   Senate Majority Leader Bob Dole, the leading candidate for the Republican presidential nomination, says he will try to add a medical savings account provision to the health insurance reform bill.

April 18   Senate rejects medical savings account amendment.

April 22   New federal government study shows accelerating losses in Medicare hospital trust fund.

April 23   Senate unanimously passes health insurance reform bill; Senate also passes bill requiring equivalent coverage of mental health.

April 25   Senator Kennedy accuses Senate Majority Leader Bob Dole of trying to defeat health insurance reform by insisting on medical savings account provision.

May 14   Congressional Budget Office says that a significant number of people could lose health insurance because of higher premiums if mental health mandated to be covered equally with physical health.

May 21   Bipartisan consensus on welfare and Medicaid reform among the nation's governors appears to be dissolving.

May 22   Congressional Republican leaders make new effort to meet some of President Clinton's objections on welfare and Medicaid reform.

May 28   Health and Human Services report that spending on health care in 1994 grew at slowest rate since 1960.

June 6   Medicare Hospital Fund trustees confirm that Medicare will go bankrupt by 2001.

June 9   President Clinton threatens veto of health insurance reform bill if it includes medical savings account provision; House Majority Leader Dick Armey dares the president to veto the bill.

June 10   Congressional Republicans agree on health insurance bill and President Clinton does not automatically dismiss bill.

July   Republicans drop Medicaid reform from welfare-reform bill.

July 19   House Republicans tell television stations that AFL-CIO ads about House Speaker Newt Gingrich's speech on Medicare is a lie and that showing the ad could result in libel suits.

July 21   Letter in *New York Times* by AFL-CIO head John Sweeney accuses Gingrich of stretching truth on AFL-CIO ad.

July 25   Senator Kennedy and Representative Bill Archer, chairman of House Ways and Means Committee, announce compromise allowing limited experiment with medical savings account in health insurance reform bill.

July 30   Kaiser Family Foundation/Harvard School of Public Health survey finds no commanding view on health insurance portability among the public.

July 31   Senate and House leaders agree on health insurance reform, including medical savings account experiment.

August 1   House overwhelmingly approves health insurance reform.

August 2   Senate overwhelmingly approves health insurance reform.

August 17	President Clinton charges that Bob Dole's 15 percent tax cut proposal might force significant cuts in Medicare.
August 21	Clinton signs health insurance reform bill.
August 24	Dole denies that tax cut plan will hurt Medicare.
September 9	House Minority Leader Richard Gephardt warns that if Republicans retain control of Congress, Medicare will be the subject of serious cuts.
September 19	House and Senate leaders announce agreement on maternity insurance coverage and equal coverage of mental health.
September 21	Republican presidential nominee Bob Dole says that Clinton's comprehensive health care reform proposal shows the president's dedication to big government programs.
October 31	Dole attacks Clinton for criticism of Republican plans on Medicare.
November 5	Clinton reelected president, with 49 percent of vote; Republicans increase majority slightly in Senate and retain control of House, though with reduced majority.
November 10	Clinton administration considering incremental health care policy reform, focusing on uninsured children, families between jobs, and Medicaid costs, bipartisan commission on Medicare. Senate Majority Leader Trent Lott accuses Democrats of demagoguery on Medicare, wants administration to come up with Medicare proposal rather than bipartisan commission.
November 12	Gingrich and Lott say there is no rush to form bipartisan commission on Medicare.

Sources:

Drew, Elizabeth. 1996. *Showdown: The Struggle between the Gingrich Congress and the Clinton White House.* New York: Simon & Schuster.

Rovner, Julie. 1995. "Congress and Health Care Reform." In *Intensive Care: How Congress Shapes Health Policy,* ed. Thomas E. Mann and Norman J. Ornstein (Washington, D.C.: American Enterprise Institute and Brookings Institution).

New York Times Index.

REFERENCES

Aaron, Henry J., Thomas E. Mann, and Timothy Taylor, eds. 1994. *Values and Public Policy.* Washington, D.C.: Brookings Institution.

Allen, Jodie T. 1996. "The Budget: Another Slice of Baloney." *Washington Post National Weekly Edition* 13, no. 14 (February 5–11): 23.

Altman, Drew E. 1995. "The Realities Behind the Polls." *Health Affairs* 14, no. 1 (Spring): 24–26.

Altman, Robert H., and Stanford L. Weiner. 1978. "Regulation as a Second Best Choice." In *Competition in the Health Care Sector: Past, Present and Future,* ed. Bureau of Economics, U.S. Federal Trade Commission, 421–27. Washington D.C.: Government Printing Office.

"An Analysis of the AFDC-Related Medicaid Provisions in the New Welfare Law." 1996. Center on Budget and Policy Priorities, Washington, D.C. September 19. [http://www.handsnet.org/medicaid/cbpp.html].

Apple, R.W. Jr. 1995. "G.O.P. Blitzkreig on Health Care Shakes Capitol Hill." *New York Times,* September 23.

"A Survey of Health Care: Surgery Needed." 1991. *The Economist,* July 6, 4–5.

Aumente, Jerome. 1995. "A Medical Breakthrough." *American Journalism Review* 17, no. 10: 27–33.

Bachrach, Peter, and Morton Baratz. 1962. "Two Faces of Power." *American Political Science Review* 56, no. 4: 947–52.

———. 1963. "Decisions and Nondecisions: An Analytical Framework." *American Political Science Review.* 57, no. 3: 632–42.

Bader, John B. 1996. *Taking the Initiative: Leadership Agendas and the "Contract with America."* Washington, D.C.: Georgetown University Press.

Baker, Peter. 1996. "An All-Time High for Ballot No-Shows." *Washington Post National Weekly Edition* 14, no. 2 (November 11–17): 11–12.

Baker, Ross K. 1995. *House and Senate.* 2nd ed. New York: Norton.

Ball, Robert M. 1975. "Background of Regulation in Health Care." In *Controls on Health Care,* ed. Institute of Medicine, 3–22. Washington, D.C.: National Academy of Sciences.

Balz, Dan, and Ronald Brownstein. 1996. *Storming the Gates: Protest Politics and the Republican Revival.* Boston: Little, Brown.

Bandow, Doug, and Michael Tanner. 1995. *The Wrong and Right Ways to Reform Medicare.* Policy Analysis No. 230. Washington, D.C.: CATO Institute. June 8. [Http://www.cato.org/pubs/pas/pa230.html]

Barber, James David. 1972. *The Presidential Character.* Englewood Cliffs, N.J.: Prentice Hall.

Bauer, Raymond, Ithiel Pool, and Lewis Dexter. 1963. *American Business and Public Policy.* New York: Atherton Press.

Baumgartner, Frank R., and Bryan D. Jones. 1993. *Agendas and Instability in American Politics.* Chicago: University of Chicago Press.

Baumgartner, Frank R., and Jeffery C. Talbert. 1995. "From Setting a National Agenda on Health Care to Making Decisions in Congress." *Journal of Health Politics, Policy and Law* 20, no. 2 (Summer): 437–45.

Beach, William W. 1995. The *Cost to States of Not Reforming Medicaid.* The Heritage Foundation. F.Y.I. No. 63. September 26. [Http://townhall.com/heritage/library/categories/healthwel/fyi63.html]

Bennefield, Robert L. 1995. *Health Insurance Coverage: 1994.* Washington D.C.: Bureau of Census, U.S. Department of Commerce, 60–190.

Bennett, Lance W. 1988. *News: Politics of Illusion.* 2nd ed. New York: Longman.

———. 1996. *The Governing Crisis: Media, Money, and Marketing in American Elections,* 2nd ed. New York: St. Martin's Press.

Bennett, William J. 1994. *The Index of Leading Cultural Indicators: Facts and Figures on the State of American Society.* New York : Simon & Schuster.

Bentley, Arthur F. 1908. *The Process of Government: A Study of Social Pressures.* Chicago: University of Chicago Press.

Berelson, Bernard, Paul Lazarsfield, and William McPhee. 1954. *Voting.* Chicago: University of Chicago Press.

Berk, Marc L. 1944. "Should We Rely on Polls?" *Health Affairs* 13, no. 1 (Spring): 299–300.

Berke, Richard L. 1995. "Republicans Rule Lobbyists' World with Strong Arm." *New York Times,* March 20.

Berry, Jeffrey M. 1997. *The Interest Group Society,* 3rd ed. New York: Longman.

Bilchik, Gloria S. 1996. "Under Scrutiny." *Hospitals and Health Networks* 70, no. 9 (May 5): 24–31.

Bilheimer, Linda T., and Robert D. Reischauer. 1995. "Confessions of the Estimators: Numbers and Health Reform." *Health Affairs* 14, no. 1 (Spring): 37–55.

Bipartisan Commission on Entitlement and Tax Reform. 1994. "Report of the Bipartisan Commission on Entitlements and Tax Reform." (August) Washington, D.C.

"Bipartisan Consumer Health Bill Turned into Partisan Bill Harmful to the Consumers." 1996. Families USA Special Report, Washington, D.C. Families USA. (April). [http://epn.org/families/fabipa.html]

Birnbaum, Jeffrey H., and Alan S. Murray. 1987. *Showdown at Gucci Gulch: Lawmakers, Lobbyists, and the Unlikely Triumph of Tax Reform.* New York: Random House.

Blendon, Robert J. 1995. "Health-Care Reform: The Press Failed to Inform Public of Alternatives." *Nieman Reports,* Fall, 17–19.

Blendon, Robert J., Drew E. Altman, John Benson, Mollyann Brodie, James Matt, and Gerry Chervinsky. 1995. "Health Care Policy Implications of the 1994 Congressional Elections." *Journal of the American Medical Association* 273, no. 8 (February 22): 671–74.

Blendon, Robert J., Mollyann Brodie, and John Benson. 1995. "What Happened to Americans' Support for the Clinton Health Plan?" *Health Affairs* 14, no. 2 (Summer): 7–23.

Blendon, Robert J., and Karen Donelan. 1990. "The Public and the Emerging Debate over National Health Insurance." *New England Journal of Medicine* 323, no. 3 (July 19): 208–12.

———. 1991. "The Public and the Future of U.S. Health Care System Reform." In

System in Crisis: The Case for Health Care Reform, ed. Robert J. Blendon and Jennifer N. Edwards. New York: Faulkner & Gray.

Blendon, Robert J., Tracey S. Hyams, and John M. Benson. 1993. "Bridging the Gap between Expert and Public Views on Health Care Reform." *Journal of the American Medical Association* 269, no. 19 (May 19): 2573–79.

Blendon, Robert J., Robert Leitman, Ian Morrison, and Karen Donelan. 1990. "Satisfaction with Health Systems in Ten Nations." *Health Affairs* 9, no. 2 (Summer): 185–92.

Blendon, Robert J., et al. 1992. "The Implications of the 1992 Presidential Election for Health Care Reform." *Journal of American Medical Association* 268, no. 23 (December 16): 3371–75.

———. 1994. "The Beliefs and Values Shaping Today's Health Reform Debate." *Health Affairs* 13, no. 1 (Spring): 274–84.

Blendon, Robert J., et al. 1995. "Who Has the Best Health Care System? A Second Look." *Health Affairs* 14, no. 4 (Winter): 220–30.

Bolce, Louis, Gerald D. Maio, and Douglas Muzzio. 1996. "Dial-in Democracy: Talk Radio and the 1994 Elections." *Political Science Quarterly* 111, no. 3 (Fall): 457–81.

Bowermaster, David. 1996. "News You Can Use: A Last Try at Health Reform." *U.S. News & World Report,* May 6. [http://usnews.com/issue/health.html]

Bowman, Karlyn H. 1994. *The 1993–1994 Debate on Health Care Reform: Did the Polls Mislead the Policy Makers?* Washington, D.C.: AEI Press.

———. 1995. "Learning from the Imperfect Debate." *Health Affairs* 14, no. 1 (Spring): 27–29.

Brace, Paul, and Barbara Hinckley. 1992. *Follow the Leader: Opinion Polls and the Modern Presidents.* New York: HarperCollins.

Brady, David W., and Kara M. Buckley. 1995. "Health Care Reform in the 103d Congress: A Predictable Failure." *Journal of Health Politics, Policy and Law* 20, no. 2 (Summer): 447–54.

Breyer, S. 1979. "Analyzing Regulatory Failures: Mismatches, Less Restrictive Alternatives and Reform." *Harvard Law Review* 92, no. 1: 549–609.

Broder, David S. 1996a. "No Friends among Foes." *Washington Post National Weekly Edition* 13:36 (July 1–7): 4.

———. 1996b. "Power to Both Parties." *Washington Post National Weekly Edition* 14, no. 2 (November 11–17): 7–8.

Brodie, Mollyann. 1996. "Americans' Political Participation in the 1993–1994 Health Care Reform Debate." *Journal of Health Policy and Law* 21, no. 1 (Spring): 99–128.

Brodie, Mollyann, and Robert J. Blendon. 1995. "The Public's Contribution to Congressional Gridlock on Health Care Reform." *Journal of Health Politics, Policy and Law* 20, no. 2 (Summer): 403–10.

Brooks, Durad, David R. Smith, and Ron J. Anderson. 1991. "Medical Apartheid: An American Perspective." *Journal of the American Medical Association* 266, no. 9 (November 20): 2746–47.

Brown, Lawrence D. 1992. "The Politics of Health-Care Reform." *Current History* 91, no. 564 (April): 173–75.

Burner, Sally T., and Daniel R. Waldo. 1995. "National Health Expenditure Projections, 1994– 2005," *Health Care Financing Review* 16, no. 4 (Summer): 221–42.

Burns, James McGregor. 1978. *Leadership.* New York: Harper & Row.

Butler, Stuart M. 1995. "The Conservative Agenda for Incremental Reform." *Health Affairs* 14, no. 1 (Spring): 150–60.

———. 1996. *Urgent Action Needed on Medicare.* F.Y.I. No. 110. Washington, D.C.: Heritage Foundation. June 17. [http://www.townhall.com/heritage/library/categories/healthwel/fyi110.html]

Canaham-Clyne, John P. 1995. "Clinton's Folly—The Health Care Debacle," *New Politics* 5, no. 2 (Winter): 27–34.

Cappella, Joseph N., and Kathleen Hall Jamieson. 1997. *Spiral of Cynicism: The Press and the Public Good.* New York: Oxford University Press.

Caraley, Demetrios. 1996. "Dismantling the Federal Safety Net: Fictions versus Realities." *Political Science Quarterly* 111, no. 2 (Summer): 225–58.

Carmines, Edward G., and James A. Stimson. 1989. *Issue Evolution : Race and the Transformation of American Politics.* Princeton: Princeton University Press.

Case, Tony. 1994a. "No Dearth of Health Care Coverage." *Editor and Publisher* 127, no. 40 (October 1): 14–15, 37.

———. 1994b. "Health News with Tabloid Appeal." *Editor and Publisher* 127, no. 40 (October 1): 15, 37.

Cassata, Donna. 1995. "GOP Retreats on Hatfield, But War Far from Over." *Congressional Quarterly Weekly Report* 53, no. 10 (March 11): 729–31.

Chubb, John E., and Paul E. Peterson, eds. 1985. *The New Direction in American Politics.* Washington, D.C.: Brookings Institution.

Clancy, Carolyn M.; and Charlea T. Massion. 1992. "American Women's Health Care: A Patchwork Quilt with Gaps." *Journal of the American Medical Association* 268, no. 14 (October 24): 1918–20.

"Clinton: How Will He Handle Specific Problems." 1993. *Gallup Poll Monthly,* no. 320 (January): 25.

Cloud, David S. 1994a. "Democrats Band Together to Repel Assault on Employer Mandate." *Congressional Quarterly Weekly Report* 52, no. 24 (June 18): 1615–19.

———. 1994b. "House Moderates Offer Plan." *Congressional Quarterly Weekly Report* 52, no. 32 (August 13): 2550.

———. 1994c. "Mitchell Trying to Find a Graceful Exit." *Congressional Quarterly Weekly Report* 52, no. 37 (September 24): 2693–95.

Clymer, Adam. 1995a. "2 Senators Offer New Health Bill." *New York Times,* July 14.

———. 1995b. "Organized Labor Goes on the Offensive, and the Republicans Cry Foul." *New York Times,* July 20.

———. 1995c. "Wary of Congress on Medicaid, Governors Seek a United Front." *New York Times,* July 31.

———. 1995d. "With Political Discipline, It Works Like Parliament." *New York Times,* August 6.

———. 1995e. "2 Political Parties Turn to Airwaves for Medicare Debate." *New York Times,* August 16, B10.

———. 1995f. "G.O.P. Lawmakers Scramble to Pass a Medicare Plan." *New York Times,* October 19.

———. 1995g. "House Votes to Curb Costs on Medicare by $270 Billion; President Promises a Veto." *New York Times,* October 20.

———. 1996a. "Senate Defeats Dole Revision to Health Bill." *New York Times,* April 19.

———. 1996b. "Senate Passes Health Bill with Job-to-Job Coverage." *New York Times,* April 24.

———. 1996c. "Clinton-Dole Fight on Health Bill Is Preview of Campaign to Come." *New York Times,* April 25.

———. 1996d. "Kennedy Says Dole Is Trying to Sabotage Insurance Bill." *New York Times,* April 26.

———. 1996e. "Health Care Bill Fails over Dispute between Parties." *New York Times,* June 8.

———. 1996f. "Union Attacks, and Republicans Cry Foul." *New York Times,* July 20.

————. 1996g. "Clinton and Congress: Partnership of Self-Interest." *New York Times,* October 2.

————. 1997. "White House and the G.O.P. Announce Deal to Balance Budget and to Trim Taxes." *New York Times,* July 29.

Cobb, Roger W., and Charles D. Elder. 1982. *Participation in American Politics: The Dynamics of Agenda-Building.* 2nd ed. Baltimore: Johns Hopkins University Press.

Cohen, Bernard. 1963. *The Press and Foreign Policy.* Princeton: Princeton University Press.

Cohen, Richard E. 1995. "Lobbying Reform Targets GOP Foes." *National Journal* 27, no. 36 (September) 9): 2234.

Cohen, Richard E., and William Schneider. 1995. "Epitaph for a Era." *National Journal* 27, no. 2 (January 14): 83–86.

Cohn, Victor. 1993. "We've Come a Long Way Since Covering Blue Cross." *Nieman Reports* 47, no. 4 (Winter): 3–5.

Conti, Delia B. 1995. "Reagan's Trade Rhetoric: Lessons for the 1990s." *Presidential Studies Quarterly* 25, no. 1 (Winter): 91–108.

Cook, Timothy E. 1990. "Show Horses in House Elections: The Advantages and Disadvantages of National Media Visibility." In *Media Power in Politics,* 2nd ed., ed. Doris A. Graber, 193–204. Washington, D.C.: CQ Press.

Cowley, Geoffrey. 1996. "Flunk the Gene Test and Lose Your Insurance." *Newsweek* CXVIII, no. 26 (December 23). 48–50.

Craig, Stephen C. 1993. *The Malevolent Leaders: Popular Discontent in America.* Boulder, Colo.: Westview Press.

Czitrom, Daniel. 1982. *Media and the American Mind.* Chapel Hill: University of North Carolina Press.

Dahl, Robert. 1956. *A Preface to Democratic Theory.* Chicago: University of Chicago Press.

————. 1961. *Who Governs?* New Haven: Yale University Press.

————. 1967. *Pluralist Democracy in the United States: Conflict and Consent.* Chicago: Rand McNally.

Davis, Karen. 1995. "Health and Society, 1965–2000: President's Message from the 1995 Annual Report." Commonwealth Fund. [http://www.cmwf.org/presmes.html]

Democratic National Committee. 1996. "GOP Extremists Plan to Slash Medicare." *Bottom Line.*

"Dems Health Care Campaign: Grassroots Nixed, Air War Starts." 1994. *Campaign and Elections* 15, no. 2 (May): 11.

Dentzer, Susan. 1990. "America's Scandalous Health Care," *U.S. News & World Report,* March 12, 25–30.

"Details of Constitution Escape Many." 1997. *Springfield News-Leader,* September 16.

Dewar, Helen, and Eric Planin. 1996. "A Switch in Time That May Have Saved the GOP." *Washington Post National Weekly Edition* 13, no. 40 (October 7–13): 9–10.

Diamond, Edwin. 1991. *The Media Show: The Changing Face of the News, 1985–1990.* Cambridge, Mass.: MIT Press.

Diamond, Edwin, and Stephen Bates. 1992. *The Spot: The Rise of Political Advertising on Television.* 3rd ed. Cambridge, Mass: MIT Press.

Diamond, Edwin, Steven Katz, and Cara Matthews. 1994, "Conflict v Context in Covering . . . Clinton's Health Care Proposal." *National Journal* 26, no. 47 (November 19): 2738–39.

Disch, Lisa. 1996. "Publicity-Stunt Participation and Sound Bite Polemics: The Health Care Debate 1993–1994." *Journal of Health Politics, Policy and Law* 21, no. 1 (Spring): 3–33.

Dodd, Lawrence C. 1996. "Re-Envisioning Congress: Some Reflections on the Coming of the Republican Revolution." Paper prepared for presentation at the annual meeting of the American Political Science Association, San Francisco, August 29–September 1.

Dodd, Lawrence C., and Bruce I. Oppenheimer. eds. 1993. *Congress Reconsidered.* 5th ed. Washington, D.C.: CQ Press.

Donham, Carolyn S., Arthur L. Sensenint, and Stephen K. Heffler. 1995. "Health Care Indicators." *Health Care Financing Review* 16, no. 4 ((Summer): 243–72.

Donovan, Beth. 1994a. "Democrats as Divided as Ever on Eve of First Markup." *Congressional Quarterly Weekly Report* 52, no. 8 (February 26): 475, 478.

———. 1994b. "Details of Kennedy Plan." *Congressional Quarterly Weekly Report* 52, no. 19 (May 14): 1222.

———. 1994c. "Panel Strikes Surprising with Benefits, Cost Concept." *Congressional Quarterly Weekly Report* 52, no. 20 (May 21): 1299–1300.

———. 1994d. "Senate Labor First Out of Gate with Approval of Overhaul Bill." *Congressional Quarterly Weekly Report* 52, no. 23 (June 11): 1522–24.

———. 1994e. "Betting Big on Public Backing, Clinton Stands Firm on Veto." *Congressional Quarterly Weekly Report* 25, no. 25 (June 25): 1703–6.

Donovan, Beth, and Alissa J. Rubin. 1994a. "Dingell Outline Softens Clinton Plan to Lure Energy Panel Democrats." *Congressional Quarterly Weekly Report* 52, no. 12 (March 26): 738–39.

———. 1994b. "Bipartisan Deal on Benefits Gives Boost to Overhaul." *Congressional Quarterly Weekly Report* 52, no. 20 (May 21): 1298.

Dorfman, Lori, Helen Halpin Schauffler, John Wilkerson, and Judith Feinson. 1996. "Local Television News Coverage of President Clinton's Introduction of the Health Security Act." *Journal of American Medical Association* 275, no. 15 (April 17): 1201–5.

Dorsey, Leroy G. 1995. "The Frontier Myth in Presidential Rhetoric: Theodore Roosevelt's Campaign for Conservation." *Western Journal of Communication* 59, no. 1 (Winter): 1–19.

"Downsizing of America, The." 1996. Seven Part Series. *New York Times,* March 3–10. For an expanded discussion, see also *New York Times.* 1996. *The Downsizing of America.* New York: Random House.

Drew, Elizabeth. 1996. *Showdown: The Struggle between the Gingrich Congress and the Clinton White House.* New York: Simon & Schuster.

Dreyfuss, Robert, and Peter H. Stone. 1996. "Medikill." *Mother Jones* 21, no. 1 (January/February): 22–27, 77–81.

Drucker, Peter. 1980. *Managing in Turbulent Times.* London: Pan Paperbacks.

———. 1990. "Behind Japan's Success." *Harvard Business Review* 68, no. 4 (July/August): 163, 83–90.

Durenberger, David F. 1982. "Politics of Health." In *Competition in the Marketplace: Health Care in the 1980s,* ed. James R. Gay and Barbara J. Sax Jacobs. New York: Spectrum Publications.

Durr, Robert H. 1993. "What Moves Policy Sentiment?" *American Political Science Review* 87, no. 1 (March): 158–70.

Dye, Thomas R., and Harmon Zeigler. 1987. *The Irony of Democracy: An Uncommon Introduction to American Politics.* Monterey, Calif.: Brooks/Cole.

Easton, David. 1953. *The Political System.* New York: Knopf.

———. 1965a. *A Framework for Political Analysis.* Englewood Cliffs, N.J.: Prentice Hall.

———. 1965b. *A Systems Analysis of Political Life.* New York: Wiley.

Eckholm, Erik. 1991. "Health Benefits Found to Deter Job Switching." *New York Times* September 26.

Edelman, Murray. 1964. The Symbolic Uses of Politics. Urbana: University of Illinois Press.

Edwall, Thomas B. 1996. "It Doesn't Always Take a Party." *Washington Post National Weekly Edition* 13, no. 44 (August 26–September 1): 11–12.

Edsall, Thomas Byrne, and Mary D. Edsall. 1991. *Chain Reaction: The Impact of Race, Rights and Taxes on American Politics.* New York: Norton.

Edwards, George C. III. 1989. *At the Margin: Presidential Leadership in Congress.* New Haven: Yale University Press.

Ehrenhalt, Alan. 1991. *The United States of Ambition: Politicians, Power, and the Pursuit of Office.* New York: Times Books.

Ehrenreich, Barbara. 1990. "Our Health-Care Disgrace." *Time,* December 10, 1–12.

Ellis, Richard, and Aaron Wildavsky. 1989. *Dilemmas of Presidential Leadership: From Washington Through Lincoln.* New Brunswick, N.J.: Transaction Books.

———. 1991. " 'Greatness' Revisited: Evaluating the Performance of Early American Presidents in Terms of Cultural Dilemmas." *Presidential Studies Quarterly* 21, no. 1 (Winter): 22–23.

Ellwood, Paul M. 1971. "Health Maintenance Strategy." *Medical Care* 9 (May/June): 291–98.

———. 1975. "Alternative to Regulation: Improving the Market." In *Control on Health Care,* ed. Institute of Medicine, 49–72. Washington, D.C.: National Academy of Sciences.

Engelbert, Stephen. 1995. "Conflict of Interest Is Cited in Regulatory Bill Lobbying." *New York Times,* April 5.

Enthoven, Alain. 1978a. "Consumer Choice Health Plans." *New England Journal of Medicine* 298, no. 12 (March 23): 650–58.

———. 1978b. "Consumer Choice Health Plans." *New England Journal of Medicine* 298, no. 13 (March 30): 709–20.

———. 1980. *Health Plan: The Only Practical Solution to the Soaring Cost of Medical Care.* Reading, Mass.: Addison-Wesley.

———. 1988. "Managed Competition of Alternate Delivery System." *Journal of Health Politics, Policy and Law* 13, no. 2 (Summer): 305–21.

———. 1991. "Universal Health Insurance Through Incentives Reforms." *Journal of American Medical Association* 265, no. 19 (May 15): 2532–36.

———. 1993a. "The History and Principles of Managed Competition." *Health Affairs* 12 (Supplement): 24–48.

———. 1993b. "Testimony on Managed Competition. The Jackson Hole Approach: Achieving Effective Cost Control in Comprehensive Health Care Reform." *Caring: National Association for Home Care Magazine* 12, no. 6 (June 1): 16.

———. 1994. "Why Not the Clinton Health Plan?" *Inquiry* 31, No. 2 (Summer): 129–35.

Enthoven, Alain, and Richard Kronick. 1989a. "A Consumer-Choice Plan for the 1990s: Universal Health Insurance in a System Designed to Promote Quality and Economy." Part 1. *New England Journal of Medicine* 320, no. 1 (January 5): 29–37.

———. 1989b. "A Consumer-Choice Plan for the 1990s: Universal Health Insurance in a System Designed to Promote Quality and Economy." Part 2. *New England Journal of Medicine* 320, no. 2 (January 12): 94–101.

Evans, Lawrence C. 1995. "Committees and Health Jurisdictions in Congress." In *Intensive Care: How Congress Shapes Health Policy,* ed. Thomas E. Mann and Norman J. Ornstein, 25–51. Washington, D.C.: American Enterprise Institute and Brookings Institution.

Ewen, Stuart. 1988. *All Consuming Images: The Politics of Style in Contemporary Culture.* New York: Basic Books.

Falkson, Joseph L. 1980. *HMOs and the Politics of Health Service Reform.* Chicago: American Hospital Association and Robert J. Brady.

Fallows, James. 1995. "A Triumph of Misinformation," *Atlantic Monthly*, 277, no. 1 (January). [http://www.The Atlantic.com/atlantic/election/connection/HealthCa/hcfallow.htm.]

Families USA. 1996a. "Health Legislation Enacted by the 104th Congress." Washington, D.C.: Families USA. [http://epn.org/families/fah104.html]

————. 1996b. "The New Republican Medicaid Bill: A Chip Off the Old Block Grant." Washington, D.C.: Families USA [http://epn.org/families/fachip.html]

Fan, David P., Hans-Bernd Brosius, and Mathias Hans. 1994. "Predictions of the Public Agenda from Television Coverage." *Journal of Broad and Electronic Media* 38, no. 2 (Spring): 163–77.

Feder, Judith M. 1977. *Medicare: The Politics of Federal Hospital Insurance.* Lexington, Mass.: D.C. Heath.

Fein, Esther B. 1995. "Public Hospitals Facing Deep Cuts in Medicare Bill." *New York Times,* October 21.

Ferguson, Thomas. 1995. *Golden Rule: The Investment Theory of Party Competition and the Logic of Money-Driven Political Systems.* Chicago: University of Chicago Press.

————. 1996. "Bill's Big Backers." *Mother Jones* 21, no. 6 (November/December): 60–66.

Ferrara, Peter. 1996. *The Establishment Strikes Back: Medical Savings Accounts and Adverse Selection.* Cato Briefing Paper, No. 26, April 4. Washington, D.C.: CATO Institute.

Fineman, Howard, and Bill Turque. 1996. "How He Got His Groove." *Newsweek,* September 2, 21–25.

Fiorina, Morris. 1992. *Divided Government.* New York: Macmillan.

Fishkin, James. 1992. *Democracy and Deliberation.* New Haven: Yale University Press.

Fraley, Collette. 1995a. "States Guard Their Borders as Medicaid Talks Begin." *Congressional Quarterly Weekly Report* 53, no. 23 (June 10).

————. 1995b. "Health Plans That Can Put Cash into Workers' Pockets Are Finding Favor." *New York Times,* August 29.

————. 1995c. "GOP Plows Ahead on Medicaid with Small Concessions." *Congressional Quarterly Weekly Report* 53, no. 38 (September 30): 3002.

Freudenheim, Milt. 1990. "Business and Health: Most Want U.S. to Pay the Bill." *New York Times,* July 3.

Fritsch, Jane. 1995. "The Grass Roots, Just a Free Phone Call Away." *New York Times,* June 23.

Gallup, Alex, and Lydia Saad. 1993. "America's Top Health Care Concerns." *Gallup Poll Monthly,* no. 333 (June): 2–3.

Gelderman, Carol. 1995. "All the Presidents' Words." *Wilson Quarterly* 19, no. 2 (Winter): 68–79.

Ghorpade, Shailendra. 1986. "Agenda Setting: A Test of Advertising's Neglected Function." *Journal of Advertising Research* 25, no. 23–27.

Gillespie, Ed, and Bob Schellhas, eds. 1994. *Contract with America.* New York: Random House.

Ginzberg, Eli. 1990. "High Tech Medicine and the Rising Health Care Costs." *Journal of American Medical Association* 263, no. 13 (April 4): 1820–22.

Gitlin, T. 1980. *The Whole World Is Watching.* Berkeley: University of California Press.

Glaberson, William. 1993. "Struggling to Bring the Health-Care Debate Home to Readers." *New York Times,* May 25.

Goldberg, Mark A. 1995. "Public Judgement and the Prospects for Reform." *Health Affairs* 14, no. 1 (Spring): 30–32.

Goodman, John C. 1980. *The Regulation of Medical Care: Is the Price Too High?* San Francisco: Cato Institute.

Goodman, John C., and Gerald L. Musgrave. 1994. *Patient Power: The Free-Enterprise Alternative to Clinton's Health Plan.* Washington, D.C.: CATO Institute.

Gottlieb, Martin. 1995. "Health Lobbyists Win Adjustments to Medicare Plan." *New York Times,* December 10.

Gottlieb, Martin, and Robert Pear. 1995. "Beneath Surface, New Health Bills Offer Some Boons." *New York Times,* October 15.

Graber, Doris A. 1988. *Processing the News: How People Tame the Information Tide.* 2nd ed. New York: Longman.

———. 1989. *Mass Media and American Politics.* 3rd ed. Washington, D.C.: CQ Press.

Gray, Jerry. 1996. "Congress and White House Finally Agree on Budget, 7 Months into Fiscal Year." *New York Times,* April 25.

Greenberg, Mark, and Steve Savner. 1996. "A Brief Summary of Key Provisions of the Temporary Assistance for Needy Families Block Grant of H.R. 3734" (Center for Law and Social Policy, Washington, D.C., August 13. [http://epn.org.clasp.-clbskp.html].

Greenstein, Robert, and Richard Kogan. 1996. "A Kinder, Gentler Budget? How Deep Are the Republican Budget Reductions?" Center on Budget and Policy Priorities, Washington, D.C., May 15.

Greenstein, Fred I. 1993. "The Presidential Leadership Style of Bill Clinton: An Early Appraisal." *Political Science Quarterly* 108, no. 4 (Winter): 589–601.

———. 1994a. "The Hidden-Hand Presidency: Eisenhower as Leader." *Studies Quarterly* 24, no. 2 (Spring): 233–41.

———. 1994b. "The Two Leadership Styles of William Jefferson Clinton." *Political Psychology* 15, no. 2 (1994): 351–61.

Grossman, Lawrence K. 1995. *The Electronic Republic: Reshaping Democracy in the Information Age.* New York: Viking.

Grumbach, Kevin, and Thomas Bodenheimer. 1990. "Reins or Fences: A Physician's View of Cost Containment." *Health Affairs* 9, no. 4 (Winter): 120–26.

Hacker, Jacob S. 1996. "National Health Care Reform Debate: Part I." Press Release. University of Pennsylvania, Philadelphia, July 18.

Hafner-Eaton, Chris. 1993. "Will the Phoenix Rise, and Where Should She Go? The Women's Health Agenda." *American Behavioral Scientist* 36, no. 6 (July/August): 841–56.

Hager, George. 1995. "Clinton Shifts Tactics, Proposes Erasing Deficit in 10 Years." *Congressional Quarterly Weekly Report* 53, no. 24 (June 17): 1715–20.

Hager, George, and Alissa J. Rubin. 1995. "Last-Minute Maneuvers Forge a Conference Agreement." *Congressional Quarterly Weekly Report* 53, no. 25 (June 24): 1814–19.

———. 1996. "GOP Plan Gets Token Praise but Little Hope for Success." *Congressional Quarterly Weekly Report* 54, no. 19 (May 11): 1283–87.

Havemann, Judith. 1995. "Blocking the Path to Big Budget Cuts." *Washington Post National Weekly Edition* 12, no. 37 (July 17–23): 27.

———. 1996. "President Signs Insurance Portability Bill into Law. *Washington Post,* August 22.

Health Insurance Association of America. 1995. *Source Book of Health Insurance Data.* Washington, D.C.: HIAA.

"Health Legislation Enacted by the 104th Congress." 1996. Families USA, Washington, D.C. December. [http://epn.org/families/fah104.html], 3/20/96.

Hennessy, Bernard. 1985. *Public Opinion.* 5th ed. Monterey, Calif.: Brooks/Cole.

Heclo, Hugh. 1978. "Issue Networks and the Executive Establishment." In *The New American Political System,* ed. Anthony King, 87–124. Washington, D.C.: The American Enterprise Institute.

Heinz, John P., Edward O. Lawmann, Robert L. Nelson, and Robert H. Salisbury. 1993. *The Hollow Core: Private Interests in National Policy Making.* Cambridge, Mass.: Harvard University Press.

Hernandez, Debra Gersh. 1995. "The Public Monitors Congress." *Editor and Publisher* 128, no. 37 (September 16): 24–25.

Herson, Lawrence J.R. 1984. *The Politics of Ideas: Political Theory and American Public Policy.* Pacific Grove, Calif.: Brooks/Cole.

"Hillary Clinton and Health Care Task Force." 1993. *Gallup Poll Monthly,* no. 329 (February): 4.

House, Robert J., William D. Spangler, and James Woycke. 1991. "Personality and Charisma in the U.S. Presidency: A Psychological Theory of Leader Effectiveness." *Administrative Science Quarterly* 36, no. 3 (September): 364–96.

Hudson, William E. 1995. *American Democracy in Peril.* Chatham, N.J.: Chatham House.

Hunter, James Davison. 1991. *Culture Wars: The Struggle to Define America.* New York: Basic Books.

"Hurting Real People: The Human Impact of Medicaid Cuts." 1995. Families USA, Washington, D.C. [http://epn.org/families/fahurt.html]

Iglehart, John K. 1995. "Health Policy Report: Republicans and the New Politics of Health Care." *New England Journal of Medicine* 332, no.14 (April 6): 972–75.

Immerwahr, John, and Jean Johnson. 1994. *Second Opinions: Americans' Changing Views on Healthcare Reform.* New York: Public Agenda.

Iyengar, S., and D.R. Kinder. 1995. "A Summer of Discontent: Press Coverage of Murder and Medical Care Reform." *Journal of Health Politics, Policy and Law* 20, no. 2 (Summer): 493–501.

Jacobs, Lawrence R. 1992. "The Recoil Effect: Public Opinion and Policymaking in the U.S. and Britain." *Comparative Politics* 24, no. 2 (January): 199–217.

———. 1993. "Health Reform Impasse: The Politics of American Ambivalence toward Government." *Journal of Health Politics, Policy and Law* 18, no. 3 (Fall): 629–55.

Jacobs, Lawrence R., and Robert Y. Shapiro. 1994a. "Studying Substantive Democracy." *PS: Political Science and Politics* 28, no. 1 (March): 9–17.

———. 1994b. "Public Opinions' Tilt Against Private Enterprise." *Health Affairs* 13, no. 1 (Spring 1): 285–98.

———. 1995. "Don't Blame the Public for Failed Health Care Reform." *Journal of Health Politics, Policy and Law* 20, no. 2 Summer (1995): 411–23.

———. 1997. "The Myth of Pandering and Public Opinion During President Clinton's First Term." Mimeographed.

Jacobson, Gary C. 1990. *The Electoral Origins of Divided Government: Competition in U.S. House Elections, 1946–1988.* Boulder, Colo.: Westview Press.

———. 1996. "The 1994 House Elections in Perspective." In *Midterm: The Elections of 1994 in Context,* ed. Philip A. Klinkner. Boulder, Colo.: Westview Press.

Jajich-Toth, Cindy, and Burns W. Roper. 1990. "American's Views on Health Care: A Study in Contradictions." *Health Affairs* 9, no. 4 (Winter): 149–57.

Jamieson, Kathleen H., and Karlyn Kohrs Campbell. 1992. *The Interplay of Influence:*

News, Advertising, Politics and the Mass Media. 3rd ed. Belmont, Calif.: Wadsworth.
———. 1994a. "The Role of Advertising in the Health Care Reform Debate: Part One. Press Release. University of Pennsylvania, Philadelphia, July 18.
———. 1994b. "The Role of Advertising in the Health Care Reform Debate: Part Two. Press Release. University of Pennsylvania, Philadelphia, July 25.
Jamieson, Kathleen, and Joseph N. Cappella. 1994. *Media in the Middle: Fairness and Accuracy in the 1994 Health Care Reform Debate.* Philadelphia: Annenberg Center for Public Policy, University of Pennsylvania. [Http://www.asc.upenn.edu/research/rwj/toc.htm]. 12/29/95.
Johnson, Haynes, and David S. Broder. 1996. *The System: The American Way of Politics at the Breaking Point.* Boston: Little, Brown.
Johnson, Jean, and Adam Kernan-Schloss. 1992. *Faulty Diagnosis: Public Misconceptions About Health Care Reform.* New York: Public Agenda Foundation.
Jones, Charles O. 1989. "Congress and the Constitutional Balance of Power." In *Congressional Politics,* ed. Christopher J. Deering. Chicago: Dorsey Press.
———. 1990. "The Separated Presidency—Making It Work in Contemporary Politics." in *The New American Political System,* ed. Anthony King. Washington, D.C.: AEI Press.
———. 1991. "The Diffusion of Responsibility: An Alternative Perspective for National Policy Politics in the U.S." *Governance* 4 (April).
Joyce, Philip G. 1996. "Congressional Budget Reform: The Unanticipated Implications for Federal Policy Making." *Public Administration Review* 56, no. 4 (July/August): 317–25.
Judis, John B. 1995. "Abandoned Surgery: Business and the Failure of Health Care Reform." *The American Prospect,* no. 21 (Spring): 65–73. [http://epn.org/prospect/21/21judi.html]
Kaiser Commission on the Future of Medicaid. 1994. *Health Reform Legislation: A Comparison of Major Proposals.* Washington, D.C.: Henry J. Kaiser Family Foundation.
"Kassebaum-Kennedy Health Insurance Bill Clears Congress." 1996. Families USA, Washington, D.C. August. [http://epn.org/families/fakcka.html]
Katz, Jeffrey L. 1994. "Clinton Urged to Slow Down." *Congressional Quarterly Weekly Report* 52, no. 3 (January 22): 119.
Kellner, Douglas. 1990. *Television and the Crisis of Democracy.* Boulder, Colo.: Westview Press.
Kerbel, Robert M. 1995. *Remote and Controlled: Media Politics in a Cynical Age.* Boulder, Colo.: Westview Press.
Kernell, Samuel. 1986. *Going Public: New Strategies of Presidential Leadership.* Washington, D.C.: CQ Press.
Kettering Foundation. 1991. *Citizens and Politics: A View from Main Street America.* Dayton, Ohio: Kettering Foundation.
Key, V.O., Jr. 1961. *Public Opinion and American Democracy.* New York: Knopf.
King, Anthony. 1997. *Running Scared: Why America's Politicians Campaign Too Much and Govern Too Little.* New York: Free Press.
Kingdon, John W. 1995. *Agendas, Alternatives and Public Policies,* 2nd ed. New York: HarperCollins.
Klapper, Joseph. 1960. *The Effects of Mass Communication.* New York: Free Press.
Klinkner, Philip A. 1996. *Midterm: The Elections of 1994 in Context.* Boulder, Colo.: Westview Press.
Kolbert, Elizabeth. 1993. "New Arena for Campaign Ads: Health Care." *New York Times,* October 21, A1.
———. 1995. "Public Opinion Polls Swerve with the Turns of a Phrase." *New York Times,* June 5, 1 and 6.

Kosicki, Gerald M. 1993. "Problems and Opportunities in Agenda-Setting Research." *Journal of Communication* 43, no. 2 (Spring): 100–27.

Kosterlitz, Julie. 1991. Agenda-Setting . . . Again." *National Journal,* January 19, 187.

———. 1994a. "Journalist, Heal Thyself." *National Journal* 26, no. 13 (March 26): 748.

———. 1994b. "Harry, Louise and Doublespeak." *National Journal* 26, no. 26 (June 25): 1542.

Koszczuk, Jackie. 1996. "Clinton Embraces GOP Rhetoric." *Congressional Quarterly,* January 27, 211.

Kraft, Michael E. 1996. "Environmental Policy in Congress: Revolution, Reform, or Gridlock?" In *Environmental Policy in the 1990s,* ed. Norman J. Vig and Michael E. Kraft. 3rd ed. Washington, D.C.: CQ Press.

Kressel, Neil J., ed. 1993. *Political Psychology: Classic and Contemporary Readings.* New York: Paragon House.

Kristol, William. 1994. "How to Oppose the Health Plan—and Why." *Wall Street Journal,* January 11.

Krugman, Paul. 1994. *The Age of Diminished Expectations: U.S. Economic Policy in the 1990s.* Revised and updated. Cambridge, Mass.: MIT Press.

Kurtz, Howard. 1996. *Hot Air: All Talk, All the Time: An Inside Look at the Performers and the Pundits.* New York: Times Books.

Latham, Bryan W. 1983. *Health Care Costs: There Are Solutions.* New York: American Management Association.

Lav, Iris J. 1996. "MSA Provision in Health Care Reform Bill Creates Tax Shelter and Casts Doubt on Expansion of Insurance Coverage." Center on Budget and Policy Priorities, Washington, D.C., March 27.

Lazare, Daniel. 1996. *The Frozen Republic: How the Constitution Is Paralyzing Democracy.* New York: Harcourt, Brace.

Lazarsfeld, Paul, Bernard Berelson, and Hazel Gaudet. 1948. *The People's Choice.* New York: Columbia University Press.

Lee, Ronald. 1995. "Humility and the Public Servant: Jimmy Carter's Post-Presidential Rhetoric of Virtue and Power." *Southern Communication Journal* 60, no. 2 (Winter): 120–30.

Lemov, Penelope. 1995. "The Medicaid Numbers Game." *Governing,* May, 27–28.

Levit, Katherine R., Gary L. Olin, and Suzanne W. Letsch. 1992. "American's Health Insurance Coverage, 1980–1991." *Health Care Financing Review* 14, no. 1 (Fall): 31–57.

Levit, Katharine R., et al. 1996. "Data View: National Health Expenditures, 1994." *Health Care Financing Review* 17, no. 3 (Spring): 205–42.

Lewis, Anthony. 1991. "A Sick System." *New York Times,* June 3.

———. 1996a. "Key Changes Needed in the Governor's Medicaid Proposal." Heritage Foundation, F.Y.I., No. 89. (March 12). [http://townhall.com/heritage/library/vategories/healthwel/fui89.html]

———. 1996b. "A Guide to Kassebaum-Kennedy." Issue Bulletin No. 222. Heritage Foundation, Washington, D.C., March 22.

Lewis, Anthony, and Robert E. Moffit. 1996. *Issues '96: The Candidate's Briefing Book.* Ch. 10. Heritage Foundation, Washington, D.C. [http://www.townhall.com/heritage/issues96/chapt10.html].

Lichter, Robert S., Stanley Rothman, and Linda S. Lichter. 1986. *The Media Elite: America's New Powerbrokers.* New York: Hastings House.

Lieberman, Trudy. 1993. "Covering Health Care Reform Round One: How One Paper Stole the Show." *Columbia Journalism Review* 32, no. 3 (September–October): 33–35.

————. 1994. "The Selling of 'Clinton Lite.'" *Columbia Journalism Review* 32, no. 6 (March–April): 20–22.

Light, Paul. 1997. *A Delicate Balance: An Essential Introduction to American Government.* New York: St. Martin's Press.

Lindblom, Charles E., and Edward J. Woodhouse. 1993. *The Policy Making Process,* 3rd ed. Englewood Cliffs, N.J.: Prentice Hall.

Lindsey, Brink. 1993. *Patient Power: The CATO Institute's Plan for Health Care Reform.* Briefing Paper No.19. Cato Institute, Washington, D.C.

Lippman, Walter. 1922. *Public Opinion.* New York: Harcourt, Brace.

Liu, John C. 1995. "August Insider—Robbing Peter to Pay Grandma." Heritage Foundation, Washington, D.C., August. [http://www.townhall.com/heritage/library/categories/healthwel/inauglin2.html]

Liu, John C., and Robert E. Moffit. 1996. "Health Care." In *Issues 96: The Candidates' Briefing Book,* ed. Stuart M. Butler and Kim R. Holmes. Washington, D.C.: The Heritage Foundation. [http://www.heritage.org/heritage/issues96]

Long, Stephen H., and Susan M. Marquis. 1993. "Gaps in Employer Coverage: Lack of Supply or Lack of Demand?" *Health Affair* 12 (Supplement): 282–93.

Loomis, Burdett A., and Allan J. Cigler, eds. 1991. "Introduction: The Changing Nature of Interest Group Politics." In *Interest Group Politics.* 3rd. ed. Allan J. Cigler and Burdett A. Loomis, 1–32. Washington, D.C.: CQ Press.

Lowi, Theodore J. 1964. "American Business, Public Policy, Case-Studies, and Political Theory." *World Politics* 16, no. 4 (July): 677–715.

————. 1979. *The End of Liberalism.* 2nd ed. New York: Norton.

————. 1985. *The Personal President: Power Invested, Promise Unfulfilled.* Ithaca, N.Y.: Cornell University Press.

Luttbeg, Norman R., and Michael M. Gant. 1995. *American Electoral Behavior 1952–1992.* 2nd ed. Itasca, Ill.: F.E. Peacock.

McCaughey, Elizabeth. 1994. "No Exit: What the Clinton Plan Will Do for You." *New Republic* 210, no. 6 (February 7): 21–26.

McClure, Walter. 1981. "Structural and Incentive Problems in Economic Regulation of Medical Care." *Milbank Memorial Quarterly/Health and Society* 59, no. 2: 107–44.

McComb, Maxwell E., and Donald L. Shaw. 1993. "The Evolution of Agenda-Setting Research: Twenty-Five Years in Marketplace of Ideas." *Journal of Communication* 43, no. 2 (Spring): 58–67.

McGregor, Maurice. 1981. "Hospital Costs; Can They Be Cut?" *Milbank Memorial Fund Quarterly/Health and Society* 59, no. 1 (Winter): 89–98.

McMannus, Leo E. 1993. "Presidential Rhetoric: Clinton Replaces Bush." *English Today* 36 (October): 13–17.

McQuail, Denis. 1990. "The Influence and Effects of Mass Media." In *Media Power in Politics,* 2nd ed., ed. Doris A. Graber. Washington, D.C.: CQ Press.

Madrick, Jeffrey. 1995. *The End of Affluence: The Causes and Consequences of America's Economic Dilemma.* New York: Random House.

Maioni, Antonia. 1995. "Nothing Succeeds Like the Right Kind of Failure: Postwar National Health Insurance Initiatives in Canada and the United States." *Journal of Health Politics, Policy and Law* 20, no. 1 (Spring): 5–30.

Makin, John H., and Norman J. Ornstein. 1994. *Debt and Taxes: How America Got into Its Budget Mess and What to Do about It.* New York : Times Books.

Mann, Cindy. 1995. "A Medicaid Block Grant Is Likely to Lead to an Inequitable Distribution of Federal Funds." Center for Budget and Policy Priorities, Washington, D.C. [http://epn.org/cbpp/cbineq.html]

Mann, Cindy, and Kogan, Richard. 1995. "Comparing the Options for Achieving Federal Medicaid Savings." Washington, D.C.: Center on Budget and Policy Priorities. [http://epn.org/cbpp/cbsavi.html]

Mann, Thomas E., and Norman J. Ornstein, eds. 1995. *Intensive Care: How Congress Shapes Health Policy.* Washington, D.C.: American Enterprise Institute and Brookings Institution.

Maraniss, David. 1994. "Clinton's Past as Prologue." *Washington Post National Weekly Edition* 12, no. 5 (December 5–11): 6–7.

———. 1995a. "Bill Clinton's Private War: The Rhodes Scholar Wrestled With the Conflict Between Duty and Ambition." *Washington Post National Weekly Edition* 12, no. 14 (February 6–12): 6–7.

———. 1995b. "The Boy With His Eyes on a Political Prize." *Washington Post National Weekly Edition* 12, no. 14 (February 6–12): 8.

———. 1995c. "The Call to Higher Office—and Whether to Answer." *Washington Post National Weekly Edition* 12, no. 14 (February 6–12): 9.

Maraniss, David, and Michael Weisskopf. 1996. *Tell Newt to Shut Up.* New York: Touchstone Books.

Marmor, Theodore. 1973. *The Politics of Medicare.* Chicago: Aldine.

———. 1994a. *Understanding Health Care Reform.* New Haven: Yale University Press.

———. 1994b. "The Politics of Universal Health Insurance: Lessons from Past Administration?" *PS: Political Science & Politics* 27, no. 2 (June): 194–98.

———. 1994c. The National Agenda for Health Care Reform: What Does It Mean for Poor Americans?" *Brooklyn Law Review* 60, no. 1 (Spring): 83–103.

———. 1995. "A Summer of Discontent: Press Coverage of Murder and Medical Care Reform." *Journal of Health Politics, Policy and Law* 20, no. 2 (Summer): 493–501.

Marmor, Theodore, Donald A. Wittman, and Thomas C. Heagy. 1983. "The Politics of Medical Inflation." In *Political Analysis and American Medical Care,* ed. Theodore Marmor, 61–75. Cambridge, England: Cambridge University Press.

Marmor, Theodore, Jerry L. Mashaw, and Philip L. Harvey. 1990. *America's Misunderstood Welfare State: Persistent Myths, Enduring Realities.* New York: Basic Books.

Martin, Cathie J. 1995. "Stuck in Neutral: Big Business and the Politics of National Health Reform." *Journal of Health Politics, Policy and Law* 20, no. 2 (Summer): 431–36.

Mayhew, David R. 1991. *Divided We Govern: Party Control, Lawmaking, and Investigations 1946–1990.* New Haven: Yale University Press.

Mills, C. Wright. 1956. *The Power Elite.* New York: Oxford University Press.

Mitchell, Alison. 1995. "The Tactics of His Old Foes Help Clinton to Fight G.O.P." *New York Times,* October 13, A1.

Monroe, Alan D. 1979. "Consistency between Public Preferences and National Policy Decisions." *American Politics Quarterly* 7, no. 1 (January): 3–19.

———. 1983. "American Party Platforms and Public Opinion." *American Journal of Political Science* 27, no. 1 (February): 27–42.

Moon, Marilyn. 1996. *Medicare Now and in the Future.* 2nd ed. Washington, D.C.: Urban Institute Press.

Moon, Marilyn, and Karen Davis. 1995. "Preserving and Strengthening Medicare." *Health Affair* 14 (Winter): 31–46.

Moon, Marilyn, Len M. Nichols, and Susan Wall. 1996. *Medical Savings Accounts: A Policy Analysis.* Washington, D.C.: Urban Institute Press.

Moore, David W. 1994a. "Desire for Health Care Reform Remains Strong." *Gallup Poll Monthly,* no. 343 (April): 7–11.

———. 1994b. "Public Firm on Health Reform Goals." *Gallup Poll Monthly,* no. 346 (July): 12–31.

————. 1995a. "Clinton's Re-election Chances Improve." *Gallup Poll Monthly*, no. 358 (July): 6–7.

————. 1995b. "Budget Dispute Helps Democrats." *Gallup Poll Monthly*, no. 362 (November): 10–11.

Moore, David W., and Lydia Saad. 1993. "Most People Satisfied with Own Health Insurance." *Gallup Poll Monthly*, no. 332 (May): 14–15.

————. 1996. "Budget Battle Now a Political Standoff." *Gallup Poll Monthly*, no. 364 (January): 15–17.

Morin, Richard. 1990. "Americans Want Health Care to Save Lives Whatever the Cost." *Washington Post National Weekly Edition*, February 5–11, 38.

————. 1995. "Looking Again—and Liking What They See." *Washington Post National Weekly Edition* 12, no. 14 (February 6–12): 37.

————. 1996. "The Shortsightedness of Focus Groups." *Washington Post National Weekly Edition* 13, no. 53 (October 28–November 3): 35.

————. 1997. "Which Comes First, the Politician or the Poll?" *Washington Post National Weekly Edition* 14, no. 15 (February 10): 35.

Morone, James A. 1990. *The Democratic Wish: Popular Participation and the Limits of American Government*. New York: Basic Books.

————. 1994. "The Politics of Health Care Reform." *Rhode Island Medicine* 77, no. 9 (September): 310–11.

————. 1995. "Nativism, Hollow Corporations, and Managed Competition: Why the Clinton Health Care Reform Failed." *Journal of Health Politics, Policy and Law* 20, no. 2 (Summer): 391–98.

Morrow, David J. 1996. "High Cost of Plugging the Gaps in Medicare." *New York Times*. May 12.

Mosca, Gaetano. 1939. *The Ruling Class*. New York: McGraw-Hill.

Muir, William K. 1992. *The Bully Pulpit: The Presidential Leadership of Ronald Reagan*. San Francisco: Institute for Contemporary Studies Press.

Muller, Charlotte. 1990. *Health Care and Gender*. New York: Russell Sage Foundation.

Nardulli, Peter F. 1995. "The Concept of a Critical Realignment, Electoral Behavior, and Political Change." *American Political Science Review* 89, no. 1 (March): 10–22.

National Academy on Aging, 1995. "Fact On . . . Medicare: Hospital Insurance and Supplementary Medical Insurance." Washington, August. [http://epn.org/aging/agmedi.html]

Navarro, Vicente. 1995a. "The Politics of Health Care Reform in the United States, 1992–1994: A Historical Review." *International Journal of Health Services* 25, no. 2: 185–201.

————. 1995b. "Why Congress Did Not Enact Health Care Reform." *Journal of Health Politics, Policy and Law* 20, no. 2 (Summer): 455–62.

Nelson, Michael, ed. 1993. *The Elections of 1992*. Washington, D.C.: CQ Press.

Neustadt, Richard E. 1990. *Presidential Power and the Modern Presidents: The Politics of Leadership From Roosevelt to Reagan*. New York: Free Press.

Newport, Frank. 1993. "Health Care, Crime Escalate as 'Most important Problem.' " *Gallup Poll Monthly*, no. 336 (September): 4–5.

Newport, Frank, and David Moore. 1993. "After the Health Care Address: Clinton Job Approval Jumps." *Gallup Poll Monthly*, no. 336 (September): 7–9.

Newport, Frank, David Moore, and Lydia Saad. 1995. "Mixed Reaction to Republican Budget Cuts." *Gallup Poll Monthly*, no. 356 (May): 2–3.

Newport, Frank, and Lydia Saad. 1993. "Americans Support Broad-Based Benefits of Health Care Plan." *Gallup Poll Monthly*, no. 338 (November): 5–9.

"New Republican Medicaid Bill, The: A Chip Off the Old Block Grant." 1996. Washington, D.C.: Families USA. [http://epn.org/families/fachip.html]

New York Times. 1996. *The Downsizing of America.* New York: Times Books.

Nimo, Dan, and James E. Combs. 1993. *Mediated Political Realities.* 2nd ed. New York: Longman.

Noll, Roger C. 1975. "The Consequences of Public Utility Regulation of Hospitals." In *Control on Health Care,* ed. Institute of Medicine, 23–48. Washington D.C.: National Academy of Sciences.

Odegard, Peter. 1958. "A Group Basis of Politics: A New Name for Ancient Myth." *Western Political Quarterly* 11: 692–702.

Office of Management and Budget. 1995. *Budget of the United States Government, Fiscal Year 1996.* Washington D.C.: Government Printing Office.

————. 1996. *Historical Tables: Budget of the United States Government, Fiscal Year 1997.* Washington, D.C.: Government Printing Office.

Oliver, Thomas R. 1991. "Ideas, Entrepreneurship, and the Politics of Health Care Reform." *Stanford Law and Policy Review* 3 (Fall): 160–80.

Olson, Mancur. 1982. *The Rise and Decline of Nations: Economic Growth, Stagflation, and Social Rigidities.* New Haven, Conn.: Yale University Press.

"Opinion Outlook." 1996. *National Journal* 28, no. 43 (October 26): 2313.

Orient, June M. 1994. "What NBC Didn't Tell You about Health-Care Reform." *Freeman* 44, no. 11 (November 1): 598–99.

Page, Benjamin I. 1994. "Democratic Responsiveness? Untangling the Links between Public Opinion and Policy." *PS: Political Science and Politics* 28, no. 1 (March): 25–29.

Page, B., and R. Shapiro. 1992. *The Rational Public: Fifty Years of Trends in Americans' Policy Preferences.* Chicago: University of Chicago Press.

Parenti, Michael. 1993. *Inventing Reality: The Politics of New Media,* 2nd ed. New York: St. Martin's Press.

Patel, Kant, and Mark E. Rushefsky. 1995. *Health Care Politics and Policy in America.* Armonk, N.Y.: M.E. Sharpe.

Patterson, Thomas E. 1990. "Views of Winners and Losers." In *Media Power in Politics.* 2nd ed., ed. Doris A. Graber, 176–83. Washington, D.C.: CQ Press.

————. 1997. *The American Democracy.* 3rd ed. New York: McGraw-Hill.

Pear, Robert. 1994. "Gaps in Coverage for Health Insurance." *New York Times,* March 29.

————. 1995a. "Another Set of Dire Warnings on Social Security and Medicare Trust Funds." *New York Times,* April 4.

————. 1995b. "Soaring Costs in Medicaid Push Congress toward a Major Overhaul of the Program." *New York Times,* June 12.

————. 1995c. "Clinton Proposes U.S. Rules for Private Health Insurance." *New York Times,* June 15.

————. 1995d. "G.O.P. Proposing Greater Choices about Medicare." *New York Times,* July 17.

————. 1995e. "G.O.P. Announces Plan to Overhaul Medicare System." *New York Times,* September 15.

————. 1995f. "House G.O.P. Plan Doubles Premiums under Medicare." *New York Times,* September 22.

————. 1995g. "Familiar Ring to the G.O.P. Medicare Plan? It's What Clinton Talked About." *New York Times,* September 26.

————. 1995h. "Senate G.O.P. Plan for Medicare Uses Benefit Cutbacks." *New York Times,* September 28.

————. 1995i. "A.M.A. Has Objections to Limits on Fees in G.O.P. Medicare Plan." *New York Times,* October 4.

————. 1995j. "Retirees and Doctors Attack Republican Medicare Plan." *New York Times,* October 6.

————. 1995k. "Doctors' Group Backs Plan on Republicans on Medicare." *New York Times,* October 11.

————. 1995l. "Doctors' Group Says G.O.P. Agreed to Deal on Medicare." *New York Times,* October 12.

————. 1995m. "Health Industry Leads a Lobbying Stampede." *New York Times,* October 24.

————. 1995n. "G.O.P. Emphasizes Similar Estimates in Medicare Plans." *New York Times,* December 11.

————. 1996a. "With or Without a Budget Pact, The G.O.P.'s Fiscal Squeeze Is On." *New York Times,* February 1.

————. 1996b. G.O.P. Plans Its Own Health Insurance Bill." *New York Times,* March 5.

————. 1996c. "House Panel Approves Bill to Close an Insurance Gap." *New York Times,* March 20.

————. 1996d. "House Panel Approves Bill on Insurance." *New York Times,* March 21.

————. 1996e. "Politics and the Health Care Bill." *New York Times,* March 24.

————. 1996f. "Democrats Object to a Health Plan by G.O.P. in House." *New York Times,* March 29.

————. 1996g. "For President, Health Bill of G.O.P. May Go too Far." *New York Times,* March 30.

————. 1996h. "In Congress, Leaders Agree on Insurance Plans." *New York Times,* September 20.

————. 1997. ". . . As Congress Touches the Third Rail and Lives." *New York Times,* August 4.

Pearlstein, Steven, and Clay Chandler. 1995. "Splitting the Budget Difference." *Washington Post National Weekly Edition* 12, no. 52 (October 30–November 5): 14.

"People Trends." 1996. *New York Times,* March 3.

Peters, Ronald M. Jr. 1996. "The Republican Speakership." Paper prepared for presentation at the annual meeting of the American Political Science Association, San Francisco, August 29–September 1.

Peterson, Mark A. 1992. "Momentum Toward Health Care Reform in the U.S. Senate." *Journal of Health Politics, Policy and Law* 17, no. 2 (Fall): 553–73.

————. 1993. "Political Influence in the 1990s: From Iron Triangles to Policy Networks." *Journal of Health Politics, Policy and Law* 18, no. 2 (Summer): 395–438.

————. 1995. "The Health Care Debate: All Heat and No Light." *Journal of Health Politics, Policy and Law* 20, no. 2 (Summer): 426–30.

Phillips, Kevin P. 1970. *The Emerging Republican Majority.* New York: Doubleday/Anchor.

————. 1990. *The Politics of Rich and Poor: Wealth and the American Electorate in the Reagan Aftermath.* New York: Random House.

Pika, Joseph A., and Norman C. Thomas. 1992. "The Presidency Since Mid-Century." *Congress and the Presidency* 19, no. 1 (Spring): 29–46.

"Poll Shows Most Against Cuts in Medicare, Social Security." 1997. *Palm Beach Post,* March 29.

Princeton Survey Research Associates. 1993. *US News & World Report Poll.* Storrs, Conn: Roper Center for Public Opinion Research, January 12.

Pritchard, David, and Dan Berkowitz. 1993. "The Limits of Agenda-Setting: The Press and the Political Responses to Crime in the United States, 1950–1980." *International Journal of Public Opinion Research* 5, no. 1 (Spring): 87–91.

Protess, David L., and Maxwell McCombs. 1991. *Agenda Setting: Readings on Media, Public Opinion, and Policymaking.* Hillsdale, N.J.: Erlbaum.

Public Papers of the Presidents of the United States—William J. Clinton—1993. Vols. 1 and 2. Washington, D.C.: Government Printing Office, 1994.

Purdum, Todd S. 1996. "White House Report Foresees a Sharp Decline in the Deficit." *New York Times,* July 17.

Rasell, Edith. 1995. "Unworkable Schemes for Cutting Medicare: Proposal to Trim Program Risk Serious Damage to the System." Issue Brief No. 107, Economic Policy Institute. [http://epn.org/economy/epmedi.html]

Rauch, Jonathan. 1996. "The End of Government." *National Journal* 28, no. 36 (September 7): 1890–95.

Reinhardt, Uwe E. 1995. "Turning Our Gaze from Bread and Circus Games." *Health Affairs* 14, no. 1 (Spring): 33–36.

Reinhold, Robert. 1993. "A Health-Care Theory Hatched in Fireside Chats." *New York Times,* February 10.

Renshon, Stanley A. 1994. "A Preliminary Assessment of the Clinton Presidency: Character, Leadership, and Performance." *Political Psychology* 15, no. 4 (June 1): 375–94.

Rieselbach, Leroy N. 1995. *Congressional Politics: The Evolving Legislative System,* 2nd ed. Boulder, Colo.: Westview Press.

Ripley, Randall B., and Grace A. Franklin. 1982. *Bureaucracy and Policy Implementation.* Homewood, Ill.: Dorsey Press.

Roberts, Marilyn, and Maxwell McCombs. 1994. "Agenda Setting and Political Advertising: Origins of the News Agenda." *Political Communication* 11, no. 3 (July–September): 249–62.

Rockman, Bert A. 1995. "The Clinton Presidency and Health Care Reform." *Journal of Health Politics, Policy and Law* 20, no. 2 (Summer): 399–402.

Rogers, Everett M., and James W. Dearing. 1988. "Agenda Setting Research: Where Is It Going?" in *Communication Yearbook II,* ed. James A. Anderson. Beverly Hills, Calif.: Sage.

Rogers, Everett M., James W. Dearing, and Dorine Bregman. 1993. "The Anatomy of Agenda-Setting Research." *Journal of Communication* 43, no. 2 (Spring): 68–84.

Rose, Richard. 1991. *The Postmodern President.* Chatham, N.J.: Chatham House.

Rosenbaum, David E. 1995a. "The Medicare Brawl: Finger-Pointing, Hyperbole and the Facts Behind Them." *New York Times,* October 1.

———. 1995b. "Savings and Smoke." *New York Times,* September 15.

Rothman, David. 1993. "A Century of Failure: Health Care Reform in America." *Journal of Health Politics, Policy and Law* 18, no. 2 (Summer): 271–86.

Rowland, Diana, Barbara Lyons, Alina Salaganicoff, and Peter Long. 1994. "A Profile of the Uninsured in America." *Health Affairs* 13, no. 2 (Spring): 283–89.

Rubin, Alissa J. 1993. "The Gatekeepers." *Congressional Quarterly Weekly Report* 51, supplement to 38 (September 25): 37–40.

———. 1994a. "Two Ideological Poles Frame Debate over Reform." *Congressional Quarterly Weekly Report* 52, no. 1 (January 8): 23–28.

———. 1994b. "The Plans: Clinton vs. Cooper." *Congressional Quarterly Weekly Report* 52, no. 5 (February 5): 251.

———. 1994c. "CBO Turns Budget Spotlight on Health-Care Overhaul." *Congressional Quarterly Weekly Report* 52, no.6 (February 12): 290–91.

———. 1994d. "GOP Seeks Unity to Bargain With Democrats." *Congressional Quarterly Weekly Report* 52, no. 9 (March 5): 550.

———. 1994e.'Stark's Bill Modeled on Medicare." *Congressional Quarterly Weekly Report* 52, no. 10 (March 12): 609.

———. 1994f. "Clinton's Main Tenets Drive New Movement on Health." *Congressional Quarterly Weekly Report* 52, no. 12 (March 26): 737–42.

———. 1994g. "Bad News for Cooper-Breaux Bill." *Congressional Quarterly Weekly Report* 52, no. 18 (May 7): 1125.

———. 1994h. "Slow Pace of Overhaul Frustrates Democrats." *Congressional Quarterly Weekly Report* 52, no. 21 (May 28): 1387–88.

———. 1994i. "Deadline Pressure Forces Talk of Compromise." *Congressional Quarterly Weekly Report* 52, no. 24 (June 18): 1611–14.

———. 1994j. "Moderates on Senate Finance Panel Offer a '95 Percent' Solution." *Congressional Quarterly Weekly Report* 52, no. 25 (June 25): 1707–8.

———. 1994k. "GOP Senators Backing Dole Plan." *Congressional Quarterly Weekly Report* 52, no. 26 (July 2): 1799.

———. 1994l. "Leaders Using Fervent Approach to Convert Wavering Members." *Congressional Quarterly Weekly Report* 52, no. 30 (July 30).

———. 1994m. "A Mixed Review from CBO." *Congressional Quarterly Weekly Report* 52, no. 32 (August 13): 2347.

———. 1994n. "Chafec Group Unveils Last-Minute Plan." *Congressional Quarterly Weekly Report* 52, no. 33 (August 20): 2459.

———. 1994o. "Details of Bipartisan Bill." *Congressional Quarterly Weekly Report* 52, no. 37 (September 24): 2694.

———. 1996. "A Gentler Hand with Medicare." *Congressional Quarterly Weekly Report* 54, no. 19 (May 11): 1286.

Rubin, Alissa T., and Beth Donovan. 1994. "Two Ideological Poles Frame Debate over Reform." *Congressional Quarterly Weekly Report* 52, no. 1 (January 8): 23–28.

———. 1994. "Leaders Tell Clinton Measure Must Have Slower Approach." *Congressional Quarterly Weekly Report* 52, no. 29 (July 23): 2041–42.

———. 1994. "With Outcome Still Uncertain, Members Face Critical Vote." *Congressional Quarterly Weekly Report* 52, no. 31 (August 6): 2201–8.

Rubin, Irene S. 1990. *The Politics of Public Budgeting: Getting and Spending, Borrowing and Balancing.* Chatham, N.J.: Chatham House.

Rushefsky, Mark E. 1981. "Energy Policy." In *Congress, the President, and Foreign Policy,* ed. John Spanier and Joseph Nogee, 161–88. New York: Pergamon Press.

———. 1996. *Public Policy in the United States: Toward the Twenty-First Century.* 2nd ed. Chicago: Harcourt, Brace.

Saad, Lydia. 1994. "Public Has Cold Feet on Health Care Reform." *Gallup Poll Monthly,* no. 347 (August): 2–7.

———. 1995. "Budget Standoff Not Welcomed by Most Americans." *Gallup Poll Monthly,* no. 362 (November): 5–7.

Sabato, Larry J. 1991. *The Feeding Frenzy: How Attack Journalism Has Transformed American Politics.* New York: Free Press.

Sabato, Larry J., and Glenn R. Simpson. 1996. *Dirty Little Secrets: The Persistence of Corruption in American Politics.* New York: Times Books.

Samuelson, Robert J. 1995a. *The Good Life and Its Discontents: The American Dream in the Age of Entitlements.* New York: Times Books.

———. 1995b. "The Spigot of Last Resort." *Newsweek* 126 (January): 45.

Samuelson, Robert J. 1997a. "The Budget: A Model of Muddling." *Washington Post National Weekly Edition* 14, nos. 37 and 38 (July 28): 28.

———. 1997b. "Balancing Act." *Newsweek* CXXX, no. 6 (August 11): 24–27.

Scarlett, Thomas. 1994. "Killing Health Care Reform." *Campaigns and Elections* 15, no. 10 (October–November): 34–37.

Schattschneider, E.E. 1960. *The Semi-Sovereign People.* New York: Holt.

Schear, Stuart. 1994. "Covering Health Care: Politics of People?" *Columbia Journalism Review* 33, no. 1 (May-June): 36–37.

Schick, Allen. 1995. "How a Bill Did Not Become a Law." In *Intensive Care: How Congress Shapes Health Policy,* ed. Thomas E. Mann and Norman J. Ornstein, 227–72. Washington, D.C.: American Enterprise Institute and Brookings Institution.

Schlesinger, Mark, and Tae-ku Lee. 1993. "Is Health Care Different? Popular Support of Federal Health and Social Policies." *Journal of Health Politics, Policy and Law* 18, no. 3 (Fall): 551–628.

Schneider, William. 1994. "Clinton: The Reason Why." *National Journal* 26, no. 46 (November 12): 2630–32.

———. 1995a. "Who's Really Medicare's Best Friends?" *National Journal* 27, no. 18 (May 6): 1138.

———. 1995b. "Spin Control on Medicare and Taxes." *National Journal* 27, no. 42 (October 21): 2622.

———. 1996. "The Two Worlds of American Politics." *National Journal* 28, no. 50 (December 14): 2723.

Schram, Martin. 1990. "The Great American Video Game." In *Media Power in Politics.* 2nd ed., ed. Doris A. Graber, 184–92. Washington, D.C.: CQ Press.

Schwartz, John E. 1988. *America's Hidden Success: A Reassessment of Public Policy from Kennedy to Reagan.* Rev. ed. New York: Norton.

"Search for the Perfect President, The." 1995. *The Economist.* 337, no. 6 (November 18): 1993–95.

Segal, David. 1995. "Business Is on the Bandwagon for Medicare Cuts." *Washington Post National Weekly Edition* 14, no. 2 (November 13–19): 17.

"Senate Panel Passes Health Insurance Bill." 1995. *New York Times,* August 3.

Serafini, Marilyn Werber. 1995a. "Going for the Gold." *National Journal* 27: 13 (April 1): 804–8.

———. 1995b. "Senior Schism." *National Journal* 27, no. 28 (May 6): 1089–93.

———. 1995c. "No Strings Attached!" *National Journal* 27, no. 20 (May 20).

———. 1995d. "Who's in Charge Here?" *National Journal* 27, no. 26 (July 1): 1710–13.

———. 1995e. "Turning Up the Heat." *National Journal* 27, no. 32 (August 12): 2051–54.

———. 1995f. "How an Insurance Cure Has Been Revived." *National Journal* 27, no. 45 (November 11): 2809–11.

———, 1995g. "Newtral Actions." *National Journal* 27, no. 47 (November 25): 2918–22.

———. 1996a. "Swift Path to Health Bill?" *National Journal* 28, no. 7 (February 17): 378.

———. 1996b. "Motherhood, Apple Pie and Medicare." *National Journal* 28, no. 43 (October 26): 2293–94.

———. 1997a. "Medicare Crooks." *National Journal* 29, no. 29 (July 19): 1458–60.

———. 1997b. "Brave New World." *National Journal* 29, no. 33 (August 16): 1636–39.

Shaw, Donald, and Shannon Martin. 1992. "The Function of Mass Media Agenda Setting." *Journalism Quarterly* 69, no. 4 (Winter): 902–20.

Shaw, Donald, and Maxwell McCombs, eds. 1977. *The Emergence of American Political Issues: The Agenda-Setting Function of the Press.* St. Paul, Minn.: West.

Shear, Jeff. 1995. "The Big Fix." *National Journal* 27, no. 12 (March 25): 734–38.

———. 1996. "Going for the Silver." *National Journal* 28, no. 42 (October 19): 2219–22.

Shogan, Robert. 1991. *The Riddle of Power: Presidential Leadership from Truman to Bush.* New York: Dutton.

Silvia, John. 1996/5. "Is the Contract Good Economics? A Scorecard." *National Review* 47, no. 2 (February 6): 34.

Skocpol, Theda. 1994. "From Social Security to Health Security? Opinion and Rhetoric in U.S. Social Policy Making." *PS: Political Science and Politics* 28, no. 1 (March): 21–25.

———. 1995. *Social Policy in the United States: Future Possibilities in Historical Perspective.* Princeton: Princeton University Press.

———. 1996. *Boomerang: Clinton's Health Security Effort and the Turn Against Government in U.S. Politics.* New York: Norton.

Smith, Craig A., and Kathy B. Smith. 1994. *The White House Speaks: Presidential Leadership as Persuasion.* Westport, Conn.: Praeger.

Smith, Hedrick. 1988. *The Power Game: How Washington Works.* New York: Ballantine Books.

Smith, Mark D., et al. 1992. "Taking the Public's Pulse on Health System Reform." *Health Affairs* 11, no. 2 (Summer): 125–33.

Smith, Steven S. 1993. *The American Congress.* Boston: Houghton Mifflin.

———. 1995. "Commentary—The Role of Institutions and Ideas in Health Care Policy." *Journal of Health Politics, Policy and Law* 20, no. 2 (Summer): 385–89.

Social Security Administration. 1995. *Status of the Social Security and Medicare Programs: A Summary of the 1995 Annual Report.* Washington, D.C.: Government Printing Office. [http://www.ssa.govt/policy/trustecssummary1995.html]

Spangler, William D., and Robert J. House. 1991. "Presidential Effectiveness and the Leadership Motive Profile." *Journal of Personality and Social Psychology* 60, no. 3 (March): 439–55.

Spanier, John, and Joseph Nogee, eds. 1981. *Congress, the President, and Foreign Policy.* New York: Pergamon Press.

"Special Issue: Ageism on the Agenda." 1997. *EXTRA! The Magazine of Fair* 10, no. 2 (March/April).

Sparrow, Malcolm K. 1996. *License to Steal: Why Fraud Plagues America's Health Care System.* Boulder, Colo.: Westview.

Spicer, Michael W. 1995. *The Founders, the Constitution, and Public Administration: A Conflict in World Views.* Washington, D.C.: Georgetown University Press.

Spragins, Ellyn. 1996. "Does Your HMO Stack Up?" *Newsweek,* June 24, 56–63.

Starobin, Paul. 1993. "The Big Story." *National Journal* 25, no. 41 (October 9): 2420–24.

———. 1995. "Right Fight." *National Journal* v. 27, no. 49 (December 9): 3022–26.

Starr, Paul. 1982. *The Social Transformation of American Medicine.* New York: Basic Books.

———. 1992. *The Logic of Health Care Reform.* New York: Penguin Books, 1992.

———. 1995. "What Happened to Health Care Reform?" *American Prospect,* no. 20 (Winter): 20–31.

———. 1995. "Look Who's Talking Health Care Reform Now." *New York Times Magazine,* September 3, 42–43.

Steinmo, Sven, and Jon Watts. 1995. "It's the Institutions Stupid! Why Comprehensive National Health Insurance Always Fails in America." *Journal of Health Politics, Policy and Law* 20, no. 2 (Summer): 329–72.

Stern, Philip M. 1992. *Still The Best Congress Money Can Buy.* Rev. ed. Washington, D.C.: Regnery Gateway.

Stillman, Richard J. II. 1984. "The Changing Patterns of Public Administration Theory in America." In *Public Administration: Concepts and Cases,* ed. Richard J. Stillman II. 3rd ed., 5–24. Boston: Houghton Mifflin.

————. 1991. *Preface to Public Administration: A Search for Themes and Direction.* New York: St. Martin's Press.

Stimson, James A. 1991. *Public Opinion in America: Moods, Cycles, & Swings.* Boulder, Colo.: Westview Press.

Stimson, James A., Michael B. MacKuen, and Robert S. Erikson. 1994. "Opinion and Policy: A Global View." *PS: Political Science and Politics* 27, no. 1 (March): 29–35.

Stockman, David A. 1987. *The Triumph of Politics: The Inside Story of the Reagan Revolution.* New York: Avon Books.

Stone, Deborah. 1997. *Policy Paradox: The Art of Political Decision Making.* New York: Norton.

Stone, Peter H. 1995. "Madison Avenue Comes to Capitol Hill." *National Journal* 27, no. 7 (February 18): 457.

Stout, Hilary. 1994. "Many Don't Realize It's the Clinton Plan They Like." *Wall Street Journal* (March 10).

Strahan, Randall. 1996. "Leadership in Institutional and Political Time: The Case of Newt Gingrich and the 104th Congress." Paper prepared for presentation at the annual meeting of the American Political Science Association, San Francisco, Calif., August 29–September 1.

Sundquist, James L. 1988. "Needed: A Political Theory for the New Era of Coalition Government in the United States." *Political Science Quarterly* 103 (Winter): 613–35.

Sutherland, Max, and John Galloway. 1981. "Role of Advertising: Persuasion or Agenda Setting?" *Journal of Advertising Research* 21: 25–29.

Swoboda, Frank. 1991. "The Mercury Rises for Health Care Costs." *Washington Post National Weekly Edition* (February 4–10): 21.

Sylvia, Ronald D. 1995. "Presidential Decision Making and Leadership in the Civil Rights Era." *Presidential Studies Quarterly* 25, no. 3 (Summer): 391–411.

Talbert, Jeffrey. 1995. "Congressional Partisanship and the Failure of Moderate Health Care Reform." *Journal of Health Politics, Policy and Law* 20, no. 4 (Winter): 1033–50.

Tanner, Michael. 1995. *Medical Savings Accounts: Answering the Critics.* Policy Analysis No. 228. CATO Institute, Washington, D.C., May 25.

Taylor, Humphrey. 1990. "U.S. Health Care: Built for Waste." *New York Times,* April 17.

Taylor, Paul. 1990. *See How They Run: Electing President in an Age of Mediocracy.* New York: Knopf.

Thomas, John. 1995–96. "The Clinton Health Care Reform Plan: A Failed Dramatic Presentation." *Stanford Law and Policy Review* 7, no. 1: 83–104.

Thomas, Rosita M. 1992. *Health Care in America: An Analysis of Public Opinion.* CRS Report for Congress 92–769 GOV. Washington, D.C.: Congressional Research Service, October 26.

Thurber, James A. 1991. *Divided Democracy: Cooperation and Conflict between the President and Congress.* Washington, D.C.: CQ Press.

————. 1996. *Rivals for Power: Presidential-Congressional Relations.* Washington, D.C.: CQ Press.

Times Mirror Center for the People & the Press. 1993a. *The Vocal Minority in American Politics.* New York: Times Mirror Center for the People & the Press.

————. 1993b. *Cautious Support for Clinton Plan.* New York: Times Mirror Center for the People & the Press.

————. 1995a. "Media Coverage of the Health Care Reform: A Final Report." Supplement to *Columbia Journalism Review* 33, no. 6 (March/April): 1–8.

————. 1995b. *Strong Support for Minimum Wage Hike and Preserving Entitlements.* New York: Times Mirror Center for the People & the Press.

————. 1995c. *Medicare Debate Gets More Attention Than Bosnia, Dole on Hollywood, and Even OJ.* New York: Times Mirror Center for the People & the Press.

Tolchin, Susan J. 1996. *The Angry Americans: How Voter Rage Is Changing the Nation.* Boulder, Colo.: Westview Press.

Toner, Robin. 1994a. "Ads Are Potent Weapon in Health Care Struggle." *New York Times,* February 1, 14.

————. 1994b. "The Clinton's Health Care Nemesis: The Man Behind 'Harry and Louise.' *New York Times,* April 6, 18.

————. 1995. "This Time, Clinton Tries a Selective Health Care Strategy." *New York Times,* June 14.

Tocqueville, Alexis de. 1988. *Democracy in America.* Vols. 1 and 2. Translated by Henry Reeve. New York: Schocken.

Trevino, Fernando, Eugene M. Moyer, Burciaga R. Valdez, and Christine A. Stroup-Benham. 1991a. "Health Insurance Coverage and Utilization of Health Services by Mexican Americans, Mainland Puerto Ricans, and Cuban Americans." *Journal of American Medical Association* 265, no. 2 (January 9): 233–37.

————. 1991b. "Hispanic Health in the United States." *Journal of the American Medical Association* 265, no.2 (January 9): 248–52.

Truman, David B. 1951. *The Governmental Process: Political Interests and Public Opinion.* New York: Knopf.

Tulis, Jeffrey K. 1987. *The Rhetorical Presidency: The Pursuit of Popular Support.* Princeton: Princeton University Press.

Turner, Thomas. 1994. "Still Another Hidden Hand Presidency? The Presidential Leadership Styles of Abraham Lincoln and Dwight Eisenhower." *Quarterly Journal of Ideology* 17, nos. 1/2: 35–59.

Uchitelle, Louis, and N.R. Kleinfield. 1996. "The Downsizing of America: On the Battlefields of Business, Millions of Casualties." Part 1 of 7. *New York Times,* March 3.

U.S. Department of Health and Human Services. 1991. *Health Status of Minorities and Low-Income Groups.* 3rd ed. Washington, D.C.: Government Printing Office.

U.S. General Accounting Office. 1996. *Health Insurance for Children: Private Insurance Coverage Continues to Deteriorate.* Washington, D.C.: Government Printing Office, June 17. GAO/HEHS-96–129.

Valdez, Burciaga R, Hal Morgenstern, Richard E. Brown, Roberta Wyn, Wang Chao, and William Cumberland. 1993. "Insuring Latinos Against the Costs of Illness." *Journal of the American Medical Association* 269, no. 7 (February 17): 889–94.

Victor, Kirk. 1995. "Astroturf Lobbying Takes a Hit." *National Journal* 27, no. 38 (September 23): 2359–60.

Virts, John R., and George W. Wilson. 1984. "Inflation and Health Care Prices." *Health Affairs* 3, no. 1 (Spring): 88–100.

Vladeck, Bruce C. 1981. "The Market vs. Regulation: The Case for Regulation." *Milbank Memorial Fund Quarterly/Health and Society* 59, no. 2 (Spring): 209–23.

Vobejda, Barbara, and Spencer Rich. 1995. "Here Comes the Hard Part." *Washington Post National Weekly Edition* 12, no. 36 (July 3–9): 15.

Walsh-Childers, Kim. 1994. "Newspaper Influence on Health Policy Development." *Newspaper Research Journal* 15, no. 3 (Summer): 89–104.

Wanta, Wayne. 1991. "Presidential Approval Rating as a Variable in the Agenda-Building Process." *Journalism Quarterly* 68, no. 4 (Winter): 672–79.

Watt, James H., Marry Mazza, and Leslie Snyder. 1993. *Communication Research* 20, no. 3 (June): 408–35.

Waxman, Judy, and Joan Alker. 1996. "The Impact of Federal Welfare Reform on

Medicaid." *Families USA*, Washington, D.C., August 19. [http://www.hadnsnet .org/medicaid/impct.html]

Weaver, David. 1994. "Media Agenda Setting and Elections: Voter Involvement or Alienation?" *Political Communication* 11, no. 4: 347–56.

Weaver, Paul H. 1994. *News and the Culture of Lying: How Journalism Really Works.* New York: Free Press.

Weaver, R. Kent, and Bert A. Rockman, eds. 1993. *Do Institutions Matter? Government Capabilities in the United States and Abroad.* Washington, D.C.: Brookings Institution.

Weiner, Stephen M. 1982. "On Public Values and Private Regulation: Some Reflections on Cost Containment Strategy." *Milbank Memorial Fund Quarterly/Health and Society* 59, no. 2: 269–96.

Weinstein, Michael M. 1994. "Fear-Mongering on Health Care Reform: The Clinton Plan Misrepresented." *New York Times*, February 6, E16.

Weisskopf, Michael, and David Maraniss. 1996. "Behind the Stage: Common Problems." *Washington Post National Weekly Edition* 13, no. 14 (February 5–11): 9–10.

West, Darrell M., Diane Heith, and Chris Goodwin. 1996. "Harry and Louise Go to Washington: Political Advertising and Health Care Reform." *Journal of Health Politics, Policy and Law* 21, no. 1 (Spring): 35–68.

White, Joseph. 1995a. "Commentary — The Horses and the Jumps: Comments on the Health Care Reform Steeplechase." *Journal of Health Politics, Policy and Law* 20, no. 2 (Summer): 373–83.

————. 1995b. "Budgeting and Health Policymaking." In *Intensive Care: How Congress Shapes Health Policy,* ed. Thomas E. Mann and Norman J. Ornstein, 55–78. Washington, D.C.: American Enterprise Institute and Brookings Institution.

————. 1995c. *Competing Solutions: American Health Care Proposals and International Experience.* Washington, D.C.: Brookings Institution.

White, Theodore. 1973. *The Making of the President, 1972.* New York: Bantam Books.

Wildavsky, Ben. "Who's Entitles?" *National Journal* 29, no. 30 (July 26): 1509–11.

Wilson, James Q. 1980. "The Politics of Regulation." In *The Politics of Regulation,* ed. James Q. Wilson, 357–94. New York: Basic Books.

Wines, Michael. 1995. "White Accedes to G.O.P. on 7–Year Deficit Cut's Details." *New York Times*, December 6.

————. 1996a. "In New 6–Year Budget Plan With Gentler Reductions, Republicans Ease Toward Center." *New York Times*, May 9.

————. 1996b. "Minor Differences, Vast Distinctions." *New York Times*, May 12.

————. 1996c. "New Senate Chief Dresses Down Colleagues." *New York Times*, July 12.

Woodward, Bob. 1994. *The Agenda: Inside the Clinton White House.* New York: Simon & Schuster.

Yagade, Aileen, and David M. Dozier. 1990. "The Media Agenda-Setting Effects of Concrete versus Abstract Issues." *Journalism Quarterly* 67, no. 1 (Spring): 3–10.

Yankelovich, Daniel. 1995. "The Debate That Wasn't: The Public and the Clinton Plan." *Health Affairs* 41, no. 1 (Spring): 7–23.

Zernicke, Paul H. 1990. "Presidential Roles and Rhetoric." *Political Communication and Persuasion* 7, no. 4, 231–35.

Zhu, Jian-Hu, James H. Watt, Leslie B. Snyder, Jingtao Yan, and Yansong Jiang. 1993. "Public Issue Priority Formation: Media Agenda-Setting and Social Interaction." *Journal of Communication* 43, no. 1 (Winter): 8–29.

INDEX

I

ABOUT THE AUTHORS

Mark E. Rushefsky, Ph.D. SUNY/Binghamton, is a professor of political science at Southwest Missouri State University. He is the author of *Making Cancer Policy* (1986) and *Public Policy in the United States: Toward the Twenty-First Century,* 2nd ed. (1996), and coauthor of *Health Care Politics and Policy in America* (1995). He has also contributed articles and chapters on health care and environmental policies.

Kant Patel, Ph.D. University of Houston, is a professor of political science and department head at Southwest Missouri State University. He is the coauthor of *Health Care Politics and Policy in America.* He has published numerous articles in the field of health care, public policy, and American politics.